FOOD PEDAGOGIES

Critical Food Studies

Series Editor
Michael K. Goodman, Kings College London, UK

The study of food has seldom been more pressing or prescient. From the intensifying globalization of food, a world-wide food crisis and the continuing inequalities of its production and consumption, to food's exploding media presence, and its growing re-connections to places and people through 'alternative food movements', this series promotes critical explorations of contemporary food cultures and politics. Building on previous but disparate scholarship, its overall aims are to develop innovative and theoretical lenses and empirical material in order to contribute to – but also begin to more fully delineate – the confines and confluences of an agenda of critical food research and writing.

Of particular concern are original theoretical and empirical treatments of the materializations of food politics, meanings and representations, the shifting political economies and ecologies of food production and consumption and the growing transgressions between alternative and corporatist food networks.

Other titles in the series include:

Careful Eating: Bodies, Food and Care
Edited by Emma-Jayne Abbots, Anna Lavis and Luci Attala
9781472439482

Food Transgressions
Making Sense of Contemporary Food Politics
Edited by Michael K. Goodman and Colin Sage
9780754679707

Doing Nutrition Differently
Critical Approaches to Diet and Dietary Intervention
Edited by Allison Hayes-Conroy and Jessica Hayes-Conroy
9781409434795

Geographies of Race and Food
Fields, Bodies, Markets
Edited by Rachel Slocum and Arun Saldanha
9781409469254

Food Pedagogies

Edited by

RICK FLOWERS and ELAINE SWAN

University of Technology, Sydney, Australia

Routledge
Taylor & Francis Group
LONDON AND NEW YORK

First published 2015 by Ashgate Publishing

2 Park Square, Milton Park, Abingdon, Oxfordshire OX14 4RN
711 Third Avenue, New York, NY 10017

Routledge is an imprint of the Taylor & Francis Group, an informa business

First issued in paperback 2018

British Library Cataloguing in Publication Data
A catalogue record for this book is available from the British Library

The Library of Congress has cataloged the printed edition as follows:
Food pedagogies / edited by Rick Flowers and Elaine Swan.
pages cm. -- (Critical food studies)
Includes bibliographical references and index.
ISBN 978-1-4094-6504-1 (hardback)
1. Food habits--Study and teaching. 2. Food--Study and teaching.
3. Nutrition--Study and teaching. I. Flowers, Rick. II. Swan, Elaine, 1961-

GT2860.F67 2015
394.1'2071--dc23

2015019278

ISBN: 978-1-4094-6504-1 (hbk)
ISBN: 978-1-138-54739-1 (pbk)

Contents

List of Tables		*vii*
Notes on Contributors		*ix*
Acknowledgements		*xix*
1	Food Pedagogies: Histories, Definitions and Moralities *Rick Flowers and Elaine Swan*	1

PART I: EMBODIMENT AND IDENTITY

2	Where's the Pleasure? Exploring the Meanings and Experiences of Pleasure in School-based Food Pedagogies *Emma Rich and John Evans*	31
3	Potatoes in the Rice Cooker: Family Food Pedagogies, Bodily Memories, Meal-time Senses and Racial Practices *Rick Flowers and Elaine Swan*	49
4	'You Are What You Eat!'?: Crafting the (Food) Consuming Subject through Cooking Shows *Seline Szkupinski-Quiroga, Jennifer A. Sandlin, and Robin Redmon Wright*	75

PART II: TRANSFORMATION AND AFFECT

5	Food and Passion: Technologies of Self-transformation in *Jamie's Kitchen* *Lyn Harrison, Peter Kelly and Perri Campbell*	95
6	The *Loi Evin*: A Pedagogical Experiment in Responsible Drinking *Julie Robert*	113
7	If I Am What I Eat, Who Am I? How Critical Shopping Teaches Adults about Food, Identity and Social Change *Kaela Jubas*	131

PART III: GOVERNANCE AND AUTHORITY

8 'Making it Local': The Rural Consumer, the Supermarket and Competing Pedagogical Authority 149
Bronwyn Isaacs and Jane Dixon

9 'Just Say No to Pies': Food Pedagogies, Health Education and Governmentality 169
Deana Leahy and Jo Pike

PART IV: ETHICS AND CRITIQUE

10 What Do Food Labels Teach People about Food Ethics? 185
Heather J. Bray and Rachel A. Ankeny

11 Learning to Eat with Attitude: Critical Food Pedagogies 201
Jennifer Sumner

12 Food Consciousness: Teaching Critical Theory through Food Narratives 215
Meredith E. Abarca

13 Of Dialectical Food Pedagogies and Political Economies: Taking Debates Forward in an Afterword 229
Michael K. Goodman

Index *241*

List of Tables

2.1 Schools sample 33
6.1 The *Loi Evin* in brief 116

Notes on Contributors

Meredith E. Abarca is an Associate Professor in the Department of English at the University of Texas, El Paso. She is the author of *Voices in the Kitchen* (Texas A&M Press, 2006, reprinted in 2008 and reissued as an e-book in 2013). She co-edited *Rethinking Chicana/o Literature through Food* (Palgrave, 2013), and acted as guest co-editor for a Special Issue for the journal *Food & Foodways* on '*Cocinas Publicas*: Food Border Consciousness' (published by Routledge, 2007). Her work has appeared in *Food & Foodways*, *Food, Culture & Society*, and in edited collections such as *Taking Food Public: Redefining Foodways in the Changing World* (Routledge, 2011) and *The Routledge Companion to U.S. Latino Studies* (2012). Her research interests are Food Studies, US Latina/o Literature, Cultural and Literary Theory, and Mexican-American Folklore. She has lectured at community and academic settings, such as the Southern Foodways Alliance Symposium in Oxford, Mississippi and the University of Gastronomical Sciences in (Colormo) Parma, Italy. She has been influenced by Carole Mm Counihan, Gary Paul Nabhan, Lisa Helkde, David Sutton. She is planning to develop a monograph that explores how african and amerindian culinary practices give way to a latina/o gastronomical *mestizaje*. Whilst this is in the beginning stages of research, she has already published an article on the topic. Her favourite meal is 'Los Chilaquiles': fried corn tortillas (cut into small size bites) and onions, simmered with a tomato-chilli sauce and served with cream and fresh Mexican cheese. This is a dish she grew up eating which her mother referred to as 'la comida de los pobres' (the food of the poor). Her first food studies article published is called, 'Los Chilaquiles de mi 'ama: The Language of Everyday Cooking' (2001).

Rachel A. Ankeny is Professor of History at the University of Adelaide. Her research interests cross several areas and fields: the history and philosophy of science particularly biomedical/ biological sciences, bioethics and science policy, food studies, and migration history. In food studies, Rachel's research interests include food ethics, food habits of women and children, food habits in the Italian diaspora, and the relationship of science to food habits. She received an Australian Research Council Discovery Project grant (2011–13) entitled *What Shall We Have for Tea? Toward a New Discourse of Food Ethics in Contemporary Australia* which supported the research associated with this article, and among her next project is a whole of value chain examination of animal welfare in Australia's livestock industry. Her favourite meal involves anything 'exotic' that makes her young son happy, most recently an excursion to a Nonya restaurant in a Singapore business park.

Heather J. Bray is a science communicator and researcher in agriculture and food at the University of Adelaide. She is fascinated by both the science in agriculture and the social aspects of food production in contemporary Australia. Her background is in agricultural and animal science (BScAgr (Hons), PhD (Veterinary Science)) and she has worked as a research scientist in both Australia and the Netherlands. After completing a Graduate Diploma in Science Communication, she worked for 10 years developing education and community engagement programmes for agricultural research centres that use complex and controversial technologies, as well as a range professional development programmes for young and developing scientists. More recently her research has focused on exploring community understandings of and attitudes to science in food production. Simple pasta dishes are among Heather's favourite meals, eaten outdoors at sunset with a glass of wine.

Perri Campbell is a Research Fellow in the Faculty of Arts and Education at Deakin University in Geelong, Australia. She is also the recipient of an Alfred Deakin Postdoctoral Fellowship at Deakin University. Perri is the author of *Digital Selves: Iraqi Women's Weblogs and the Limits of Freedom* (Common Ground, 2014); and journal papers, including: '"Don't be a Smart Arse": Transitional Labour Market Programs as Neo-liberal Technologies of the Self' (*British Journal of Sociology of Education*, 2014), 'Fractured Lives, Digital Selves: Writing the Self in Post-Invasion Iraq' (*Journal of Sociology*, 2013). Dr Campbell's research is concerned with the lives of young men and women in contemporary society, their transitions into adulthood, and use of digital communication technologies. Her work is influenced by critical social theorists, such as Judith Butler, Donna Haraway, Rosi Braidotti and Michel Foucault. Perri's current research investigates new forms of political practice and selfhood emerging in relation to the use of social media in countries around the world. Perri's favourite meal is the classic chocolate soufflé.

Jane Dixon is a Senior Fellow at the National Centre for Epidemiology and Population Health at the Australian National University. She has published six books, including: *When Culture Impacts Health: Global Lessons for Effective Health Research* (Elsevier Science, 2013), *The Weight of Modernity: An Intergenerational Study of the Weight of Modernity* (Springer Publishing, 2012) and *The Changing Chicken: Chooks, Cooks and Culinary Culture* (University of New South Wales Press, 2002). Her work appears in *Agriculture & Human Values, Food Policy, Journal of Sociology, British Food Journal* and the *International Journal of Epidemiology*. Jane's core research interests involve power in food systems, the nutrition transition fostered by supermarket chains, and the cultural dynamics underpinning social change and public health. She has been influenced by political and cultural economists and sociologists including Karl Marx, Scott Lash, Harriet Friedman, Philip McMichael and David Goodman. Her current research programme involves investigating the way labour markets shape culinary cultures, how the retail transition underway in Thailand and other Asian countries is having an impact on food security, and the contribution that poultry systems can make to the cultural and political economies of low- and middle-income countries. Her favourite meal centres on a 'shared table' laden with dishes made from fresh ingredients of known origin, where respect is paid to the ingredients and their biosphere, the cooks and their inputs. However, this reflection should not dominate the meal, and there should be plenty of lively discussion about matters of importance to all and sundry! It would be a bonus if my co-author, Bronwyn Isaacs, could be present.

John Evans is Professor of Sociology of Education and Physical Education in the School of Sport, Exercise and Health Sciences, Loughborough University. He has edited and written many books and journal papers in the sociology of education including (with Emma Rich, Brian Davies and Rachel Allwood) *Education, Disordered Eating and Obesity Discourse: Fat Fabrications* (Routledge, 2008). John is also founding editor of the international research journal *Sport, Education and Society*. His research interests centre on equity, inclusion and embodiment in education and Physical Education. He favours large chips, a big Mac and a ciggy, preferably sitting down.

Rick Flowers is a Senior Lecturer in the School of Education, Faculty of Arts and Social Sciences, University of Technology Sydney. He was Director of the Centre for Popular Education at the University of Technology, Sydney from 1999 to 2007 which undertook research in environmental education and advocacy, community cultural development, health education and community development, the pedagogy and politics of working with young people, union and community organising, and community leadership. Rick is currently collaborating with Elaine Swan. Drawing on Rick's research on collective action and learning, and Elaine's work on whiteness, gender and public pedagogies, they are developing a major research programme on food pedagogies. They have edited a special issue on Food Pedagogies for the *Australian Journal of Adult Learning* (2012), and written journal papers about food activism, culinary tour guiding, the Internet and food multiculturalism. Rick plans to extend a research agenda which focuses on everyday, cultural and public pedagogies. His work has been influenced by scholarship in the field of popular education. One of Rick's favourite dishes is Hainanese chicken rice – where the chicken has been gently poached in a master stock matured over years, the rice steamed in the same stock with pandan leaves, and served with chilli sauce.

Michael K. Goodman is Professor of Geography (Environment and Development) in the Geography and Environmental Science Department, University of Reading. He is broadly interested in the cultural politics of food, environment and development and is slowly (and hopefully) prying open the study of celebrity culture, politics and materialities to new and different interdisciplinary audiences. Food is central to these concerns and so current research is focused on the powerful mediations of food, eating and sustainability by celebrity chefs and other forms of contemporary food media cultures; both will figure heavily in forthcoming special issues of the journals *Geoforum* and *Food, Culture and Society*. Recent publications include *Alternative Food Networks* (Routledge, 2012 with David Goodman and Melanie DuPuis), a co-edited volume with Colin Sage entitled *Food Transgressions* (Ashgate, 2014) that explores the multiple and contentious boundary-crossings of food, and also the co-edited volume *Consuming Space* (Ashgate, 2010; David Goodman and Michael Redclift). He edits the Critical Food Studies book series with Ashgate and, with David Goodman, co-edits a second book series entitled Contemporary Food Politics with Bloomsbury. His scholarly influences are cosmopolitan and legion, from political ecologists such as Arturo Escobar and Michael Watts, to 'materialist' theorists like Latour and Jane Bennett, to the geographers David Harvey, Derek Gregory and Gill Valentine, to critical pedagogy scholars such as Paolo Freire and Henry Giroux, to consumption scholars like Zygmunt Bauman, critical theorists such as Foucault, Gramsci, Stuart Hall, Elspeth Probyn and Raymond Williams and more recent media/cultural studies types such as Lillie Chouliaraki, Jo Littler and Bev Skeggs. A veritable smorgasbord really that at some level does actually make sense (to him at least). As for foods, well let's just say he is ecstatic that there are burrito shops opening up on every other corner in London and other parts of the UK these days and they do their very best to replicate the justifiably world-conquering San Francisco burrito. That said, adding curry to burrito rice – while satisfying the aphorism of 'becoming local to a place' – does nothing for him. Weirdly, lemon drops are also a favourite as they remind him of the mysteriously ever-full handbag of his grandmother who would apportion the lemon drops out with the same liberal nature as her mindset. And pizza.

Lyn Harrison is Associate Head of Research in the School of Education at Deakin University, Victoria, Australia. She is the co-author of two books: *Working in Jamie's Kitchen: Salvation, Passion and Young Workers* (2009) and *Smashed! The Many Meanings of Intoxication and Drunkenness* (2011). She also co-authored a major monograph *Sexuality Education Matters: Preparing Pre-service Teachers to Teach Sexuality Education* in 2013. Lyn has published articles in *The British Journal of Sociology of Education, Health, Risk and Society, Sport, Education and Society and Culture, Health and Sexuality* amongst others. Lyn's core interests are in Critical Youth Studies, Health and Well-being and Sexuality Education. Michel Foucault and poststructuralist feminist scholars including Emma Renold and Judith Butler have influenced her work. She is in the latter stages of an Australian Research Council (ARC) Linkage project researching a Social Enterprise Transitional Labour Market Program in the hospitality industry and in 2014 begins another ARC Linkage project *Engaging Young People in Sexuality Education* focusing on student voice. Share plates with family and friends – Italian, Thai or Spanish – are her favourite meals.

Bronwyn Isaacs is a doctoral candidate in Anthropology at Harvard University. She has published articles in *The Asia Pacific Journal of Anthropology, Public Health Nutrition, Journal of Sociology, Agriculture and Human Values,* and *Food Policy* and contributed to the collective volume *Street Food: Culture, Economy, Health and Policy.* Inspired by the work of anthropologists including Michael Herzfeld, Bruce Kapferer and Saba Mahmood, Bronwyn's research interests are located in political anthropology, performances of selfhood and sincerity and models of morality. These themes are contributing to her current research in Thailand. Bronwyn's favourite meal would be shared among friends on a long evening accompanied by sticky rice, crispy catfish, papaya salad served with hot chillies and a cool Thai beer.

Kaela Jubas is an Assistant Professor in Adult Learning at University of Calgary, Alberta, Canada. Her book *The Politics of Shopping: What Consumers Learn about Identity, Globalization, and Social Change* discusses her doctoral study of shopping as long-lasting, politically charged learning. She has published in journals such as *International Journal of Lifelong Education*, *Review of Education*, *Pedagogy*, and *Cultural Studies, Adult Education Quarterly*, *Studies in Continuing Education*, *Social Identities*, *Studies in the Education of Adults*, and *International Journal of Qualitative Methods*. Informed by Antonio Gramsci's concepts and more recent feminist, critical theory and postmodern writing, Kaela explores public pedagogy, identity, work and learning, and health care-related learning. Ongoing projects include studies about Alberta's Undergraduate Nurse Employee programme, conducted with nursing colleagues, and work in the neoliberal academy. Her favourite meals include good conversation, ambiance and food (meat-free, sourced as sustainably and ethically as possible!). Mezes on an Istanbul terrace, wine and cheese with colleagues at her British Columbia home, and locally caught fish north of Powell River, on Haida Gwaii and in Fort Bragg are memorable treats!

Peter Kelly is the Deputy Head for Research and Innovation in the School of Education, RMIT University Melbourne. He is a social theorist/social researcher who has published extensively on young people, the practice of Youth Studies; social theory and globalisation, and the ways in which youth transitions – and the family, employment, study and peer relationships shaped by these processes of transition – are being remade by the emergence of a globalised knowledge economy. His new book *The Self as Enterprise: Foucault and the Spirit of Twenty-First Century Capitalism* suggests that twenty-first century, flexible capitalism creates new demands for those who work to acknowledge that the cultivation of the self as an enterprise is the life-long activity that should give meaning, purpose and direction to a life. His 2009 book (with Lyn Harrison) *Working in Jamie's Kitchen: Salvation, Passion and Young Workers* used the manufactured drama of the TV series *Jamie's Kitchen* and *Jamie's Kitchen Australia* to examine the ways in which marginalised young people are required to transform themselves into the type of person who can secure a tenuous form of salvation in the globalised labour markets of the twenty-first century. His favourite meal would involve tapas, wine, a good view, good company and good music.

Deana Leahy is a Senior Lecturer in the Faculty of Education at Monash University, Australia. Her research interests are framed by her concerns about the political and moral work that is 'done' under the guise of improving the health of children and young people in educational settings. Her research draws from Foucauldian and post-Foucauldian inspired writings on governmentality to consider the various mentalities that are assembled together in policy and curriculum and how they are translated into key pedagogical spaces. Deana has published in a range of national and international scholarly journals as well as several book chapters in edited collections. She is currently working on a co-authored book entitled *School Health Education in Changing Times: Policies, Pedagogies and Partnerships*. The book will be published by Routledge in 2015. Deana's favourite meal varies, but usually involves pasta and wine.

Jo Pike is currently a Lecturer in Childhood Studies at the University of Leeds, UK. Her research relates to the ways in which space is implicated in the production of children as self-governing healthy subjects with a particular focus upon school-based foodscapes. Her work, to date, has generally followed a Foucauldian-inspired trajectory while her interest in spatiality has resulted in publications in journals such as *Children's Geographies.* Her most recent publications include 'Beyond Jamie's School Dinners: The Moral Geographies of Young People and Food' with Peter Kelly (2014) and 'Young People and Food: The Moral Project of the Healthy Self', in P. Kelly and A. Kamp (eds), *A Critical Youth Studies for the Twenty-First Century* (2014). While writing this brief biography in the midst of a particularly sombre UK winter, she confesses: 'my favourite food item to be the traditional British mince pie. I found it impossible to "say no" to these over Christmas.'

Emma Rich is a Senior Lecturer in the Department of Health at the University of Bath. She is author of *The Medicalization of Cyberspace* (2008, Routledge, with Professor Andy Miah) *Education, Disordered eating and Obesity Discourse: Fat Fabrications* (2008, Routledge, with Professor John Evans) *and Debating Obesity: Critical Perspectives* (2011, Palgrave, with Monaghan and Aphramor). She has published articles in a range of international peer-reviewed journals including *British Educational Research Journal*, *Discourse: Studies in the Cultural Politics of Education*, *'Health': An Interdisciplinary Journal for the Social Study of Health, Illness and Medicine*, *International Studies in Sociology of Education*, and *Sociology of Health and Illness*. Her future research focuses on the people's experiences and understandings of health through emerging technologies such as social media. Her favourite meal is a roast dinner – wholesome, filling favourite throughout her childhood!

Julie Robert is a Senior Lecturer of Cultural and International Studies at the University of Technology, Sydney. Her research covers areas pertaining to medical and public health discourses in the construction of national identities in both France and Canada, responsible drinking initiatives, embodied philanthropy and the cultural representations of alcohol. She has published work on these topics in *Social Semiotics*, *Portal* and the *Cultural Studies Review*. Her work is interdisciplinary and draws on scholars in a number of fields, including linguistic anthropology, cultural and literary studies, history and medical humanities. She is currently undertaking further research on popular embodied philanthropy initiatives, including those aimed at promoting and utilising responsible drinking strategies. Hard-pressed to name a favourite meal due to a tendency for palate fatigue and a love of variety, she concedes that breakfast cereal is the one dish she could eat for a fortnight without tiring of it.

Jennifer A. Sandlin is an Associate Professor in the School of Social Transformation at Arizona State University in Tempe, where she teaches courses focused on consumption and education, social and cultural pedagogy, and public pedagogy. Her research interests include public pedagogy, popular culture, informal learning, and various sites of ideological education for children, youth and adults. Her recent work investigates consumer education, broadly defined, and she is especially interested in sites of public pedagogy, informal learning, and anti-consumption social activism that question the norms of consumption, create resistance to consumer culture, and focus on 'unlearning' consumerism. She recently edited, with Jake Burdick and Michael O'Malley, *Problematizing Public Pedagogy* (2013, Routledge), and is currently working on an edited volume (with Julie Maudlin) focused on the curricula and pedagogy of the Walt Disney Company. She co-edits, with Will Letts, the *Journal of Curriculum and Pedagogy*, and her work has appeared in various outlets including *Journal of Consumer Culture*, *Qualitative Inquiry*, *International Journal of Qualitative Studies in Education*, *Teachers College Record*, *Adult Education Quarterly*, *International Journal of Lifelong Education*, and *Studies in the Education of Adults*. She loves the all you can eat vegetarian Indian buffet at her favourite restaurant (Udupi Cafe) in Tempe, Arizona, eats way more French fries than she should, and is currently trying to grow lots of kale and parsley in her garden.

Jennifer Sumner is a lecturer in Adult Education and Community Development at OISE/University of Toronto. She has authored and co-edited the following books: *Sustainability and the Civil Commons: Rural Communities in the Age of Globalization* (author) and *Critical Perspectives in Food Studies* (co-editor). She has published in various journals, including *Agriculture and Human Values*, *Journal of Sustainable Agriculture*, *Studies in Social Justice*, *Studies in the Education of Adults*, *Adult Education Quarterly* and *Canadian Journal for the Study of Adult Education*. Her core research interests include sustainable food systems, food and cooperatives, critical pedagogy, globalization and organic agriculture. Jennifer's work has been deeply influenced by David Harvey, Patricia Allen and Julie Guthman. Her research plans include continuing to investigate the parameters of a sustainable food system, and the role of cooperatives within such a system. And her favourite meal involves Lebanese food. 'Although I've never been to Lebanon, something about the food appeals deeply to me – the choice of spices, the uniquely smooth flavours and the wide array of vegetarian options.'

Elaine Swan is a Senior Lecturer in the School of Communication Faculty of Arts and Social Sciences, at the University of Technology, Sydney. She is the author of *Worked up Selves* (Palgrave) on the interface between therapeutic cultures and the workplace and *Gender and Diversity in the Workplace* (with Caroline Gatrell, Sage). Recent papers include 'Cooking up a Storm: Politics, Labour and Bodies' in a Special Issue of *Leisure/Loisir* on Food and Leisure, 'States of White Ignorance, and Audit Masculinity in English Higher Education' (Social Politics), 'Commodity Diversity and Smiling Faces' (Organization). With Rick Flowers, she has been researching food pedagogies under the umbrella of a programme on everyday, cultural and public pedagogy out of which they have published 'Eating the Asian Other? Pedagogies of Food Multiculturalism in Australia' (*Portal Journal of Multidisciplinary International Studies*) and 'Teaching People to Suck Eggs: Pedagogies and Food Activists' (*Australian Journal of Adult Learning*), and co-edited a Special Issue of the *Australian Journal of Adult Learning* on Food Pedagogies. Her work is underpinned by the concept of 'pedagogy', inspired by Carmen Luke's wonderful book *Feminism and the Pedagogies of Everyday Life*, and always influenced by many critical race theorist and feminist writers, including Sara Ahmed, Catriona Elder, Charles Mills, Celia Lury and Beverly Skeggs. Working with Rick, she is starting research on multiculturalism as work, which will examine unpaid labour and pedagaogies with case studies on food tours, food festivals and food social enterprises. Her favourite food usually begins with two cocktails, preferably with a tiny umbrella and a little plastic monkey on the side of a very large glass, followed by tiddly giddiness and meals which include rice, garlic and chilli, but no meat. When she has no ingredients at home, she will cook spaghetti and aglio olio. But she has also relished her co-researcher's rösti, many portions of which have nourished the writing and editing of this book.

Seline Szkupinski-Quiroga is Faculty Research Affiliate at the Southwestern Interdisciplinary Research Center of Arizona State University, and Principal Consultant of Culture Cures Consulting. Her work has been published in the *Journal of Family Practice*, *Archives of Family Medicine*, *Journal of Health Care for the Poor and Underserved*, *Hypatia: A Journal of Feminist Philosophy*, and *Latino Studies*. Her research focuses on health disparities, the lived experience of illness among vulnerable populations as revealed through narratives, and the intersection of food and culture. She is influenced by the work of Michel Foucault, and critical race theorists. Her current projects are developing a culturally informed metric of food environments, and an intervention promoting healthy eating. She was unable to come up with one favourite meal, though chiles en nogada, pierogi, morcilla, and barbeque ribs were all contenders. What these dishes have in common is that they carry memories of friends and family.

Robin Redmon Wright is currently an Assistant Professor of Adult Education at Penn State, Harrisburg. She holds both a BA and an MA in English Literature from the University of Tennessee and a PhD in Adult Education from Texas A&M University. Her research interests reflect a critical perspective on adult identity development, feminist identity development, popular culture and informal adult learning and development, and adult learning, educational access and socio-economic class. Recent publications include articles in the *International Journal of Lifelong Education, Adult Education Quarterly, Journal of Transformational Education, Journal of Studies in International Education*, and *The Journal of Curriculum and Pedagogy*. Dr. Wright's work is influenced by theorists in the critical tradition such as Michel Foucault, Antonio Gramsci, Herbert Marcuse, and Jurgen Habermas; critical feminists like Simone de Beauvoir, Julia Kristeva, and Judith Butler; and cultural theorists like Henry Giroux, bell hooks, Stuart Hall, and Edward Said. She is currently working on a critical analysis of the proliferation of working-class reality TV shows in the US. 'My favourite meal is dependent on my mood and the season, but almost everything I cook contains hot peppers of various kinds that I grow each summer. I like food spicy!'

Acknowledgements

We'd like to acknowledge the financial support we have received for undertaking research and travel from the Cosmopolitan Civil Societies Research Centre, Faculty of Arts and Social Sciences and Creative Practices, Cultural Economy Research Centre – all at the University of Technology, Sydney.

We'd like to extend our gratitude to all of the contributors for their ideas, and for taking the time to revise chapters. In addition, and we are grateful to our colleagues Elaine Lally, Julie Robert and Kate Barclay, members of the research programme we convened entitled Everyday, Cultural and Public Pedagogies, for their intellectual insights. As part of this programme, we organised a full-day workshop on Pedagogies with Anna Hickey-Moody, Valerie Harwood, Greg Noble, and Megan Watkins to provide feedback on the group's research. We would like to thank Anna, Valerie, Greg, and Megan for their interest and advice.

Rick would like to thank Franziska Trede, his wife and Toni, Jesse and Tascha, their children for supporting and encouraging his research. Franziska has been generous, loving and respectful of his efforts.

He would also like to say how rewarding and special the research of the last three years has been, undertaken with Elaine Swan who came from Lancaster University to the University of Technology, Sydney. He recognises and acknowledges her commitment to nurturing a deeply collaborative research relationship, her fierce intelligence, ability to eloquently cut swathes through dense theorising, voracious appetite for reading and friendship.

Elaine would like to thank Steve Fox for his unstinting encouragement and Jo Bu at UTS for her support, and administrative skills over the past three years.

She must thank Reno the mule for the famous mule ride down the Grand Canyon. Finally, she would like to express her gratitude to Rick for the research collaboration over the past three years. From their first reading of David Sutton on food and the senses and Jane Kenway on skin pedagogies, it has been a stimulating, challenging, vital partnership. In Rick, she found a co-researcher and special friend who is intellectually incisive, imaginative, curious, open, patient, thoughtful, pro-feminist and mercurially witty. With him, she has learned so much about the research 'object' of food in all its guises; research methodologies; goalkeeping and kayaking; scholarship and importantly, conviviality over food.

Chapter 1

Food Pedagogies: Histories, Definitions and Moralities

Rick Flowers and Elaine Swan

From the *Slow Food Movement* to the *World Street Food Congress* and Jamie Oliver's *Ministry of Food* and the 'healthy eating' campaigns of government and non-government agencies, efforts to 'teach' us about food have intensified. In this book we apply the concept of 'food pedagogies' to analyse the proliferation of teaching and learning about food, the diversification of food educational processes, the rise of new food pedagogues and the shift in expertise and knowledge about food. In essence, in this collection the term food pedagogies denotes a congeries of educational, teaching and learning ideologies and practices carried out by a range of agencies, actors, institutions and media which focus variously on growing, shopping, cooking, eating and disposing of food. This definition points to various forms, sites and processes of formal, informal and incidental education and learning, inside and beyond the classroom. Scholars in the field of adult education use the adjectives formal, informal and incidental to typologise, roughly speaking, the degree to which learning is programmatic; led by teachers; and undertaken purposely by learners (Flowers, Guevara and Whelan 2009). Examples of formal food pedagogies include cooking masterclasses, health education in schools, nutrition workshops in food security programmes, and permaculture courses; instances of informal food pedagogies are food programmes on television, community gardening, and social marketing campaigns led by food social movements or supermarkets; and incidental food pedagogies cover learning from social occasions, eating and drinking with friends, families and on holidays.

As these examples suggest, food pedagogies entail significant and asymmetrical relations of power, authority and expertise. They reproduce 'moral economies' (Coveney 2006) of knowledge and food practices reproducing categories of 'good' and 'bad' mothers/eaters/consumers: those who look after their health and those who put their children's health at risk; those who have refined taste and those who eat indiscriminately; those who care about animal welfare and environmentalism and those who buy cheap food regardless of where it comes from; those who have cosmopolitan sensibilities and try new ethnic foods and those who are unadventurous, even racist, in their eating. Often classist, sexist and racist, food pedagogies are grounded in the assumption that the main determinant of 'bad' food choice is lack of knowledge, ignoring the social, political and cultural complexities of food in people's lives (Guthman 2008a and b; Hayes-Conroy 2009).

As a result, food pedagogies position women as bad mothers and cooks; responsibilise individuals and ignore wider structural inequalities and social hierarchies; perpetuate universalist assumptions about what constitutes 'good food'; overemphasise nutritional scientific knowledge; and privilege bodily health over mental well-being (Coveney 2006; Guthman 2008a/b; Berlant 2010; Hayes-Conroy and Hayes-Conroy 2014).

Food pedagogies elevate those 'in the know' and their 'good intentions'; and shame classed and racialised forms of food knowledge, lifestyle and embodiment. Moreover, middle-class food pedagogies such as permaculture workshops and cooking classes, voluntarily paid for as leisure pursuits, reproduce status distinction and consolidate classed and racialised hierarchies of taste, 'healthism' and 'doing good' (Guthman 2008a and b; Flowers and Swan 2012c). Indeed, garnering new knowledge about food constitutes the core of middle-class foodie, locavore and food adventurer identities (De Solier 2013; Johnston and Baumann 2010).

The proliferation and intensification of food pedagogies means that there is a plethora of pedagogues with a mission to 'educate' us about food:

- farmers and small food producers;
- cultural intermediaries, such as celebrity chefs, cookbook and food writers, food bloggers, lifestyle and nutritional practitioners, and food marketing, public relations and advertising professionals;
- school teachers, doctors and nurses, health educators;
- activists in diverse social movements from animal welfare, food justice, permaculture, slow food and organic farming;
- government bodies, local councils, and health agencies with their policy instruments such as national food plans, school curricula reform, labelling and nutrition guidelines;
- large corporate food producers and retailers.

Some of these clearly have extensive economic and cultural power to define meanings about 'good' food, health, and ways of consuming, and authors in this collection, in particular, discuss the politics of the food pedagogies of supermarkets, school teachers and health educators.

This list of food pedagogues underlines how wide the range of food pedagogies circulating across different sites is, and gives us a sense of the heterogeneity of their curricula including their specific educational aims, content, pedagogical relations, and learning processes. In spite of the power of pedagogues and the intensive, even invasive, nature of food pedagogies, we should not underestimate the agency of targeted 'learners'. As this book shows in detailing the effects and efficacies of various food pedagogies, learners do not simply slurp up the lessons on offer. Whether it is supermarkets trying to instil certain food lifestyles, shoppers reading labels, viewers watching food programmes on TV, school pupils being given nutritional edicts, French consumers of alcohol advertising, authors suggest that pedagogies can 'fail'.

The Pedagogical Turn

Having outlined the nature and extent of food pedagogies, in this next section we introduce how the concept of pedagogy has been used in education studies, the 'turn' to pedagogy as an analytic in cultural studies, and three approaches within this 'turn'. Narrowly speaking then, 'pedagogy' is a foundational concept in education studies, deployed to characterise teaching, learning and assessment practices in schools, colleges and universities (Lingard 2009; Hickey-Moody, Savage and Windle 2010a/b). Thus, educational theorist, Bob Lingard (2009) states that in its most traditional usage, pedagogy refers to 'teachers in classrooms': i.e. instruction, teaching, and curricula. He calls, however, for pedagogy to be extended to the social and political context of classroom practices including macro discourses of learning, teaching and assessment. For feminist educational theorists, analysis of pedagogy must include how gender underpins the context of the classroom and wider educational discourses (Luke and Gore 1992; Kenway and Modra 1992).

A burgeoning body of work outside education studies has turned to the concept of pedagogy to analyse the educational effects of cultural and social processes beyond the classroom (Luke 1996; Giroux 2004a; Watkins, Noble and Driscoll 2015; Hickey-Moody, Savage and Windle 2010; Flowers and Swan 2012; Kenway and Bullen 2011; Swan 2012). Thus, Jennifer Sandlin, Michael O'Malley and Jake Burdick make clear that pedagogy:

> involves learning in institutions such as museums, zoos and libraries; informal educational sites such as popular culture, media, commercial spaces and the Internet; and through figures and sites of activism, including public intellectuals and grassroots social movements. (2011: 338–9)

Broadly speaking, theorists use pedagogy to study, in particular, cultural and social processes which attempt to modify, or transform how we act, feel and think (Noble 2012; Watkins, Noble and Driscoll 2015). Anna Hickey-Moody, Glen Savage and Joel Windle (2010) gloss this body of work as 'pedagogy writ large' to underline the extension of pedagogy as an analytic to a diversity of cultural practices from health promotion, screen technologies, food activism, Disney films, marketing and advertising to children, reality TV, cosmetic surgery, through to shopping and community arts; and to highlight the range of theoretical traditions and methodological approaches being used in these analyses (Hickey-Moody, Savage and Windle 2010; Sandlin, Schultz and Burdick 2010; Sandlin and McLaren 2010).

To trace the development of this body of work, in this next section, we demarcate and describe three distinct, but related approaches: 'public pedagogy'; 'pedagogies of everyday life' and 'cultural pedagogy'.

Public Pedagogy

Fundamentally, for theorists who examine public pedagogy: 'culture *can* and *does* operate in pedagogical ways' (Hickey-Moody, Savage and Windle 2010: 227). Although there are various lineages in the scholarship on public pedagogy, it is mainly a Northern American body of work based on neo-Marxist ideology-critique and heavily influenced by Henry Giroux (Hickey-Moody et al. 2010; Sandlin et al. 2011; Watkins et al. 2015). Using the term 'public pedagogy' first in 1998, Giroux a prolific writer, sees his project as putting an analysis of pedagogy in dialogue with cultural studies (1998, 1992, 2004a/b). More concretely, he deploys public pedagogy, first, to challenge what he sees as the educative project of capitalism transmitted through popular culture; and secondly, to refer to public intellectuals such as writers, journalists and artists who can teach citizens to transform the oppressive conditions in which they live. Thus, for Giroux, public pedagogy can be repressive *and* resistive; popular culture a site of social reproduction, and contestation. For example, he writes:

> the media, as well as the culture they produce, distribute, sanction, have become the most important educational force in creating citizens and social agents capable of putting existing institutions into question and making democracy work – or doing just the opposite. (2005: 45)

Studying a diverse range of cultural and social practices from Disney films, Calvin Klein and Benetton advertising, rap music and media coverage of Abu Graib, his recent work focuses on the repressive power of public pedagogy: how popular media 'teach neoliberalism' and corporations extend their influence on public spaces and 'harness the resources of "the public" for corporate gain' (Hickey-Moody 2013: 28).

Studies of public pedagogy, however, are not limited to Giroux or ideology critique. North Americans, Jake Burdick and Jennifer Sandlin, by far the most prolific synthesisers of the field, edited a *Handbook of Public Pedagogy* (2010) with 65 chapters and a smaller volume entitled *Problematising Pedagogy* (2014). These go beyond Giroux's approach by expanding the range of cultural sites studied, extending the role of public intellectuals to include social activists, grassroots organisations, and artist collectives; and drawing on post-structuralist theories of power. Burdick and Sandlin's extensive scholarship does important definitional work in the field and builds on the Girouxian view that public pedagogy can be about resistance as well as social reproduction (Sandlin, O'Malley and Burdick 2011).

Their frustration (like others) is that theorising on public pedagogy does not make clear what makes a space or process 'pedagogical'. Thus, pedagogy is cited frequently 'without adequately explicating its meaning, its context, or its location' (Sandlin, O'Malley and Burdick 2011: 339). Accordingly, they argue 'more work needs to be conducted on how the various sites, spaces, products and places identified as public pedagogy actually operate as pedagogy' (2011: 359). As a result, their more recent work turns to the topic of pedagogical processes: what they defined as 'the mechanisms and interactions that enable an individual's capacity to learn' (Burdick and Sandlin 2013: 143). Surveying literature on pedagogy, they chart (2013) three 'schools': transfer, relational and post-human – and identify the pedagogical processes associated with each. *Transfer* pedagogies are humanist and thus reproduce a view of learners as autonomous, susceptible to the transmission of meanings and ideology in culture from mechanisms such as images, music, dialogue and sounds. Influenced by feminist arts scholarship, *Relational* pedagogies emphasise non-cognitive learning such as embodiment, movement, sensations and aesthetics. Finally, *Post-human* pedagogies challenge 'anthropocentric liberal subjectivity' centring animals, nature and the 'fabulous', rupturing modernist ideas of individual autonomy and control and dissolving binaries of sense/cognition and nature/culture/animal (2013: 167–8). This work is significant for researching food pedagogies on several counts. First, it elaborates a range of pedagogical processes outside transmission models of education; secondly, it challenges the idea that public pedagogy operates hypodermically, with culture as an 'educational force' working on unsuspecting humans; and thirdly, it shows how learning can be unpredictable, dynamic and relational. In sum, their work prises open the category of pedagogy, showing how people learning about food goes beyond cognitive, information transfer or ideological influence, and calls for more attention to be given to the concrete processes and interactions through which people transform how they cook, shop, and eat, and including senses, emotions, bodies and non-humans.

Pedagogies of Everyday Life

Not all pedagogy studies focus on public pedagogy. At the same time as Giroux started his writing on public pedagogy, Australian educationalist Carmen Luke, edited an interdisciplinary feminist book in 1996 to examine how the domestic and private sphere work pedagogically to teach children and women about gender, class and race. Influenced by feminist and Foucauldian theories of power and discourse rather than neo-Marxian ideology critique, and somewhat overshadowed in accounts of public pedagogy, Luke describes the aim of her project as the interrogation of the 'pedagogical project of everyday life' (1996: 1). In the collection, authors explore popular culture in the home, from television programmes, computer games, parenting magazines, and toys; and discuss how friendship, mothering, and parenting constitute pedagogical relations. Her work matters for food pedagogy scholarship because contra Girouxian writing on the public sphere as a site of pedagogy, the book emphasises the salience of the domestic sphere as an arena of pedagogical relations and activities; and provides feminist detailed empirical studies of the relations between everyday life, learning, and identity formation in the home. In a prescient study of the everyday before the recent 'turn to the everyday' in social theory, her work augments feminist food studies on feeding work in the domestic because of its clear focus on pedagogy in the home. The book reminds us that everyday relations like friendships and mothering, activities such as reading magazines and playing with toys, and using objects such as computer games all teach. Whilst written some 20 years ago, and with cultural analysis of the everyday and domestic objects being much more widespread, Luke's book is important for food pedagogy studies because of the range of domestic objects and pedagogical relations it details, and the ways in which the authors show how popular culture in the home and intimate everyday practices are sites of learning and negotiation about class, gender and race.

Cultural Pedagogy

The third body of pedagogy studies derives from recent Australian scholarship by authors such as Gregory Noble, Megan Watkins, Catherine Driscoll, Glen Savage, Joel Windle and Anna-Hickey-Moody, who badge their work as 'cultural pedagogy', to distance their approach from North American public pedagogy literature. For example, in a special issue on pedagogy, Hickey-Moody, Savage and Windle (2010) provide a detailed rationale for their use of the category cultural pedagogy. First, they argue that Giroux's take on public pedagogy is too North American, and assumes that all publics, regardless of local context, respond to American popular culture uniformly. Secondly, they suggest that Giroux sees pedagogy like socialisation, reproducing an idea of stable social systems transmitting pre-formed norms from society to individual; rather than taking as a starting point that society is structured by conflict, and that norms are developed and contested. Thirdly, his understanding of power is too narrow and repressive because he views public pedagogy as 'negative ideological forces that … act upon and corrupt individuals'; and furthermore, ignores the significance of affect, bodies and desire (Savage 2010: 109). Moreover, authors suggest that Giroux does not make clear how critical pedagogues are immune to the corrupting, monolithic forces of public pedagogy (Savage 2010; Noble 2004). In sum, these theorists recognise the contribution of Giroux but are critical of what they see as his deterministic, broad-brushed, and overly negative approach which gives little attention to learners (Hickey-Moody, Savage and Windle 2010; Noble 2004; Savage 2010).

Like Burdick and Sandlin, these theorists problematise the under-researching and under-theorising of pedagogical processes. For instance, Greg Noble argues that Giroux represents pedagogy as a 'black box'; signalling 'something is done but without explaining *how* it is done' (Noble 2004: 2). Indeed, Watkins, Noble and Driscoll (2015) develop this criticism further, taking cultural studies to task for deploying the term pedagogy 'rhetorically' rather than 'analytically'. The latter entails a more in-depth, and empirical examination of what makes a cultural or social process pedagogical and the effects these processes eventuate. Thus, Noble asserts cultural studies replaced 'crude, simplistic ideas about social and cultural transmission' with more 'nuanced categories of interpellation, appropriation, embodiment, becoming and identify formation', but 'without ever adequately unpacking the pedagogic dimensions of these processes' (2004: 2). Consequently he, Watkins and Driscoll are concerned to research and theorise the processes by which cumulative changes in 'how we act feel and think' are produced using concepts of 'capacitation, habituation and embodiment' to start to pin down the durational effects of pedagogical relations and mechanisms (Noble 2004: 2; Watkins et al. 2015). Indeed, as several of the chapters in this volume argue, pedagogic processes through which conduct is 'capacitated, fashioned, regulated, re-directed and augmented' are not simply cognitive but embodied (involving the training of specific capacities) and deeply affective (Noble, 2012: 2). In forcing us to examine more closely how transformation and learning take place, Noble and colleagues develop much further than Burdick and Sandlin, the dynamics of what makes a cultural and social process pedagogical. The durational nature of pedagogies, and what they can capacitate, is of particular concern for Noble, who writes that 'learning is cumulative, accretive and iterative, and not about moments of enlightenment or liberation' (2012: 4). In foregrounding embodiment, habits and capacities, the work of Noble and colleagues can clearly contribute to food studies by encouraging us to scrutinise how forms of conduct; technical and cultural capacities; ideas; affect; and practices are acquired, shaped, fashioned and regulated discursively and materially. For example, to analyse the effects of TV cooking programmes on viewers – a popular topic in food studies – we might think more explicitly about theories of multi-modal representational processes; analyses of verbal, narrative, visual and music televisual properties; their meaning-making potential and theories of audience reception such as psychoanalytic identification or non-representational affect (Flowers and Swan 2011). Furthermore, Noble and colleagues insist that it is through close-up, concrete qualitative study that we can identify how people 'acquire' knowledge, values and skills about food, cooking, eating, gender, race and so forth. Their overall project being to prise open the black box of pedagogy and to identify, describe and analyse the pedagogical relations, techniques and practices through which subjectivity is formed; minds and bodies are shaped; and the teaching and learning of social and cultural practices.

Food Studies and Pedagogy

This brief summary of pedagogy studies raises questions about how authors in food studies have deployed the term pedagogy. Broadly speaking, we discern two core ways: rhetorically, to suggest that social and cultural practices in relation to food are educative; and analytically, to examine teaching and learning processes about food, inside and outside education institutions. Additionally, some authors write about food learning and teaching but do not use the term pedagogy. Below we introduce authors from these three approaches.

First, we turn to Jennifer Sumner, who uses the term pedagogy of food in her writing and teaching, developing the first university subject to be called Pedagogy of Food at the University of Toronto in a master's programme aimed at adult educators. Influenced by theories of adult education and sustainable education, Sumner (2008, 2013) writes of 'eating as a pedagogical act' and puts forward an argument about education, food justice and the global political economy of food. She discusses the design of her subject in more depth in her chapter in this book, in which she deploys the term pedagogy in a more traditional educational sense to describe the teaching of global food systems in the university, rather than as an analytic to examine public or cultural pedagogy.

Jessica Hayes-Conroy (2009) researches teaching and learning in school gardening and cooking programmes aimed at healthy eating in her doctoral thesis and dedicates a whole chapter to a discussion of food pedagogy. Her main aim is to examine 'taste education' in schools and how social difference produces differential access to viscerality. Like Sumner she deploys pedagogy to analyse formal education and institutional curricula and to evaluate the political potential of taste education to challenge social structures and categories. In similar vein, her sister, Alison Hayes-Conroy examines the Slow Food Movement. Together they study how bodies, sensations, moods and feelings are mobilised in alternative food activism (Hayes-Conroy, 2014). Their political project is to highlight that senses and viscera should not be romanticised as pre-social in sensory education and food activism, but rather understood as profoundly classed, gendered and racialised. On the one hand, their work is not explicitly focused on producing knowledge about public or cultural pedagogy but on the other hand, like Noble and colleagues advocate, they trace pedagogical processes in empirical detail, discussing the body's presence in learning and learning through commensality. In a similar move, Ben Highmore (2008) calls for more research on sensual pedagogies in everyday life, to examine non-mentalist 'sensual habits' and 'corporeal learning'. Examining a white working-class man eating a hot curry in the UK, he suggests the eating of the curry can be understood as having a 'pedagogical function', with the chilli being a kind of 'teacher' which educates the white body to accept new flavours and tastes. Thus, he argues that our bodies are 'in process', and eating 'foreign' foods provides us with an 'alimentary pedagogy'.

Whilst Hayes-Conroy and Hayes-Conroy show how alternative food activism produce visceral attachments, other scholars in education studies examine how health education creates affective investment in a normative ideal of a 'healthful' body. Using the concept of pedagogy, but pre-fixed by various terms such as health, body and bio, these scholars have written a body of work, focused on formal and informal pedagogies aimed at children, mothers and parents, particularly focused on healthism, nutritional science (Coveney 2012) and 'obesity discourse' (Evans, Rich, Davies and Allwood 2008). For instance, John Coveney (2006) wrote an in-depth Foucauldian analysis of the history and morality of nutritional education in his book *Food, Morals and Meaning*. In the book, Coveney uses the term pedagogy rhetorically more than analytically, to chart how Christian technologies of the self such as the confessional and abstinence influence nutritional expertise and practice. In a later paper, he uses pedagogy more analytically to extend this discussion to the discourse of the decline of cooking skills in the media (2012). Although he does not situate his work in pedagogy literature, his focus on technologies of power and of the self – highly concrete, mundane, even 'minor and petty' forms of expertise, techniques, judgements and sanctions – in relation to nutritional science and its moral subjectivities, means that scholars interested more explicitly in the pedagogical processes of health promotion campaigns in and outside schools have taken up his work (for instance, Leahy, 2010; Pike and Leahy, 2012; Rich and Evans and Leahy and Pike this volume).

Indeed the Foucauldian influence on anti-obesity health promotion pedagogy scholars is strong. For instance, since 2007, education academics Jan Wright and Valerie Harwood have coined the concept of 'bio-pedagogy' – after Foucault's term bio-power – to critique the governance and regulation of children and parents through formal school practices and informal educational initiatives aimed at normative ideals of 'healthy bodies' (Wright and Harwood 2009; Wright and Hasle 2014). Their emphasis is on going beyond 'body pedagogies' to examine how multiple pedagogical sites such as formal curricula in school, public health campaigns including websites, lifestyle reality TV programmes, billboards, posters and pamphlets attempt to govern bodies and lives. Like traditional public pedagogy theorists, they analyse a wide range of media, but influenced by Foucauldian and feminist theorists of the body, they detail how discourses, ideals and media techniques produce meanings about bodies, resources for identity formation, and advice and techniques for monitoring and surveillance. Jan Wright argues that these media are pedagogical in the sense that they attempt to increase knowledge, provide instruction, offer resources for sense-making and techniques for changing the self and others. Using the term pedagogical practices, they argue that these various media affect how children, young people and parents see themselves and others, and how they then act on themselves and others to change bodies and subjectivities (Wright 2009). In summary, they suggest that these pedagogies work as 'cultural relational practices' through which knowledge, norms, ideals, emotions and power are resisted, negotiated and reproduced (Wright 2009). Importantly, like authors in chapters in this book, they emphasise how these pedagogies produce not only ideas and knowledge but invoke emotions such as shame through positioning certain bodies and ways of eating as irresponsible and abject (Wright and Halse 2014). Their work is important in food studies as it emphasises the proliferation of anti-obesity media and analyses these in close detail, but from a pedagogy studies viewpoint, there is less scrutiny on what makes these media pedagogical and how the effects on children, teachers and parents are produced.

On the same terrain but using different conceptual resources, feminist geographers Bethan Evans, Rachel Colls, and Kathrin Horschelmann (2011) evaluate a British national anti-obesity public health campaign through the concept of relationality, locating their analysis in studies of embodied and public health pedagogies. Defining relationality as forms of 'embodied connections' between people –

inter-subjectively, inter-corporeally, inter-sectionally and inter-generationally – they argue that relationality challenges neoliberal and corporeal individualism, and concomitant notions of individual agency and responsibilisation. Most public health pedagogy campaigns, they argue, reproduce a neoliberal view of subjects and bodies as bounded and singular – what they call corporeal individualism – rather than as products of relations and multiple inter-subjectivities: what they call 'embodied-subjects'. In their view, a relational approach to health pedagogies offers a way to re-vitalise the see-saw debates on whether public pedagogies shape or meet resistance from subjects, by foregrounding the 'multiple elements of relatedness' in people's embodied lives (Rich et al., 2004, cited Evans et al. ibid.: 38). Whilst the campaign they study claims to offer an approach of society wide connectedness around food and embodiment, Evans and colleague show how it continues to individualise children's agency and mothers' responsibility, and thus does not challenge neoliberal views of embodied subjecthood in ways a relational approach can. In focusing on relational theories of bodies and food, the chapter makes an important contribution to research on anti-obesity pedagogies, particularly Foucauldian influenced studies, but is limited in the extent to which it analyses pedagogical processes and effects.

Although food education, domestic science and school gardens have been part of Western schooling since the early twentieth century, there is now a body of work showing how schools are sites of intense pedagogical interventions around food and health (Hayes-Conroy 2009; Vileisis 2008). For instance, John Evans and Emma Rich make a substantial contribution to food pedagogy scholarship because they position their work clearly in a lineage of pedagogy studies literature including Basil Bernstein (Evans, Rich and Holyroyd 2004; Evans, Rich, Davies and and Allwood 2008) and Henry Giroux and Carmen Luke (Rich 2011a/b). Moreover, they do not simply situate their analysis in this clear pedagogy studies literature but have undertaken extensive empirical research on pedagogical processes and their effects in a range of official and alternative pedagogies in schools and popular culture (see also their chapter in this book for more work in this area).

Deana Leahy too, in sole authored research and with co-researcher, Jo Pike, writes in this book, and elsewhere, of the ways in which public health concerns, school food initiatives, and legislative reforms congeal into 'pedagogical assemblages' which work affectively to shame and scare children and parents, particularly mothers, through specific forms of what she calls, 'disgusting pedagogies' (Leahy, 2009; Leahy and Pike 2012). Like Evans and Rich, their work contributes to food pedagogy studies because they offer detailed studies of pedagogical processes and interventions rather than just invoking pedagogy rhetorically.

In our own work, we draw on feminist and cultural pedagogy scholarship to examine food activism, food multiculturalism, and food social enterprises, for instance, ethnic food tours. In particular, we have attempted to examine what makes practices pedagogical: for example, we have analysed the specificities of how media such as films and websites operate pedagogically through their materialities and representational practices; and researched the racialised and gendered body work of ethnic food tour guides in 'teaching' food multiculturalism. Furthermore, in this collection, we draw on anthropological concepts of social reproduction as a way to understand pedagogies in families, drawing on important empirical scholarship on family meals and the subtle processes of informal learning through food, eating and conversation at the table (Quarmby and Dagkas 2013; Laurier and Wiggins 2011; Ochs and Shohet 2006). Keen to bring pedagogy studies in dialogue with food studies, we convened a special issue of the *Australian Journal of Adult Learning* in 2012 (Flowers and Swan 2011, 2012a/b/c).

Having described studies in which pedagogy is used as a core concept, we briefly turn to food studies writers who are interested in teaching and learning about food but do not use the term pedagogy. For example, Julie Guthman (2008a/b) has critiqued the racialised and classed politics of knowledge and learning in alternative food initiatives and university teaching; and has referred although very briefly to the term 'radical food pedagogy' in an interview (Stoneman 2009). Coming from a very different perspective, anthropologist David Sutton (2001, 2006) researches the teaching and learning of women's cooking skills through a close-up analysis of micro-practices in Greek kitchens entailing sensory memories, embodied habits, and practical know-how. In a critique of the common-place view that cooking skills are in decline, Frances Short (2006) examines learning through home-cooking, and argues that preparing pre-prepared, convenience foods requires substantial knowledge and relatively advanced cooking skills. Aya Kimura (2011) provides an important critique of Japanese food reform aimed at food choices and cooking in the home. In emphasising that food education has been reduced to food literacy, a deficit model of food knowledge and skills, which individualises and depoliticises why people choose to eat certain foods, and furthermore, puts additional pressures onto women in the home in terms of their domestic labour, Kimura's argument extends way beyond Japan.

After schools, the media represents the site of teaching and learning most researched by food studies scholars. Hence, several authors research how, and what, TV cooking programmes, celebrity chefs, actors, and musicians, websites, and cookbooks teach viewers about food, cooking and eating, and social difference (De Solier 2005, 2013; Rousseau 2012; Lewis 2008; Hollows and Jones 2010; Johnston and Baumann 2010). Whilst authors debate how much viewers learn from the media, and in particular, TV cooking programmes, there is a clear intent to educate (De Solier 2005, 2013; Johnston and Baumann 2010). In contrast to public health and body pedagogy research, much of this scholarship examines middle-class education and learning. For example, although they do not use the concept of pedagogy, in their research on foodiesm, Josee Johnston and Shyon Baumann (2010) show that interviewees define learning, and a disposition of aesthetic appreciation and knowledge acquisition as central to the foodie identity. Thus, respondents claimed that foodies needed to learn and practise cooking techniques. But also foodies seek out information about provenance, production, and sensory qualities of food, learning from newspapers, food blogs, cookbooks, cooking classes and TV and their social networks. The educational dimension of being a foodie means learning about food qualities, history, and conditions of production and consumption including highly specific and technical information and the dishes and ingredients associated with a very wide range of cuisines. What Johnston and Baumann underline is that the foodie creates status and distinction by acquiring knowledge and learning about food centred on aesthetic appreciation and deliberation.

Developing the centrality of learning in foodiesm further than Johnston and Baumann, Isabelle De Solier (2013) coins the term 'gastronomic education' to characterise how 'foodies' use their leisure time to learn about food from what she calls 'material media' such as lifestyle media, TV cooking programmes, cookbooks, restaurant guidebooks and watching peers cook. One of her arguments is that contra recent analyses of TV cooking, foodies do watch cooking shows – particularly those with a realist instructional mode – primarily to learn about what to consume and produce from professional chefs and not just to be entertained. She suggests that for the middle classes, these forms of learning about food constitute 'productive leisure' or knowledge based leisure: where productivity has been translated from work to leisure and entails 'new understandings of being productive … bound up with expressing or acquiring knowledge'. She explains in more detail that:

> this involves practices of learning and education, formal or informal. For many, it involves a material education; the acquisition and expression of knowledge of material objects, their consumption and production, from material media. (2013: 6)

Importantly for food pedagogy studies, she discusses the nature of food knowledges in ways that extend beyond nutritional science, often the main focus in public health pedagogy writing. For example, she writes that within gastronomic education, there are theoretical and practical knowledges, culinary skills, taste formations, knowledge of restaurants, chefs, cuisines, ingredients, producers, suppliers, food history, anthropology and skills in food media like photographing food.

In contrast to Johnston and Baumann, and De Solier with their focus on foodie learners, Tania Lewis (2008) researches the array of media food pedagogues such as nutritionists, health consultants, food coaches and celebrity TV chefs, and the rise of particular forms of advice, knowledge and expertise, all of which, she claims, influence our conceptions of food. More specifically she compares nutritionist experts' rationalised, psychologised and medicalised views of food, health and restraint with those of celebrity chefs such as Nigella Lawson and Jamie Oliver who draw on charismatic personality and life experiences to present food knowledge related to pleasure, aesthetics and ethics. Lawson and Oliver offer an antidote to the rationalisation of food with their focus on escapism and indulgence. Lewis' main point is that there are widely divergent and contradictory forms of advice and knowledge about in food pedagogies, sometimes embodied in one chef such as Oliver, but which condense contemporary cultural concerns and anxieties about responsibility, health, industrialisation, and risk. Whilst her book offers an important examination of different food pedagogues and their forms of expertise, she is less concerned with pedagogical processes and how consumers transform and modify their food habits.

In summary, although the term pedagogy is rarely used as an analytic, this work provides us with detailed empirical studies of food learning and food expertise across a range of media. Furthermore, they reinforce how food pedagogies are dominated by bourgeois values, knowledge and practices. As De Solier puts it:

> knowledge itself is not a neutral term … but is invested in systems of power and exclusivity, attaching different values to different types of knowledge and their possessors. (2013: 29)

In their editorial for a special issue, Josee Johnston and Mike Goodman begin to unpack what they call 'the mediating impacts' of food celebrities, arguing like other theorists that media shape and reflect food cultures, but extending this often made point to highlight a number of influencing processes such as the use of powerful and spectacular images, emulation, authenticity, elevated media voices, celebrity embodiment of lifestyle, and cultural intermediation between viewer and celebrity, all of which could be conceived of as pedagogical. In this collection, using different methods, sites, and forms of analysis, many of the chapters seek to identify, freeze-frame and describe such pedagogical processes, some focusing on media, and others, inter-personal encounters such as teaching or family meals.

Structure of the Book

Chapters in this book draw to varying degrees on literature in pedagogy studies and food studies scholarship on teaching and learning. Many of the chapters can be seen as a response to the calls in the pedagogy literature to research pedagogy in practice. To different scales, the chapters examine food pedagogical aims, curricula, processes, and learners' receptions of these, drawing from empirical studies in France, Britain, Canada, USA and Australia. The authors in the book employ a range of research methodologies including ethnography, textual and visual methods, surveys, and in-depth interviewing which enable closer attention to be given to pedagogical mechanisms and effects, than is often the case in pedagogy and food studies. To structure the book, we organise the chapters into four themes, which speak to core debates in food studies scholarship on food pedagogy, and food studies more broadly:

- embodiment and identity
- transformation and affect
- governance and authority
- ethics and critique.

Part I: Embodiment and Identity

In this first part, the chapters present analyses of different pedagogical sites in three countries – English schools, an Australian mixed-race family and American alternative TV cooking programmes, and surface how food pedagogies work through embodied practices of eating, cooking and performing. Mobilising distinct theoretical frameworks, the chapters draw on surveys, interviews and media analysis to show close-up how pedagogical processes produce bodies, subjectification and identity making.

In Chapter 2, Emma Rich and John Evans, academics in the sociology of education, health and sport, examine the pedagogical effects of public health policies designed to address a perceived crisis in obesity in schools in the UK. Drawing on surveys and interviews with teachers and pupils, they trace how pleasure in food is constructed in school curricula and teachers' and pupils' discourses. More specifically, they illustrate how 'healthy lifestyle' reforms produce 'body pedagogies' which shape how young people learn about food pleasures. They show how teachers educate young people to curb their sensory desires through pedagogical processes such as direct classroom teaching, teacher and peer feedback. Moreover, teachers and peers reward young people's talk about pleasure through self-restraint. As a result of their analysis, Rich and Evans establish that cultural anxieties about the health risk of food pleasures lead to the surveillance and pathologisation of certain populations in schools. In their summary, Rich and Evans call for a sensory food pedagogy which goes beyond narrow and moralistic food teaching and acultural, classed concepts of the senses. In relation to the theme of embodiment and identity, the chapter maintains that young people's interpretation of the school food pedagogies is sensory and corporeal as well as socio-cognitive. In other words, the school food pedagogies constitute embodied learning, affecting how the young people eat and feel. Of importance to food pedagogy studies, they emphasise that the development of sensory food pedagogies requires complex theorising of the intersection between pleasure, class, gender and race.

Following this, our own chapter analyses how family food practices work pedagogically to perform race and gender in a mixed-race Australian family. We argue that families are under-theorised as sites of racialisation and gendering in relation to food. Situating our analysis in relation to theories on cultural transmission and food racial practices, the chapter focuses on the childhood memories of two Anglo-Australian Chinese sons. Our chapter builds on sensory food studies, and Rich and Evans' point that senses are learned, to show how the cooking arrangements, smell, aesthetics, and bodily movements in the kitchen and at the dining table, taught the sons about race, gender and identity. We discuss too, how race includes whiteness. Emphasising that food memories are not always of the 'happy family meal', we work concretely through four remembered food incidents to stress that the family's pedagogical processes include a congeries of modes, objects, media, senses and skills. We emphasise that pedagogical processes should be understood as racialised and gendered, and in so doing we speak to recent calls to attend to race in food studies (Slocum and Saladhana 2013; Williams-Forson 2013).

In the final chapter of this section (Chapter 4), Seline Szkupinski-Quiroga, a health anthropologist, and two adult education academics, Jenny Sandlin and Robin Redmon Wright, contrast mainstream TV 'celebrity chef' cooking programmes shown on the US Food Network channel to 'alternative cooking programmes' shown on community channels. The alternative cooking programmes feature a vegan activist chef and a punk performance artist chef. The chapter draws our attention to the differently performed embodied pedagogies and notions of conviviality and consumption in the two cooking programmes. In the mainstream cooking programmes, the authors claim that pedagogies include 'teaching' people to aspire to consumerist lifestyles through sleek staging, celebrity branding, and charismatic presenting. In contrast, drawing on parodies of celebrity chefs, and 'lo-fi staging', Szkupinski-Quiroga, Sandlin, Redmon Wright suggest that the alternative programmes 'teach' their audience to consume in ethically and politically alternative ways, mobilising discourses of animal rights, and socio-political discussions of health and corporate agri-business. Their overall argument is that the alternative chefs offer a pedagogy of ethical-political community. Although there is a proliferation of food studies research on food TV programmes as we discussed above, with some focusing on pedagogies, this chapter makes a distinctive contribution with its examination of alternative chefs as pedagogues (De Solier 2005, 2013).

Part II: Transformation and Affect

This section explores how affect and emotion are imagined to produce transformations in habits of working; shopping; and drinking. Researching quite different pedagogical sites – reality TV, French drink advertising and food shops- the chapters analyse how emotions such as passion, pleasure and anger are mobilised by Jamie Oliver and his TV producers, the French government and self-identified radical shoppers to enable learning.

In the first chapter of this section (Chapter 5), education scholars Lyn Harrison, Peter Kelly and Perri Campbell illustrate the complexities of affect as a pedagogical mechanism. Here, they develop a Foucauldian analysis of technologies of the self in Jamie Oliver's reality-based television programme *Fifteen*. Their main argument is that passion becomes a 'pedagogical device' to educate 15 young, previously unemployed, London-based trainee chefs. Harrison, Kelly and Campbell show how Jamie Oliver's biography, his willingness to learn and work hard, and importantly, his passion for food and cooking are put together to construct a pedagogical role-model of entrepreneurial qualities of get-up and go, and self-discipline. The aim of the pedagogy is that the trainees should 'emulate' his capacity to undertake mundane, repetitive restaurant work, and his passion for slow, organic and sustainable food in order to transform their working lives. While observing that learning 'passion' opens up opportunities for the trainees to pursue alternative futures, the authors argue that the programme sidelines the trainees' own off-screen passions and realities of their work futures. Like other chapters in the book, they highlight the significance of emotion and affect in food pedagogies, but more specifically emphasise how the chefs are being taught neoliberal entrepreneurship.

In Chapter 6, Julie Robert, a cultural and international studies academic, examines the imagined power of affect-based advertising images through the lens of pedagogy. To challenge taken-for-granted assumptions about the influence of affect in drink advertising, she undertakes a close textual and visual analysis of campaigns produced under some of the world's most stringent alcohol legislation in France – known as the *Loi Evin*. The *Loi Evin* prohibits the advertising of alcoholic drinks on television and permits it only on billboards, radio and the Internet. The law set out to 're-teach' young people in France how to drink more responsibly. Images of people and lifestyles were effectively banned as it was imagined they would have dangerous affective pedagogical qualities, leading to people emulating role models in adverts and as a result, take up excessive drinking lifestyles. Hence, advertising was stripped of the 'affective pedagogy' of lifestyle images and replaced with an 'informational pedagogy' of rational drink and health messages. Robert shows how the *Loi Evin* is based on reductive assumptions about advertising's pedagogical effects and how these 'work' on drinking motivations and behaviours.

In Chapter 7 Kaela Jubas, a scholar in the field of adult learning, explores ethical food consumption, draws on 32 interviews conducted with self-identified 'radical' shoppers to argue that 'radical' food shopping 'functions pedagogically' to 'teach' people about global issues. Examining shopping as a process of informal and incidental learning, she asserts that knowledge and understanding alone do not necessarily change shoppers' actions, echoing some of the themes in other chapters. Jubas describes how 'radical' shoppers argue that their experience of emotions such as anger or pleasure work pedagogically. Hence, Jubas suggests that social change through food pedagogy is as much a process of affect as of reason. Although sensitive to the attempts of shoppers to exert individualised ethical consumption as a result of their learning, she concludes that a collective ethical pedagogy would be more politically effective.

Part III: Governance and Authority

This section extends studies of governmentality in food studies, illustrating the pedagogic authority of supermarkets and teachers. Both chapters in Part III show through detailed observation how the pedagogical authority of these pedagogues is reproduced through prevailing discourses of health. Isaacs and Dixon in their study show how pedagogical processes of information and advice giving are undertaken by the supermarkets, and Leahy and Pike reveal how pedagogical techniques of disgust and surveillance in the schools are deployed by schools. Both chapters emphasise the tactics of resistance to the pedagogical authorities mobilised by local activists in the case of Isaacs and Dixon, and pupils in the study by Leahy and Pike.

In Chapter 8, Bronwyn Isaacs, an anthropologist, and Jane Dixon, a public health scholar, offer an ethnographic study of rural supermarkets and 'pedagogical authority' in a rural Australian town. They position a range of stakeholder groups in the rural region as having pedagogical 'authority', particularly on the question of who supports 'local' food. These groups include farmers, local retail and food manufacturing businesses, growers' markets, and consumer activists. Their focus is, however, on the pedagogical authority of the two largest supermarket chains in Australia – Coles and Woolworths. Their findings suggest that people in a rural community have a strong concern for the health of their regional economy and in particular, the livelihood of local farmers. But alongside these community values, sits an appreciation of the convenience and abundance that large supermarkets offer. Isaacs and Dixon present a detailed study of the struggle that takes place between the various 'pedagogical authorities' in the region. Significantly for our thinking on pedagogues, they emphasise the weight and reach of the power of supermarkets in shaping lifestyles, values and habits: what they call 'experts in subjectivity'. They draw our attention to the variety of pedagogical strategies that are deployed, from information-giving, profiling of certain foods, and the privileging of particular types of advice about which foods are 'best' (i.e. cheap, easy, healthy and family friendly) and most 'local'.

Building on their previous work on parenting pedagogies, and governmentality studies, Deana Leahy and Jo Pike (Chapter 9) analyse three vignettes of the 'hurly-burly' of classroom teaching in school to map the 'assemblage' of knowledge, rationalities and technologies mobilised by teachers as they inculcate pupils in government policies on obesity. Although they argued that 'hybrid' knowledge about food circulates in schools, pupils find it difficult to resist the weight of the anti-obesity discourse. As an instance, they show how pupils are taught to surveil their eating behaviours through food diaries which makes it difficult to problematise expert-sanctioned, nutritional knowledges. Seeing the classroom as a 'contact point' for the take up of policy pedagogies and governmentality, they emphasise, like other chapters in this volume, that it is not just expertise being deployed in school pedagogies, but also affect. Thus, disgust and repulsion are mobilised to shape pupils' food choices, aspirations and skills. Leahy and Pike show, however, that attempts to govern and teach are messy and meet with resistance from pupils. Like other chapters, they emphasise how food pedagogies are forged from emotional and rational registers which get into your brain, heart, and sense of self (Ellsworth 1997: 6 cited in Leahy and Pike's chapter in this book).

Part IV: Ethics and Critique

In the fourth and final section, the authors in the three chapters explore pedagogies on the ethics of food production and consumption, with the first chapter asking whether food labels help shoppers make ethical decisions when choosing foods. The two following chapters offer applied case studies of teaching critical theory in universities. Informed by quite different theoretical resources, the authors discuss 'real-life' examples of using food to teach their own students about food production and consumption: with Jennifer Sumner drawing on a critical pedagogy tradition, including the work of Paulo Freire; and Meredith Abarca working with postcolonial theorists and literary works. Albeit examining quite different domains – shops and university classrooms – the three chapters reflect on the knowledge people need to make ethical decisions about what they buy, cook and eat.

Whereas in Chapter 8 Isaacs and Dixon write about the contestation between supermarkets and local actors in a rural economy, in their chapter (Chapter 10), Rachel Ankeny, an historian and Heather Bray, a scholar in science-communication, examine the specific micro-practices of reading 'ethical food' labels in supermarkets. Ankeny and Bray argue that food labels are 'boundary objects': 'not free floating bundles of information' but a form of interface between stakeholders with diverse food ethics. Drawing on their qualitative research about consumers' decision-making when shopping for meat and genetically modified foods, Ankeny and Bray question how labels work to produce knowledge. Their overall point is that education about the 'facts' of food ignores the cultural, social, moral and historical context in which people make decisions about what to buy. Their concern is that labels do not teach consumers enough about the wider and deeper issues of ethical consumption.

Based in adult education, Jennifer Sumner has been teaching a course entitled Food Pedagogy for postgraduate students in the University of Toronto, Canada since 2010. In Chapter 11, Sumner describes the design of her curriculum and assessment strategies and her pedagogical rationale in detailed, pragmatic terms. She outlines how students undertake research about topics such as unsustainable fish, fair-trade chocolate, bottled water, local food, genetically modified organisms, and the 'Western' diet. For Sumner, the aim is for students to learn about the political economy of environmentalism, food production and consumption and develop strategies to address food injustices, in what she calls, after Paulo Freire, a pedagogy of the possible.

In contrast to Sumner who teaches a subject called pedagogy of food, Meredith Abarca, who teaches womens' studies and cultural studies at the University of El Paso in Texas, USA, uses 'food narratives' to teach critical theory in humanities and social theory. She defines food narratives as personal stories, images and passages from literary works (such as novels, poems, short stories, autobiographies). Echoing previous chapters, in Chapter 12 Abarca claims that 'the analysis of food passages is not purely a cognitive process but most often it is one that begins through the sensory recollections they evoke'. A key pedagogical concept for Abarca is 'food consciousness' where 'students begin to understand that their food choices are never neutral, but governed by social, political, economic, and cultural ideologies that continuously (re)shape their individual, familial, and cultural sense of self.' Abarca's pedagogical philosophy is informed by concepts from postcolonial scholars, – bell hooks' engaged pedagogy, Louise Pratt's contact zones, M. Jacqui Alexander's pedagogies of crossing, and Gloria Anzaldua's 'meztizo' consciousness. Using the reading of texts in the classroom, together with other pedagogical processes such as sharing of food memories, collaborative thinking, and collective eating, her main aim is to enable the students to understand the complexities of critical theory and to do so by mobilising representations of food and material food practices such as cooking and eating as a resource for critique.

Conclusion

Our intention in this collection was to prise open the aims, curricula and processes in food pedagogies across a range of sites. Responding to the call in pedagogy studies to go beyond rhetorical assertions that cultural and social practices are pedagogical, chapters in the book ground their analyses in empirical research on the interactions, content and relations in pedagogical encounters. As a result various food practices, structures, institutions and pedagogical sites such as school, shopping, supermarkets, families, university classrooms and relations of knowledge, affect, embodiment, resistance, and power are brought into view.

Food pedagogies are important not only because they are proliferating but because of the social, cultural and symbolic meanings of food and 'good lives; which they reproduce. Thus, food is seen as the means through which we can (and should) improve our individual and collective lives: our physical and mental health, the happiness of children and families, our sense of community and connection, the state of the environment, and the future of the planet. Consequently, food pedagogies offer us hope that we can learn so much: about the Other, about our selves, our food producers, and the animals and plants which are our food. Many of them promise us that we can become 'fairer, kinder, healthier', and more moral, nourished, ecological and well-fed (Freidberg 2010). Pedagogues, described by authors in various chapters, reproduce culturally circulating ideas about healthism, 'doing good' and 'being good' through food. Importantly though, several chapters emphasise how food pedagogies go beyond the transmission of knowledge. They illustrate how they affect how we feel about what we eat and drink: from disgust to shame, pleasure, aspiration, pride and anger. The affective economy of food pedagogies is unevenly distributed because as we see from chapters in the book, some forms of food education are classist, racist and sexist, and shame, patronise and berate 'targeted learners' and their lives.

An important theme for many authors in the collection are the political and moral effects of food pedagogies. From the chapters, we can see how there are powerful actors who have clear 'educational' agendas to control what we eat, and how we think and feel about food: for example, supermarkets, policy makers, health authorities, nutritionists, advertisers, and celebrity chefs. There is a classed, racialised and gendered politics to who is set up as 'in the know'. Hierarchies are created of 'good' and 'bad' consumers, diets, eaters, parents, families, cooks, and foods (Flowers and Swan 2011; Swan and Flowers 2015). Scholars in this book, and elsewhere, point to the way that women and in particular, working-class mothers are targeted, responsibilised and shamed. For instance, knowledge about how to cook is imagined to be on the decline as a result of 'modern' motherhood and subject to policy and media commentary, and pedagogical intervention (Short 2006, Kimura 2011). As a result, mothers are seen to be responsible for the ill-health of their children and the nation. In particular, working-class mothers are demonised, seen as deficient and irrational in their food habits. Indeed, health focused food pedagogies – making 'healthy' school lunch boxes, shopping for local and organic ingredients, and cooking slow food – position women's place as back doing intensive and unpaid labour in the kitchen (Kimura 2011). Gender and class are vital for understanding food pedagogies but several chapters underline that age is critical, given the extent and intensity of food messages aimed at young people (Leahy and Pike in this volume; Rich and Evans in this volume; Harrison, Kelly and Campbell in this volume). Authors emphasise too how food pedagogies reproduce hetero-normativity (Rich and Evans in this volume; Robert in this volume).

Whilst the book has made inroads into researching the practices involved in food pedagogies across different social domains, there are opportunities for further research, particularly in relation to two themes: first, race and food pedagogies; and secondly, how pedagogical processes 'operate' on us, which includes how food pedagogies are encountered and negotiated by 'learners'. In their chapter, Quiroga, Sandlin and Redmon Wright show how on alternative TV programmes, issues of race, class and food are discussed, and Iranian-Guatamalan and Jewish food of the presenters' backgrounds profiled rather than white middle-class foodie cooking, and done in ways which do not exoticise but position food culture through narratives of colonial history. Our own chapter attends to the racialised nature of food pedagogies generally, and focuses in particular on the under-researched topic of food practices in mixed-race families. But in relation to racialisation, there are more questions to be answered about social justice, food inequalities and the whiteness of food pedagogies. For instance, there is growing critique of the racialised and classed inequalities of food production and consumption, and the politics of white, middle-class alternative food movements (Williams-Forson and Walker 2013; Alkon and Agyeman 2011; Paddock 2011; Slocum 2007, 2008, 2011; Guthman 2008a/b; Etmanski 2012; Walter 2012). This critique shows how sustainable and ethical food consumers make normative judgements about what constitutes 'good' food, diets and consumption and morally deride other types of food consumption. Moreover, ethical food consumption itself has become a symbolic marker of classed capital (Johnston and Baumann 2010; Paddock 2011). The financial and time resources needed to sustain these forms of consumption, and access to the 'health-giving' properties of middle-class 'good' food have been roundly challenged for being out of the reach of white and racially minoritised working classes (Guthman 2008a/b; Paddock 2011). On the racialisation of alternative food practices such as food markets and alternative agriculture, Guthman and Slocum suggest such initiatives reproduce white embodied spaces, discourses, and political aims which reconsolidate racial food inequalities and exclusionary practices. In an important redress to the sensory turn in food movements and food studies, Jessica Hayes-Conroy (2009) challenges the romanticisation of white taste and sensory education in school garden projects, emphasising that food pedagogues need to understand senses not as natural and acultural but as grounded in classed and racialised practices.

Secondly the book expands understanding of how social and cultural processes are pedagogical. Hence, chapters show that people learn about food knowledges, meanings and practices through various formal and informal processes, media and mechanisms, in cognitive, sensory, embodied, gendered, classed and racialised ways. As pedagogues promulgate across a front of media from webpages, food workshops, print media through to television, more empirical and theoretical attention needs to be given to the complex debates in cultural and media studies about how meaning is made, how media mediate. For instance, in our work on food activist films (Flowers and Swan 2011) and food tourism websites (Flowers and Swan in press), we have attended to the specificities of film and website representational practices in pedagogising food. As we noted, authors in pedagogy studies insist that we move beyond assuming food pedagogies are 'forces' which 'shape' our identities, what we think and feel, and how we act. Thus, further research should be given to theorising what the 'catalytic stuff' of food pedagogies is and how it 'works upon' or constitutes individuals, class, gender and race: examining what of us is 'shaped', and into what 'ideal endpoint' we are 'shaped' (Swan 2007, 2008). At the same time, chapters in the book illuminate that readers and viewers do not simply uncritically slurp up so-called ideological messages about food: they counter, reject and ignore food pedagogies, although the resources needed to do this against powerful pedagogues are unevenly allocated by race, class and gender. Nevertheless, as work on race and food movements points out, alternative food pedagogies from a range of activists are gaining momentum: the pedagogies of activists and social movement learning being another area ready for more research attention.

Finally, chapters in the book have begun to expand on concepts of subjectification, identification and social reproduction as ways of explicating learning and transformation, but as pedagogy studies scholars emphasise practices of embodiment, capacitation and habituation need more research. Recent theorising on senses, viscera, materialisation of race and bodies in food studies can aid this project, augmented by work by pedagogy scholars such as Hickey-Moody who investigates the pedagogy of affect: vibrations, sensation, rhythms and sounds. This would entail extending our concepts of how food pedagogies interpellate, mobilise and produce us, individually and collectively, through a plethora of bodily, intellectual, sensory and emotional 'materials': for example, cognition; the unconscious; visuality; smell; touch; habits; imagination; aspirations; fantasies; dreams and desires. What this argument emphasises, and many chapters in the book foreground, is that food pedagogies work not simply through information-giving and messages, but through emotional, ethnical, and embodied registers and attachments, which means that any activist, resistive and alternative food pedagogies should not be based on addressing what are seen as different groups' knowledge deficits: or as Guthman (2008b) succinctly puts it, the white middle-class food activist rhetoric of 'if only they knew'.

Acknowledgement

Some ideas in this chapter have been published in an earlier form in our introduction to the 2012 special issue on Food Pedagogies in the *Australian Journal of Adult Learning*.

References

Alkon, A.H. and Agyeman, J. (2011). *Cultivating Food Justice: Race, Class and Sustainability*. London: MIT Press.

Belasco, W.J. (2007). *Appetite for Change: How the Counterculture Took on the Food Industry*. New York: Cornell University Press.

Berlant, L. (2010). Risky bigness: On obesity, eating and the ambiguity of 'health'. In J.M. Metzl and A. Kirkland (eds), *Against Health: How Health Became the New Morality*. New York: NYU Press, 26–39.

Burdick, J. and Sandlin, J.A. (2013). Learning, becoming, and the unknowable: Conceptualizations, mechanisms, and process in public pedagogy literature. *Curriculum Inquiry*, 43(1), 142–77.

———, and O'Malley, M.P. (eds). (2013). *Problematizing Public Pedagogy*. New York: Routledge.

———, Sandlin, J. et al. (2010). Educational inquiry and the pedagogical other: On the politics and ethics of researching critical public pedagogies. In J.A. Sandlin, B. Schultz and J. Burdick (eds), *Handbook of Public Pedagogy: Education and Learning beyond Schooling*. London/New York: Taylor & Francis, 116–24.

Cook, S. (2009). New spaces and new places: Adult education and the creation of alternative foodscapes *Graduate Food Discussions Paper Series*, Ryerson University, Canada, 1, 19–31.

Coveney, J. (2006). *Food, Morals and Meaning: The Pleasure and Anxiety of Eating*. London: Routledge.

De Solier, I. (2005). TV dinners: Culinary television, education and distinction. *Journal of Media & Cultural Studies*, 19(4), 465–81.

——— (2013). *Food and the Self: Consumption, Production and Material Culture*. A & C Black.

Edwards, R. and Usher, R. (2007). *Globalisation and Pedagogy: Space, Place and Identity*. London: Routledge.

Etmanski, C. (2012). A critical race and class analysis of learning in the organic farming movement. *Australian Journal of Adult Learning, 52*(3), 484.

Evans, B., Colls, R. and Hörschelmann, K. (2011). 'Change4Life for your kids': Embodied collectives and public health pedagogy. *Sport, Education and Society*, 16(3), 323–34.

Evans, J., Rich, E., Davies, B., and Allwood, R. (2008). *Education, Disordered Eating and Obesity Discourse: Fat Fabrications*. London: Routledge.

Evans, J., Rich, E., and Holroyd, R. (2004). Disordered eating and disordered schooling: What schools do to middle class girls. *British Journal of Sociology of Education*, 25(2), 123–42.

Flowers, R. and Swan, E. (2011) Eating at us: Representations of knowledge in the activist documentary film Food, Inc. *Studies in the Education of Adults*, 43(2), 234–50.

——— (2012a) Eating the Asian other? Pedagogies of food multiculturalism in Australia. *Portal Journal of Multidisciplinary International Studies*, 9(2), 1–30.

——— and Swan, E. (eds). (2012b). Special Issue *Australian Journal of Adult Learning: 'Food Pedagogies'*, 52(3), 532–72.

——— and Swan, E. (2012c). Pedagogies of doing good: Problematisations, authorities, technologies and teleologies in food activism. *Australian Journal of Adult Learning*, 52(3), 532.

——— and Swan, E. (in press) Seeing Benevolently: Digital Multiculturalism and Ethnic Food Tours on the Internet, *Geoforum*.

———, Guevara, R. and Whelan, J. (2009). Popular and informal environmental education: The need for more research in an 'emerging' field of practice. *Report: Zeitschrift für Weiterbildungsforschung*, 2(2009), 36–50.

Freidberg, S. (2010). Perspective and power in the ethical foodscape. *Environment and Planning*. A, 42(8), 1868.

Freire, P. (1970). *Pedagogy of the Oppressed*, trans. Myra Bergman Ramos. New York: Continuum.

Giroux, H.A. (1988). *Teachers as Intellectuals: Toward a Critical Pedagogy of Learning*. Westport: Greenwood Publishing Group.

——— (1992). Cultural studies, resisting difference, and the return of critical pedagogy. In H. Giroux *Border Crossings: Cultural Workers and the Politics of Education*. New York: Routledge, 161–79.

——— (2004a). Cultural studies and the politics of public pedagogy: Making the political more pedagogical. *Parallax*, 10(2), 73–89.

——— (2004b). Cultural studies, public pedagogy, and the responsibility of intellectuals. *Communication and Critical/Cultural Studies*, 1(1), 59–79.

——— (2005). *Against the New Authoritarianism: Politics after Abu Ghraib*. Winnipeg: Arbeiter Ring.

Guthman, J. (2008a). Neoliberalism and the making of food politics in California. *Geoforum*, 39(3), 1171–83.

——— (2008b). Bringing good food to others: Investigating the subjects of alternative food practice. *Cultural Geographies*, 15(4), 431–47.

Hayes-Conroy, J. (2009). Visceral reactions: Alternative food and social difference in American and Canadian schools. PhD dissertation, Geography and Women's Studies, Pennsylvania State University.

Hayes-Conroy, A. and Hayes-Conroy, J. (2008). Taking back taste: Feminism, food and visceral politics. *Gender, Place and Culture*, 15(5), 461–73.

Hayes-Conroy, J. and Hayes-Conroy, A. (eds). (2014). *Doing Nutrition Differently: Critical Approaches to Diet and Dietary Intervention*. Farnham: Ashgate.

Hickey-Moody, A. (2013). *Youth, Arts and Education: Reassembling Subjectivity through Affect*. London: Routledge.

———, Savage, G. and Windle, J. (2010). Pedagogy writ large: Public, popular and cultural pedagogies in motion. *Critical Studies in Education*, 51(3): 227–36.

Highmore, B. (2008). Alimentary agents: Food, cultural theory and multiculturalism. *Journal of Intercultural Studies*, 29(4), 381–98.

Hollows, J. and Jones, S. (2010). 'At least he's doing something': Moral entrepreneurship and individual responsibility in Jamie's Ministry of Food. *European Journal of Cultural Studies*, 13(3), 307–22.

Johnston, J., and Baumann, S. (2010). *Foodies: Democracy and Distinction in the Gourmet Foodscape*. London/New York: Routledge.

Jubas, K. (2006). The trouble with shopping: Discourses, practices and pedagogies of the consumer-citizen. In M. Hagen and E. Goff (eds), *Proceedings of the 47th Annual AERC* (196–202), 19–21 May, Minneapolis, University of Minnesota.

——— (2007). Consuming fiction: Stories about consumerism, shopping and consumption. In L. Servage and T. Fenwick (eds), *Joint International 48th Annual AERC and the 26th Annual Conference of CASAE/ACÉÉA. Learning in Community* (325–30), 6–9 June, Halifax, Mount Saint Vincent University.

Kelly, P. (2009). Food, passion and marginalised young people: Technologies of the self in Jamie's kitchen, *in TASA 2009: Proceedings of the Annual Conference of The Australian Sociological Association 2009: The Future of Sociology*, 1–12, TASA, Canberra.

——— and Harrison, L. (2011). *Working in Jamie's Kitchen: Salvation, Passion and Young Workers*. Houndmills: Palgrave Macmillan.

Kenway, J., and Bullen, E. (2011). Skin pedagogies and abject bodies. *Sport, Education and Society*, 16(3), 279–94.

——— and Modra, H. (1992). Feminist pedagogy and emancipatory possibilities. In C. Luke and J. Gore (eds), *Feminisms and Critical Pedagogy*. New York: Psychology Press, 138–66.

Kimura, A.H. (2011). Food education as food literacy: Privatized and gendered food knowledge in contemporary Japan. *Agriculture and Human Values*, 28(4), 465–82.

Laurier, E. and Wiggins, S. (2011). Finishing the family meal: The interactional organisation of satiety. *Appetite*, 56(1), 53–64.

Leahy, D. (2010). What's on (or off) the menu in school?. *Text: The Journal of the Australian Association of Writing Programs* [P], 9, 1–12.
Lewis, T. (2008). *Smart Living: Lifestyle Media and Popular Expertise*, vol. 15. New York: Peter Lang.
——— and Potter, E. (eds). (2011). *Ethical Consumption: A Critical Introduction*. London: Routledge.
Lindenfeld, L. (2010). Can documentary food films like Food Inc. achieve their promise?. *Environmental Communication*, 4(3), 378–86.
Lingard, B. (2009). Towards a sociology of pedagogies. In M. Apple, S.J. Ball, and L.A. Gandin (eds), *The Routledge International Handbook of the Sociology of Education*. London: Routledge.
Long, L.M. (ed.). (2013). *Culinary Tourism*. Lexington: University Press of Kentucky.
Luke, C. (1994). Childhood and parenting. *Popular Culture in Sociology*, 30(3), 289–302.
——— (ed.) (1996). *Feminisms and Pedagogies of Everyday Life*. New York: SUNY Press.
——— and Gore, J. (eds). (1992). *Feminisms and Critical Pedagogy*. Melbourne: Psychology Press.
Mair, H., J. Sumner et al. (2008). The politics of eating: Food practices as critically reflexive leisure. *Leisure/Loisir*, 32(2), 379–405.
Meek, M. (2013). Foreword. In P. Freire and D. Macedo, *Literacy: Reading the Word and the World*. London/New York: Routledge.
Narayan, U. (1997). *Dislocating Cultures: Third World Feminism and the Politics of Knowledge*. London: Routledge.
Noble, G. (2004). Pedagogies of the Everyday. Paper presented at the Cultural Studies Association of Australasia annual conference, 9–11 December, Murdoch University, Fremantle.
——— (2012). Pedagogies of civic belonging. Unpublished paper.
Ochs, E. and Shohet, M. (2006). The cultural structuring of mealtime socialization. *New Directions for Child and Adolescent Development*, 2006(111), 35.
Paddock, J. (2011). Class, food, culture: Exploring 'alternative' food consumption. Doctoral dissertation, Cardiff University.
Palovaara-Soberg, L. and Thuv, S. (2009). 'Food pedagogy'. Paper presented at symposium, What is Food About? A New Approach for Promoting Changes in Food Related Behaviour, convened by Consumer Citizenship Network, Technical University of Berlin.
Pike, J. and Leahy, D. (2012). School food and the pedagogies of parenting. *Australian Journal of Adult Learning*, 52(3), 434.
Quarmby, T. and Dagkas, S. (2015). Informal mealtime pedagogies: Exploring the influence of family structure on young people's healthy eating dispositions. *Sport, Education and Society*, 20(3), 323–39.
Rich, E. (2011a). 'I see her being obesed!': Public pedagogy, reality media and the obesity crisis. *Health*, 15(1), 3–21.

——— (2011b). Exploring the Relationship between pedagogy and physical cultural studies: The case of new health imperatives in schools. *Sociology of Sport Journal*, 28(1), 64–84.

Rousseau, S. (2012). *Food Media: Celebrity Chefs and the Politics of Everyday Interference*. London: Bloomsbury.

Sandlin, J.A. (2010). Learning to survive the 'Shopocalypse': Reverend Billy's anti-consumption 'pedagogy of the unknown'. *Critical Studies in Education*, 51(3), 295–311.

——— and Burdick, J. (2010). (eds). *Handbook of Public Pedagogy: Education and Learning beyond Schooling*. London/New York: Taylor & Francis.

——— and McLaren, P. (2010). Exploring consumption's pedagogy and envisioning a critical pedagogy of consumption: Living and learning in the shadow of the 'Shopocalypse'. In J.A. Sandlin and P. McLaren (eds), *Critical Pedagogies of Consumption: Living and Learning in the Shadow of the 'Shopocalypse'*. London/New York: Routledge, 1–20.

——— and Milam, J.L. (2008). 'Mixing pop (culture) and politics': Cultural resistance, culture jamming, and anti-consumption activism as critical public pedagogy'. *Curriculum Inquiry*, 38(3), 323–50.

———, O'Malley, M.P., and Burdick, J. (2011). Mapping the complexity of public pedagogy scholarship 1894–2010. *Review of Educational Research*, 81(3), 338–75.

Savage, G.C. (2010). Problematizing 'public pedagogy' in educational research. In J.A. Sandlin, B. Schultz and J. Burdick (eds), *Handbook of Public Pedagogy: Education and Learning beyond Schooling*, London/New York: Taylor & Francis, 103–15.

Short, F. (2006). *Kitchen Secrets: The Meaning of Cooking in Everyday Life*. Oxford: Berg.

Slocum, R. (2006). Whiteness, space and alternative food practice. *Geoforum*, 38(3), 520–33.

——— (2008). Thinking race through corporeal feminist theory: Divisions and intimacies at the Minneapolis Farmers' Market. *Social & Cultural Geography*, 9(8), 849–69.

——— (2011). Race in the study of food. *Progress in Human Geography*, 35(3), 303–27.

——— and Saldanha, A. (eds). (2013). *Geographies of Race and Food: Fields, Bodies, Markets*. Farnham: Ashgate.

Slow Food. (2014). Slow Food Education. www.slowfood.com accessed 19 January 2014.

Stoneman, S. (2009). Interview with Julie Guthman, on globalisation, neoliberalism, obesity, local food and education. *Politics and Culture*, 2, 37–44.

Sumner, J. (2008). Eating as a pedagogical act: Food as a catalyst for adult education for sustainability. *Kursiv-Journal fuer politische Bildung*, 4, 23–37.

——— (2013). Food literacy and adult education: Learning to read the world by eating. *Canadian Journal for the Study of Adult Education*, 25(2), 79–92.

Sutton, D. (2001). *Remembrance of Repasts: An Anthropology of Food and Memory*. New York: Berg Publishing.

Swan, E. (2007) 'The missing pedagogy: Leadership development, politics and social vision'. Working paper for CEL, Lancaster.

——— (2008) Let's not get too personal: Critical reflection, reflexivity and the confessional turn. *Journal of European Industrial Training*, 32(5), 385–99.

——— (2008) You make me feel like a woman: Therapeutic cultures and the contagion of femininity. *Gender, Work and Organization*, 15(1), 88–107.

——— (2009). *Worked up Selves: Personal Development Workers, Self-Work and Therapeutic Cultures*. Basingstoke: Palgrave Macmillan.

——— (2012). Cleaning up? Transnational corporate femininity and dirty work in magazine culture. In R. Simpson (ed.), *Dirty Work: Concepts and Identities*. Basingstoke: Palgrave Macmillan.

——— and Fox, S. (2009) Becoming flexible: Self-flexibility and its pedagogies. *British Journal of Management: Challenging Management Theory and Practice*, 20(1), 149–59.

——— and Flowers, R. (2015) Clearing Up the Table: Food Pedagogies and Environmental Education – Contributions, Challenges and Future Agendas. *Australian Journal of Environmental Education*, 35, 101–18.

Trubek, A.B. (2008). *The Taste of Place: A Cultural Journey into Terroir*, vol. 20. Berkeley: University of California Press.

Trubek, A.B. and Belliveau, C. (2009). Cooking as pedagogy: Engaging the senses through experiential learning. *Anthropology News*, 50(4), 16–16.

Vidgen, H.A., and Gallegos, D. (2010). Food literacy: Time for a new term or just another buzzword? *Journal of the Home Economics Institute of Australia*, 17(2), 2–8.

Vileisis, A. (2008). *Kitchen Literacy: How We Lost Knowledge of Where Food Comes from and Why We Need to Get It Back*. New York: Island Press.

Walter, P. (2012). Educational alternatives in food production, knowledge and consumption: The public pedagogies of growing power and Tsyunhehkw. *Australian Journal of Adult Learning*, 52(3), 573.

Watkins, M., Noble, G., and Driscoll, C. (2015). *Cultural Pedagogies and Human Conduct*. London: Routledge.

Williams-Forson, P. (2008). More than just the 'big piece of chicken': The power of race, class, and food in American consciousness. In C. Counihan and P. Van Esterik (eds), *Food and Culture: A Reader*. New York: Routledge, 342–53.

Williams-Forson, P. and Walker, J. (2013). Food and race: An overview. In K. Albala (ed.), *Routledge International Handbook of Food Studies*. London: Routledge.

Wright, J. and Halse, C. (2014). The healthy child citizen: Biopedagogies and web-based health promotion. *British Journal of Sociology of Education*, 35(6), 837–55.

Wright, J. and Harwood, V. (eds). (2009). *Biopolitics and the 'Obesity Epidemic': Governing Bodies*. London: Routledge.

PART I
Embodiment and Identity

Chapter 2
Where's the Pleasure? Exploring the Meanings and Experiences of Pleasure in School-based Food Pedagogies

Emma Rich and John Evans

Introduction

Food is the stuff of life, without it our bodies wither, perish and die. However, according to Lupton (1996) the linking of food primarily (even solely) with 'health' has become one of the most dominant ways of thinking about food and eating in Western societies. Concerns borne of claims that Western societies are experiencing an 'obesity epidemic' have exacerbated this connection. In particular, children's health has become a major issue for policy makers internationally following claims about the levels and prevalence of childhood obesity. The health risks presented to children who purportedly are overweight or obese or in danger of becoming so, have led to a proliferation of policies addressing the many sites through which children learn about 'healthy lifestyles', from formal school environments through to family life (e.g. Change4Life, DoH 2008). In the UK, public health campaigns and school policies on 'food' are intimately connected to these broader concerns (Department of Health 2004; Department of Health 2008). Underpinning these policies are a variety of 'new health imperatives' prescribing the choices individuals *should* make in relation to physical activity and food in order to achieve a 'healthy lifestyle'. In the UK as elsewhere, schools have been charged with a significant role in addressing this 'problem', with increased responsibility for safeguarding children and young people from the 'risks' of obesity by eating the right types and amounts of food in an attempt to either lose weight or maintain the 'ideal weight', thus reducing health to a measurable quality. The issue of school food has thus featured heavily in public health concerns and policies, not least following the television campaign, *Jamies School Dinners* for increased government funding and better quality school dinners, fronted by celebrity chef Jamie Oliver. A number of interventions and policies in the UK are thus geared towards governing the types of food provided within schools (Pike and Leahy 2012: 434) or influencing young people's food consumption and dietary knowledge (see Rich 2011; Vander Schee and Gard 2011). Over the last decade, schools have been subject to periodic evaluations in meeting these expectations. For example, 2005 saw the introduction of official (Office for Standards in Education [Ofsted]) inspection of 'healthy school status' in England, whereby schools were, for example, expected to have 'meals, vending machines and tuckshop facilities that are nutritious and healthy and meet or exceed national standards'; monitor pupils' 'menus and food choices to inform policy development and provision' and 'consult pupils on food choices through the school day' (DH 2005: 8).

Work elsewhere (Gard and Wright 2005; Wright and Harwood 2009) has already revealed some of the fault lines inherent within obesity discourse, not least through demonstrating its role in presaging unprecedented levels of regulation of young people's bodies through a variety of school practices and interventions (Pike and Leahy 2012; Evans et al. 2008; Wright and Harwood 2009). In the UK we have explored the relationship between formal education and health discourse around obesity (Evans et al. 2008) and its refraction within particular body pedagogies. Building on this work, this book chapter takes a rather more specific focus in exploring the relationship between new health imperatives and concerns over young people's diet and food, and contemporary *food pedagogies* (Flowers and Swan 2012) in formal school contexts.

Food has become of increasing interest to the practices of schools in the current near 'global' preoccupation with 'risk factors' affecting the body's capacity for 'health' (e.g. rising obesity levels). Evaluative perceptions of young people's diets are thus framed within a broader culture of risk, derived from concerns about the impact of 'pleasurable' activities (e.g. consuming particular 'fast'/'bad' foods) on the health of young people. A preoccupation with 'risk' in public health has in effect centred attention essentially on food practices that might either restrict or enhance the capacity for health. Work elsewhere has highlighted the importance of the broader cultural and social meaning of consumption (Bell and Valentine 1997) and the relationship between food, embodiment and subjectivity (Lupton 1996). We thus acknowledge that any attention to *food pedagogies* (Flowers and Swan 2012) necessarily entails analysing the meanings of pleasure in the framing of curricular and the content and technique of pedagogues in schools.

Methodology

Specifically, this chapter examines some of the ways that young people and teachers both *represent* and *experience* pleasure, and the role this plays in the constitution of pedagogies which seek to educate young people about food. To do so, we draw on data from research examining the impact of new health imperatives on schools in the UK. The data point to an array of food pedagogies which invoke particular subject positions based on different meanings of 'pleasure'. Our data derive from a study funded by the Economic and Social Research Council (RES000-22-2003) in the UK which has investigated how health imperatives and associated curriculum initiatives were operationalised within and across a range of schools located in the English Midlands. Questionnaire responses were received from some 1,176 pupils (aged 9–16) across eight schools with varied demographics, as captured in Table 2.1.

Table 2.1 Schools sample

School name	Description	Year groups interviewed
Bentley Grammar School	Large, independent, middle-class secondary school for boys (10–18 year-olds)	Sample includes 12–13 year-olds and 15–16 year-olds (Years 8 and 11)
Fraser Preparatory School	Large, independent, middle-class, co-ed, preparatory school/feeder school for Bentley Grammar School and Grange Park High School (4–11 year-olds)	Sample includes 9–11 year-olds (Years 5 and 6)
Grange Park High School	Large, independent, middle-class secondary school for girls (11–18 year-olds)	Sample includes 12–13 year-olds and 15–16 year-olds (Years 8 and 11)
Huntington High School	Large, co-ed, lower-middle/working-class, rural state middle school (11–14 year-olds)	Sample includes 11–14 year-olds (Years 7–9)
Longcliffe High School	Large, co-ed, working-class, multicultural, state middle school (11–14 year-olds)	Sample includes 12–13 year-olds (Year 8)
Rosehill C of E Primary School	Large, co-ed, working-class, multicultural, inner-city, state primary school (3–11 year-olds)	Sample includes 9–11 year-olds (Years 5 and 6)
Westwood C of E Primary School	Very small, co-ed, middle-class, rural/village, state primary school (4–11 year-olds)	Sample includes 9–11 year-olds (Years 5 and 6)
Fielding Community College	Large, co-ed, working-class, multicultural, inner-city college (11–16 year-olds)	Sample includes 13–15 year-olds (Years 9 and 10)

90 pupils and 18 school staff were then interviewed to explore in greater detail issues raised by pupils in the questionnaires. Here, we use material essentially from interviews with pupils and teachers. Children's responses in the interviews were prompted by a set of cards with the words, 'obesity', 'body', 'school' and 'health'. Inevitably, neither the pupil nor staff voices briefly presented represent all opinions or viewpoints encountered. The voices heard in this chapter only selectively illustrate key ways in which ubiquitous health imperatives are interpreted and recontextualised through pedagogical relationships of food unique to each school, facilitating opportunities to develop particular forms of embodiment and subjectivity. Pupils subject to the same processes within particular school settings responded differently to these processes. Whilst we did not ask the young people and teachers directly about their experiences of pleasure, their talk about food and health in school and other sites alluded to the significance of 'pleasure' in their relationships with food. Different constructs of pleasure led to different

opportunities and imperatives for regulation, leading to particular ways of being and understandings of oneself and others. In our approach to the data, whilst we analyse the discourses through which the body as 'mattered' within and by culture, is constituted by various body pedagogies, so too we acknowledge its corporeality. In work elsewhere, exploring the *body made flesh* (Evans, Davies and Rich 2009) we have developed the 'corporeal device' as a 'conceptual means of addressing the significance of both body mass and mattering in the interminable, inseparable dialectic between biology and culture' (Evans, Davies and Rich, 2014: 654). We expand on this theoretical approach in the section below, specifically in relation to understanding body pedagogies.

To begin we provide a brief overview of the theoretical perspectives that frames the analysis with reference to pedagogy and pleasure. We then delineate some of the ways that teachers and young people come to constitute 'pleasure' in relation to food. Finally, we conclude by suggesting that unless pleasure, as an aspect of embodiment is more centrally registered in pedagogical relationships then we will fail to understand well enough the relationship between learning and embodiment.

Theorising Pleasure and Food Pedagogy

Various conceptualisations stating the body's importance in social theory (for example, Butler 1993; Grosz 1994, 1995; Shilling 2000, 2005, 2008) have become increasingly central to research in education which has sought to understand how the body is 'schooled' in relation to areas of the curricular focused on for example, sport, health and food. As alluded to above, contemporary perceived threats about rising levels of childhood obesity has provided the rationale for a range of school-based interventions and policies designed to 'educate' young people about healthy lifestyles (Burrows 2009; Burrows and Wright 2007; Leahy 2009; Rich 2010; Vander Schee 2009). In work with colleagues elsewhere, we have explored the role schools play within a 'knowledge economy' in nurturing and endorsing 'particular "corporeal orientations", that is to say, ascribe value, meaning and potential to the "the body" (particular bodies) in time, place and space' (Evans, Rich, Allwood and Davies 2008: 387). In our focus on 'body pedagogies', we thus refer to: 'any conscious activity taken by one person, organisation, or a State, designed to enhance an individual's understandings of their own and/or others' corporeality. Body pedagogies define the significance, value and potential of the body in time, place and space' (Evans et al. 2008). Their derivative body pedagogics (Shilling 2008) produce particular embodied subjectivities that are essentially corporeal orientations to self and others. And because they 'define whose and what bodies have status and value, they also constitute acts of inclusion and exclusion'. With reference to weight and shape, body pedagogies play a significant role in defining certain populations as 'healthy', 'good' or 'deviant', in relation to responsibility for their health and lifestyles.

Although this conceptualisation inevitably, to some extent, simplifies complex processes of cultural reproduction and transmission, it offers a useful starting point for exploring the relationship between health imperatives, food pedagogy and embodiment. Similarly, food pedagogies also work to shape an individual's understanding of corporeality, imbued with moral overtones about consumption practices and the bodies they come to define and prescribe. As Flowers and Swan (2012: 424) observe, 'through food we are taught about power, culture, bodies, gender, class, race, status, identity, pleasure, pain, labour, health, morality, our place in the world; as is often said, "who and what we are"'. Thus, food pedagogies are embedded in relations of power and social, cultural, economic, political meaning. Our interest, in this chapter, is how food pedagogies fashion particular subject/ive positions, not just in relation to food, but broader social and cultural meanings of the body. As mentioned, currently in the UK, these processes are framed within a risk culture which is shaping how we perceive the significance of food in relation to health. Whilst food pedagogies might focus on various aspects of teaching and learning about food (from how to grow it to dietary knowledge), the focus of this chapter is how meanings of pleasure in relation to food also come to define particular populations and shape corporeal orientations. The reason for this is twofold; firstly, the constitution of 'pleasure' within public health policy and school policy influence the pedagogical practices in schools and may come to define particular populations as 'risky' in relation to their consumption practices. Secondly, different meanings of 'pleasure' may not only shape the experience of eating, but also provide particular subject positions through which young people understand their own and other's embodiment and cultural identities.

Pleasure may be constituted in food pedagogies in diverse ways, given that the meanings of pleasure are historically situated and contextual, and have different meanings in different cultural contexts (Coveney and Bunton 2003). Thus, we approach pleasure, in this sense, not from the perspective of an essential, reducible psychological experience but, as variously read, experienced and situated in social, cultural, historical and economic context. There is not space here to fully explore this, but work elsewhere alludes to the cultural differences in terms of experiences and attitudes towards pleasure. For example, Rozin et al. (1999) identify that there are substantial country (and usually gender) differences in relation to attitudes towards food and health. Elsewhere, Hayes-Conroy suggests that:

> the experience of food as comforting happens at/as the interplay between conscious/intellectual mind and remembering/reacting body, where the experience of a comforting smell, or sight, or taste depends upon and recalls the learned knowledge of both the mind and body. (2009: 183–4)

Therefore, diverse social experiences, mediated by for example, class, gender, ethnicity comes to shape one's sensory experiences. Hayes-Conroy and Hayes-Conroy (2008) suggest food beliefs are 'actually already material, experienced as part of the visceral body' and in this sense, in a relationality, pleasure, sensory experience and taste are 'materially affected' (ibid.) by ones experience of the social contexts in which they live. The emergence of a growing body of feminist work which focused on the relationships between various food practices and the gendered body reflects this very process.

However, in contemporary risk culture, 'pleasure and pleasure-seeking activities are often considered to be at the root of irrational, often spontaneous actions which predisposes individuals to unhealthy, so-called risk-taking behaviours' (Coveney and Bunton 2003: 166). This is evident in contemporary obesity discourses, and Gard and Wright (2001: 539) argue that 'obesity has been constructed as an undesirable side effect of modern western life and adds to the growing list of risks that this kind of life is charged with generating'. A moral imperative is constituted through the language of risk, imparting notions of what is good and bad, risky and safe, but also in terms of the extent to which regulation and intervention might be needed to managed risk, and with it, pleasure-seeking behaviours. As Coveney (2002: viii) articulates, 'the heart of the problem it seems is that food pleasure challenges self-control'. Thus, pleasure becomes increasingly significant within an obesity discourse which sees, at least part, of the solution to be personal responsibility and choice about individual lifestyle. Consequently, some school-based food pedagogies are focused on controlling particular desires towards pleasure. As Coveney and Bunton (2003: 163) suggest, 'so many injunctions to healthy behaviours seem to be concerned with restricting or overcoming our seemingly 'natural' inclination towards certain pleasures.' In their work on food pedagogies in UK and Australian schools, Pike and Leahy (2012: 440) assert that 'this governmentalisation has worked in two ways; first by limiting individuals' fields of action, by curtailing the types of food available to pupils at school and second, by encouraging pupils to act upon themselves as healthy subjects' (Pike and Leahy 2012: 440).

Increasingly, scholars have begun to critique the fashioning of 'pleasure' within public health policy. As Coveney and Bunton (2003) suggest, 'many public health interventions attempt to promote health and well-being while simultaneously engaging with or negating pleasure-seeking activities'. Similarly, Wellard (2012: 23) attests, 'aspects of bodily pleasure are often overlooked in favour of specific health-related measures'. Using the development of religious ideas in Western cultures, Coveney and Bunton (2003: 161) identify four forms of pleasure, examining how they 'influence approaches to our understandings of health in general and interventions to public health in particular': carnal pleasure, disciplined pleasure, ascetic pleasure and ecstatic pleasure. They argue that modern health initiatives are rooted in highly disciplined and religious movements which sought to 'reform unwholesome habits, disruptive pleasures and, in the process, transform pleasures … to replace one form of pleasure (hedonistic, canal, libidinal) with another (aesthetic, ascetic, civilised)' (ibid.: 167). Thus, the self-management of health in this context also means the self-monitoring of one's pleasure. Drawing on this framework of pleasure, what follows below is an exploration of how these different meanings of pleasure are drawn upon in food pedagogies emerging to address obesity in the context of a risk culture.

We ask: Are young people's relationships with food becoming 'disembodied' (Evans 2004) and in the process less pleasurable? Given that 'food is a critical contributor to physical wellbeing, a major source of pleasure' (Rozin et al. 1999), how might the constitution of pleasure in particular ways through food pedagogies come to limit or enhance the well-being of young people? What knowledge and 'truth' about food, health, pleasure and the self are being constituted through the discourses of food pedagogies? Drawing on a poststructuralist understanding of the fragmented, multiple and contingent self, the analysis explores the relationship between these pedagogies and young people's *subjectivity*: 'the conscious and unconscious thoughts and emotions of the individual, her sense of herself, and her ways of understanding her relation to the world' (Weedon 1987: 32).

From Good Taste to Sugar Junkies

Eating is not just a practice of survival, but central to our sense of self (Lupton 1996). Whilst young people negotiate a range of discourses which come to give different meanings to food and eating, they are also feeling, sentient beings and the body is not just a conduit for discursive messages but may have a certain generative capacity (McWilliam 1999; Zembylas 2007). Most obviously, in relation to food, this might be in the form of pleasures and sensations one feels when tasting food and drink. One might then read the sensory urges as an 'act of mediation' (Ivinson and Duveen 2006: 111) through which young people's relationships with food, and their interpretation of food pedagogy is mediated by sensory and corporeal resources, not just 'socio-cognitive' resources. Coveney and Bunton (2003: 168) describe the 'carnal' pleasure of bodily basics; 'they are sensuous, and come from the senses. They are therefore often unanticipated, arising out of nowhere but calling for attention and gratification. This engagement with the sensuous aspects of food was conspicuous by its relative absence in the way young people talked about food and its relative pleasures. Some children/students, however, did emphasise the desire to experience different tastes:

> 'cause you want to have a change, you don't want to eat it every day because you'll get bored of it and tired, you want new stuff. (Fred, Bentley Grammar School, Year 8)

For others who spoke of the pleasures of particular foods, this was not simply framed as 'taking enjoyment in gustatory sensations' (Lupton 1996: 1) but, as similar to the findings of Hayes-Conroy (2009) made sense of through wider social and cultural meanings of food:

> I'm not going to stop eating chocolate, I'm addicted to it really. It's the taste really. Healthy stuff's good but the other stuff is nicer. You have them less often so … (Sunil, Bentley Grammar School, year 8)

In the above comment, Sunil understands his decision not to comply with the expectations of risk management, to avoid chocolate, through the negative construct of 'addiction'. Whilst he acknowledges the sensory pleasure of taste, he is quick to register its association with lack of control, an urge which calls for gratification, framing this within a broader discourse of 'addiction'. The discursive production of these sorts of meaning, could also be seen in the food pedagogies promoted by some of the teachers in our study. For example, Samantha, a food technology teacher clearly constructs the subject position of 'sugar junkie', a location for those individuals oriented towards particular tastes and aligns it with self-destructive connotations of a 'junkie':

> We have some lovely little bits of videos that we use about erm … the relationship between diet and behaviour … There was a very good erm … Trevor McDonald tonight that followed some children and altered their diet and got some quite drastic … and they're quite interested in that as well erm … because, you know, they put up a list of things that are … a sugar junkie … and all the erm, things that you'd expect, behaviours that you'd expect from somebody who's a sugar junkie, and yeah they all sit there 'Yeah, yeah, yeah, yeah, yeah' (laughs), and so they can really relate to that quite nicely and that works really well with them … We also talk about obesity but … it's … it's a difficult one to approach in the classroom because there is a certain political correctness erm … the powers that be do not particularly like us turning round to children and saying do you realise that you're overweight. (Samantha, Food technology teacher, Fielding Community College)

Drawing on a discursive framework of risk management, a number of teachers tended to recognise the sensuous, but described these as urges or desires that needed to be controlled through a range of interventions or self-management techniques. These were urges towards pleasures that could lead to risky behaviours, through for example, over consumption or eating the 'wrong foods'. Some teachers were aware of the generative capacity of the body, its sentient nature and ongoing maturation:

> Sometimes I've got them to fill in bits of paper as to what did I swallow in the last week – you know everything that you've drank and everything that you've ate. We've done this as a verbal thing, we do this with the Year 8s because that's where we have a major push on healthy eating because that's *when their bodies are really changing*. (Pamela, Food technology and textiles teacher, Huntington High School)

Pamela makes reference to their changing bodies; their material, flesh and blood, sentient, thinking and feeling bodies and sees the significance of this in terms of the need for regulation and intervention as pedagogic relations are mediated by growing, developing bodies located in time, place and space (we refer to this elsewhere through our conceptualisation of the 'corporeal device') (Evans, Davies and Rich, 2009). Similarly, Melissa, head of PSHE spoke of the need to work with and against these sensuous urges, in an effort to change what are seen as preferences or dispositions towards risky foods:

> Especially for Year One, it's to encourage them to try different flavours. Especially for the younger children if they're all trying they're more likely to try aren't they … It's an awareness of things that are good for them. (Melissa, Head of PSHE, Fraser Preparatory School)

For some, like Marie, these interventions led to unpleasant experiences with food:

> When we were in science we had to taste loads of fruit and I picked up the avocado, I had a bit of it and I asked Mr A what it was and he said that's avocado so I just spit it out and put it in the bin'. (Marie, Fraser preparatory school, Year 6)

The discontent of being directed to 'try' foods to which young people have an unpleasant reaction may come to be a significant affective experience which shapes future relationships with food. Lupton (1996), for example, revealed that for some people, the pleasure of food they experience as adults emerge from the contrast of the differential power relations between adults and children and having to eat foods they disliked. The possibilities for experiencing different forms of sensuous pleasure and other forms of fulfilment are thus 'materially affected' (Hayes-Conroy, 2009) and thus governed by the food pedagogies which prevailed within these schools. Food pedagogies thus construct particular social meanings which shape young people's relationships with their sentient bodies and pleasure.

Disciplined and Balanced Pleasure

In a further effort to transform pleasure, many of the teachers we spoke to across all three schools described modalities of practice which sought to encourage what Coveney and Bunton (2003: 171) refer to as a 'rationalized and disciplined pleasure' rather than 'vulgar and emotional displays of enjoyment' (Coveney and Bunton 2003: 171). The data from our research revealed how within the food pedagogies which drew on this category of 'disciplined pleasure', young people are taught to temper the need for immediate gratification and instead make reasoned decisions about food.

> Well you can do … well I could probably do it as a lesson. You do it as a lesson and you would get fruit and you would get chocolate and things and you would do it as a lesson where you would say 'oh you can eat chocolate but in moderation, you don't have a bar every single day of the week. Instead of having a chocolate bar, you have a fruit.' And it is the same with crisps. They go out and buy all the Walkers crisps, but you can buy the lights now which are better for them, they are still not really good for you because they have still got a load of stuff in them but they are better for them. So you have got to do it in a fun way for children. You can't just say "right you will not have that, you have got to have that.' I think you have got to make something that you are going to present to them as fun. An exciting thing that will get them enthused. (Donna, Health Schools Coordinator, Rosehill C of E Primary School)

As Hannah indicates, this is deemed to be in the best interests of the child or young person within a culture of risk:

> Oh yes, definitely. It was basically like a burger bar before and they would get chips and burger or a jacket potato, but that's all gone now. Children who come into the school just accept it I think given the prediction of the obesity epidemic that they're saying will happen with our children then I think it's got to be good as it's going to cut down the problems the children are going to have particularly as they get into adult life. (Hannah, Head of PSHE, Huntington High School)

These pedagogies draw on a 'rational ascetic' (Murphy 1995), as found in the broader discourse of obesity. From this perspective, pedagogical relations seek to subject the body to a systematic regime of 'rational conduct' (ibid.: 109). As Coveney and Bunton observe, pleasure is instead derived from the ability to restrain and temper one's self and food practices and 'immediate gratification is relinquished for the pleasure and satisfaction of rationalization and reason' (2003: 171). Pedagogies drawing upon this approach to pleasure attempt to encourage young people to regulate their choices, to 'discipline the body, to ensure that the body will behave (or move) in methodical and regular ways' (ibid.: 109):

> Very much eating erm … poor diet, they have no … it's very strange, with our young people particularly, they have a concept of what they should be doing but they don't seem to think that they need to necessarily do anything about that, if you ask them the question 'What should you be eating?' they'll tell you the answer but that isn't what they're actually doing … Erm, I think some of it comes down to the fact that teenagers think they're invincible (laughs) and its part of that psychology, and I think it's also down to a lot of the pressures that are on young people at the minute, everything's down to their own personal enjoyment, you know the way computer games work and everything, it's all high intensity, it's all individual one on one and so it's not so much the … you know, that they have any sense that they're part of a community, they're part of

a … you know, that they have a responsibility there for the long term health of the nation and, you know, that just doesn't seem to play with them at all, what's important is whether I like it and that's all that is … in any way bothering them. Attitudes towards sex is a big issue around here as well … and as is drugs. (Samantha, Food technology teacher, Fielding community college)

These pedagogies emphasise the 'virtues of conscientiousness – virtues that are expressed in the careful and methodical way a person pursues a task, problem, issue or calling' (ibid.: 109). As Murphy (1995) argues, this sort of approach to the body is one that prohibits certain actions, such as idleness or indulgence in certain pleasures, but also institutes methodical practices. In the comments above, Samantha draws on this discursive framework, rationalising the problems of young people's health to their focus on individual enjoyment and lack of responsibility. In this sense, some teachers perceived 'pleasure' as problematic – as weakening and in opposition to the compliance towards the dominant food pedagogies. Resulting governance of young people's bodies focus on altering this behaviour, exemplifying broader social and cultural discourses of obesity wherein individuals are encouraged to make deliberate decisions about their bodies and lifestyles to actively protect themselves from the risks associated with being overweight and/or obese. The pedagogues role is thus to 'to shape, guide, direct the conduct of others' and 'bridle the individual's passions', inducing them to control their own instincts; they 'govern themselves' (Rose 1999: 3). However, this implies a 'greater deliberateness' (Murphy 1995: 110) than that which Samantha perceives the young people currently either demonstrate or are able and/or willing to exhibit. These young people are classified as being at risk, in perpetual states of being focused on immediate and individual pleasure and therefore potentially 'unwell'. As a consequence, in some cases, teachers adopted more extreme pedagogical approaches, sanctified as being necessary in order to control and better 'educate' potentially volatile and recalcitrant students. Moreover, in the UK, where certain populations have failed to comply with the ideologies and rules of liberal individualism and healthsim (e.g. in relation to diet and exercise) there has thus been increased levels of more direct intervention into schools and family life. In one of the more extreme examples, Pamela, adopts an approach which far from engaging with any pleasurable aspect of food, highlights the palpable risks, through pedagogies which seek explicitly to promote fear and 'disgust' (Leahy 2009):

Oh yes, quite clearly. I think in food you can get away with is the wrong term, you can probe and ask questions that might sound impertinent coming from other areas, so from that point of view the children are usually very open. You just need to point out that if you want to maximise your life-span barring accidents or illnesses over which you have no control then you need to eat healthily and what the repercussions are if you don't from cancer of the colon to diverticulitis, heart attacks. Diverticulitis is where your gut stops, you know how your esophagus and your intestines, it's this action where the muscular action

> pushes the food through and if the muscles stop working you get this condition called diverticulitis where what goes in one end no longer comes out the other … I find that if you make it quite graphic they actually listen, you know your body can only get the goodness out of the foods that you put in it. The other thing that we impress upon them is that it's not enough to do that on its own, it needs to be in conjunction with exercise. Couch potato lifestyles are really, really bad. I won't expand very much because I'm not terribly PC. But I mean as a school we've removed, when I first started there were chocolate machines, coke machines – all gone. As you know we've changed the policy in the restaurant. Before Jamie Oliver was doing his school dinners programme, I mean I've been whinging on for years about how rubbish the canteen meals were … (Pamela, food technology and textiles teacher, Huntington high school)

The affective influence of such pedagogy on the embodiment of young people is clear in the response of Marie and others below. The potential for pleasure and enjoyment is significantly shaped (and curtailed) by the fears associated with the risks associated with obesity:

> Will I die because I'm overweight and you won't get any sleep because you'll be thinking about will I die or not. Some people don't sleep at all because they think that they're going to die in their sleep because they're so obese. (Marie, Fraser preparatory school, year 6)

> When I think about weight I have dreams yeah, like I become really fat and I can't move … Because if you eat too much yeah you won't have that much life to live. (Dinesh, Rosehill C of E school, year 5)

Thus, although not straightforward, food pedagogies can reach into and regulate myriad aspects of young people's lives, bodies, affects and embodiment. As another example, even the social meaning, status and value of social occasions, such as birthdays, which act as markers of childhood were regulated, influencing the potential pleasure which could be derived from them:

> Erm, so I think that's really important, I think those messages about things like birthday sweets and I'm not saying 'oh dear, birthday sweets', but when the child brings fruits 'wow look at those strawberries, and they're delicious and they're really good for us, so that's great isn't it', and really sort of trying to boost that up, and walking through the hall and saying that's a great healthy lunch box and also supporting PE coordinator, in trying to do things and taking children out to use, obviously I guess she's told you about using goals for football and supporting matches and gymnastic club to try and actually be a visible … I think that's important really and not just saying it, but walking the talk … (Sally, Head Teacher, Rosehill C of E school)

> I mean another example of that is that we have, we sort of have had a tradition here of the children have a birthday or there's a festival or some sort of celebration and they will bring in sweets to share with the class and we've … through our … we've got a whole school food policy and we've not banned that, erm, but we did say, may be fruit would be a nice alternative, or buy a book for the class or a game for class so, giving a treat but in another way rather than sweets, that seems to be the, anything good, oh we'll have sweets and again I think its about changing staff's attitudes as well so that we're not condemning them but we're saying that we don't want too many of them. Occasionally it's okay but not on a constant basis. (Samantha, Food technology teacher, Fielding Community College)

The eschewing, or restricting of what might be typically seen as pleasurable and tasty foods is significant, given their broader social and cultural meanings in ritualized social occasions such as birthdays. Food, is after all, a significant part of the cultural and social landscape, it has multiple meanings and purposes in people's lives.

Though driven by genuinely altruistic desire to improve the health of individuals and populations, when framed within an ideology of 'liberal individualism' the relationship between food pleasure and health can take on narrow connotations. New forms of normalising practices emerge and prevail in ways that have potentially limiting and damaging consequences for the well-being of young people.

Pleasure through Restraint

How young people interpret and recontextualise the meanings and principles of obesity discourse play a part in how the body is schooled through food pedagogies and thus how these pedagogies impact embodiment and subjectivity. In terms of the potential threat to well-being, the slippage from disciplined to ascetic pleasure – which involves the pleasure derived from abstinence and the 'total control of the body's natural urges' (Coveney and Bunton 2003: 172) known as 'ascetic pleasure' – is significant. The interpretive activity of young people mediates these pedagogic relations and combine with the pedagogical forces of broader culture which promote excessive regulation of the body in often powerful ways. In an attempt to manage the 'pleasures' of the students, the elements associated with disciplinary pleasures may also lead to a more 'ascetic' pursuit of pleasure and the adoption of practices which may compromise well-being and health. Elsewhere we have documented the ascetic pleasures young women with anorexia derived from self-starvation (Evans et al. 2008). Whilst the practices in these more diverse groups of young people in the abovementioned schools were not as extreme, they included; mimicking the admired eating practices of peers, not eating for long periods of time and strict dieting, all of which drew on neo-liberal discourses that celebrated self-control and constraint echoed in public health policy.

> A huge amount, particularly with girls. They all copy one another. There has been a case in school where people have stopped eating and other girls have copied or they've cut down on their lunch and I've seen girls give their food away to boys in the class. We're talking perhaps a few cases of that but it has come to my attention. (Hannah, head of PSHE, Huntington High School)

The above comments reiterate the risks of such an approach to health, as Coveney and Bunton (2003: 172) assert, 'in trying to supplant carnal pleasures with disciplined pleasures, public health always runs the risk of paralleling religious zeal which reifies ascetic pleasures'. The pursuit of health through an engagement with ascetic pleasure led to some students compromising their well-being and health (see Gard and Wright 2005; Evans et al. 2008). As the space for engaging with sensuous pleasures with food diminishes, the significance of pleasure derived from more excessive and disciplined forms of restraint may heighten. Thus, many of the young people in our research described feeling 'happy' about their demonstration of restraint, control and refusal of certain food, fully aware of its moral connotations:

> But it's a good sense. You feel righteous when you're eating the right stuff. (Tom, Bentley Grammar School, year 11)

> Yeah like how many calories is it so I can burn off and things and eat the right amount of things, don't eat too much, that's it. (Amit, Bentley Grammar school, year 8).

Pleasure, for many, was derived through a sense of self-control, restraint, self-discipline, slipping from a focus on balanced healthy eating to more excessive forms of regulation:

> I've lost quite a lot of weight since I've been eating my bananas and everything and doing my dancing … I feel really happy with myself because I've gone on a bit of a diet. This morning I didn't have any breakfast … And I didn't have any break. (Marie, Fraser preparatory school, year 6)

Rather than measured choices or a balanced approach to food, for some young people, pleasure, rather alarmingly, is derived from abstinence and the 'total control of the body's natural urges' (Coveney and Bunton 2003: 172):

> Exactly, you go over the top and you like end up eating too much vegetables and not enough of things making you smile and stuff. Another problem you'll get is you feel bad about yourself if you have two meals in a row that you don't

think are very healthy and then you've got a religious streak where you don't eat anything unhealthy for you. (James, Bentley Grammar School, Year 11)

Conclusion: The Importance of Pleasure in Pedagogies of Food

The importance of 'pleasure' in the data above raises a number of fundamental questions concerning the relationships between desire, affect, discourse and the embodied practices and discursive systems expressed through not just health policy but the food pedagogies of teachers in schools. We have barely touched upon the complexities of these relationships between food pedagogies, desire, affect and embodied subjectivity in schools and we would argue these need much further examination. Clearly, policies and pedagogies that nurture dualistic thinking and the idea that the pleasure of eating is to be disciplined, controlled and overcome, ought to rest high amongst our concerns as pedagogues and sociologists. In contexts of heightened surveillance the reductive normalising of food practices potentially threatens the potential for well-being (Wellard 2012) and current and future relationship between food and self (Lupton 1996). As Coveney and Bunton (2003: 174) warn: 'In its attempt to transform pleasures, public health always runs the risk of introducing new and unanticipated elements that may run counter to the goals of health enhancement.'

As particular forms of pleasure are fashioned and inscribed with social meaning, they prevail or diminish as legitimate experiences. For many of the young people in our study, the pleasure of food was often derived from their ability to demonstrate self-restraint. Alarmingly, the slippage from methodical and rational choice, to abstinence and strict dieting was apparent, reflecting a slippage from what Coveney and Bunton (2003) refer to as 'disciplined' to 'ascetic' pleasure. What space then is there for pedagogies that engage with the complexities of sensory experiences and encourages young people to experience, positively, taste, touch and smell of foods as part of their learning about their own and others' bodies and culture. Moreover, following Hayes-Conroy's (2009) critique of sensory pleasures in schools, we need ways to do this which move beyond the assumptions that 'students' sensory perception exists as a natural/essential category that is both prior to and distinguishable from their social experiences and intellectual development'. This may mean developing alternative pedagogies which, for example, focus on both the risks and pleasures of certain foods and their significance across different cultural contexts.

References

Bell, D. and Valentine, G. (1997). *Consuming Geographies*. London: Routledge.

Butler, J. (1993). *Bodies that Matter: On the Discursive Limits of 'Sex'*. London: Routledge.

Bunton, R. and A. Petersen. (1997). Foucault's medicine. In A. Petersen and R. Bunton (eds), *Foucault, Health and Medicine*. London: Routledge, 1–15.

Burrows, L (2009). Pedagogizing families through obesity discourse. In J. Wright and V. Harwood (eds), *Biopolitics and the Obesity Epidemic: Governing Bodies*. New York: Routledge, 127–40.

——— and Wright, J. (2007). Prescribing practices: Shaping healthy children in schools. *International Journal of Children's Rights*, 15, 1–16.

Coveney, J. (2002). *Food, Morals and Meaning: The Pleasure and Anxiety of Eating*. New York: Routledge.

——— and Bunton, R. (2003). In pursuit of the study of pleasure: Implications for health research and practice. *Health: An Interdisciplinary Journal for the Study of Health, Illness and Medicine*, 7(2), 161–79.

Department of Health (2004). *Choosing Health: Making Healthier Choices Easier* (London: DH Publications).

——— (2005). *National Healthy School Status* (London: DH Publications).

——— (2008). *Healthy Weight, Healthy Lives: A Cross Government Strategy for England* (London: DH Publications).

——— (2008). *Change4Life*. Available at: http://www.dh.gov.uk/en/News/Currentcampaigns/Change4Life/index.htm.

Evans, J. (2004). Making a difference? Education and ability in physical education. *European Physical Education Review*, 10(1), 95–109.

———, Davies, B. and Rich, E. (2009). The body made flesh: Embodied learning and the corporeal device. *British Journal of Sociology of Education*, 30(4), 389–91.

——— (2014). We/You can tell talk from matter: A conversation with Håkan Larsson and Mikael Quennerstedt. *Sport, Education and Society*, 652–65.

———, Rich, E., Davies, B. and Allwood, R. (2008). *Education, Disordered Eating and Obesity Discourse: Fat Fabrications.* London and New York: Routledge.

Flowers, R. and Swan, E. (2012). Introduction: Why food? Why pedagogy? Why adult education? *Australian Journal of Adult Learning*, 52(3), 419–33.

Gard, M. and Wright, J. (2001). Managing uncertainty: Obesity discourses and physical education in a risk society. *Studies in Philosophy and Education*, 20(6), 535–49.

——— (2005). *The Obesity Epidemic: Science, Morality, and Ideology*. New York: Routledge.

Grosz, E. (1987). Notes towards a corporeal feminism. *Australian Feminist Studies*, 5, 1–16.

——— (1994). *Volatile Bodies: Towards a Corporeal Feminism*. Sydney: Allen & Unwin.

——— (1995). *Space, Time and Perversion: The Politics of Bodies*. Sydney: Allen & Unwin.

Hayes-Conroy, A. (2009). Visceral Reactions: Alternative food and social difference in two North American schools. PhD Dissertation, Pennsylvania State University.

——— and Hayes-Conroy, J. (2008). Taking back taste: Feminism, food and visceral politics. *Gender, Place & Culture: A Journal of Feminist Geography*, 15(5), 461–73.
Howson, A. (2004). *The Body in Society*. Cambridge: Polity Press.
Ivinson, G. and Duveen, G. (2006). Children's recontextualisations of pedagogy. In R. Moore, M. Arnot, J. Beck and H. Daniels (eds), *Knowledge, Power and Educational Reform*. London: Routledge.
Leahy, D. (2009). Disgusting pedagogies. In J. Wright and V. Harwood (eds), *Biopolitics and the Obesity Epidemic*. New York: Routledge, 172–82.
Lupton, D. (1996). *Food, the Body and the Self*. London: Sage.
Jackson, P. (ed.). (2009). *Changing Families, Changing Food*. Basingstoke: Palgrave Macmillan.
McWilliam, E. (1999). *Pedagogical Pleasures*. New York: Peter Lang Publishing.
Murphy P. (1995). The body politic. In P.A. Komesaroff (ed.), *Troubled Bodies: Critical Perspectives on Postmodernism, Medical Ethics and the Body*. Durham and London: Duke University Press, 103–24.
Pike, J. and Leahy, D. (2012). School food and the pedagogies of parenting. *Australian Journal of Adult Learning*, 52(3), 434–59.
Rich, E. (2010) Obesity assemblages and surveillance in schools, *International Journal of Qualitative Studies in Education*, 23(7): 803–21.
Rich, E. (2011). 'I see her being obesed!': Public pedagogy, reality media and the obesity crisis. *Health*, 15(1), 3–21.
Rose, N. (1999). *Powers of Freedom: Reframing Political Thought*. Cambridge: Cambridge University Press.
Rozin, P., Fischler, C., Imada, S., Sarubin, A. and Wrzesniewski, A. (1999). Attitudes to food and the role of food in life in the USA, Japan, Flemish Belgium and France: Possible implications for the diet-health debate. *Appetite*, 33, 163–80.
Shilling, C. (2000). *The Body and Social Theory*. London: Sage.
——— (2005). *The Body in Culture and Society*. London: Sage Publications.
——— (2008). *Changing Bodies: Habit, Crisis and Creativity*. London: Sage.
Vander Schee, C. (2009). Fruit, root vegetables, fatness and Foucault: governing students and their families through school health policy. *Journal of Education Policy*, 24(5), 557–74.
——— and Gard, M. (2011). Editorial: Politics, pedagogy and practice in school health policy. *Policy Futures in Education*, 9(3), 307–14.
Weedon, C. (1987). *Feminist Practice and Poststructuralist Theory*. New York: Basil Blackwell.
Wellard, I. (2012). Body-reflexive pleasures: Exploring bodily experiences within the context of sport and physical activity. *Sport, Education and Society*, 17(1), 21–33.
Wright, J. and Harwood, V. (eds). (2009). *Biopolitics and the 'Obesity Epidemic': Governing Bodies*. London: Routledge.
Zembylas, M. (2007). Risks and pleasures: A Deluzian-Guattarian pedagogy of desire in education. *British Educational Research Journal*, 33(3), 331–49.

Chapter 3

Potatoes in the Rice Cooker: Family Food Pedagogies, Bodily Memories, Meal-time Senses and Racial Practices

Rick Flowers and Elaine Swan

Introduction

In this chapter, we explore how family food practices operate pedagogically in relation to race and gender. Food, of course, is freighted with meaning. It constitutes bodily nutrition but also pleasure, anxiety, labour, and morality (Rozin 1996). Family meal-times themselves are symbolic, social, religious, and material events which define, reproduce and sustain families. For example, in deciding who eats what with whom, meal-times create exclusions and inclusions, producing boundaries between family members, acquaintances and strangers. Moreover, the provisioning, preparation and cooking of food in families – most often the responsibility of women – can be simultaneously forms of care, connection, and cultural transmission (Chen 2013). Hence, through women's work, family food connects people to ethnic, racial and national identifications, demarcating 'us' from 'them' and consolidating who 'we are' because of what and how we cook and eat (Xu 2008; Bajic-Hajdukovic 2013; Lee 2000; Law 2001). Family food practices have, however, been under-researched in relation to mixed-race families (for an exception see Flowers and Swan 2012a).

To start addressing this gap we put anthropologist David Berliner's (2013) conceptualisation of 'cultural transmission' in dialogue with recent work on racial practices (Slocum 2011), ethnic food senses (Law 2001), alimentary pedagogy (Highmore 2008) and visceral pedagogy (Hayes-Conroy and Hayes-Conroy 2008, 2010) in food studies. Berliner summarises cultural transmission as the 'processes which contribute to the creative persistence of representations, practices, emotions and institutions in a society' (2013: 73). Importantly then, transmission is not simply cognitive. Of course, according to Berliner, words are powerful 'transmitters' but other powerful mediators include: 'institutions, gestures, interactions, smells, texts, silences, ordinary moments, sounds, emotions, objects and technologies' (2013: 75). Thus, Berliner is emphasising the material and sensory as well as the interactional and representational, the latter most often discussed in food pedagogy literature. This means that learning entails explicit prescriptions but also practices that 'go without saying': everyday verbal interjections, emotional expressions, insignificant gestures and tones (ibid.). Pedagogically, there is 'no fixed model of learning'; rather, 'transmission' is dynamic and heterogeneous across a congeries of media, contexts, actors, organisational forms and materialities.

Whilst we acknowledge there is critique of the notion of 'transmission' for being one-way, linear and behaviourist, we find Berliner's more anthropological conceptualisation productive on a number of counts. Firstly, it is an expansive definition that encompasses micro and macro processes; individuals and groups; emotions and cognitions; explicit and implicit practices; and the symbolic and the material. Secondly, he argues that social theorists use terms such as 'habitus' and 'socialisation' to denote cultural change and continuity but rarely research the extent and variety of discourses, practices and mechanisms which go to make up cultural change and continuity. Thirdly, Berliner explicitly links cultural transmission to ethnographies of learning dating back over 50 years of anthropology including scholars such Margaret Mead, Marcel Mauss, Jack Goody, Pierre Bourdieu and Jean Lave. All these studies moved beyond psychologistic models of learning. As a result, we think that Berliner's work on cultural transmission is highly suggestive for exploring food pedagogies in relation to race and families when augmented by the developments in sensory and visceral scholarship in food studies (Slocum 2011; Highmore 2008; Hayes-Conroy 2010, Hayes-Conroy and Hayes-Conroy 2010; Law 2001). Importantly, this work on the senses does not essentialise or individualise smell, taste, sight, hearing and touch but sees them as historical socio-culturally located practices which are performative of race, class and gender (Law 2001).

As we can see from chapters in this edited volume, there are many contexts and actors involved in food pedagogies, with institutions such as schools and the media being seen as particularly significant. But in this chapter, we turn to the institution of the family and food practices. For example, at meal-times children can learn about food rituals and moralities; acceptable codes of conduct; gendered roles and power relations; and how to make the 'family' through food (Quarmby and Dagkas 2013; Laurier and Wiggins 2011; Ochs and Shohet 2006; Gallegos et al. 2011). And importantly, as this chapter implies, it is not just children who learn but adults too. The pedagogical heterogeneity and density of meal-times is captured by Elinor Ochs and Mervac Shohet who write that in eating together, different generations and genders:

> come to learn, reinforce, undermine, or transform each other's ways of acting, thinking, and feeling in the world, sometimes through cajoling, begging, probing, praising, bargaining, directing, ignoring, or otherwise interacting with one another in the course of nourishing one's body. (2006: 47)

It is important to note, however, as feminists emphasise, that meal-times do not just provide nourishment but also teach about gendered labour, control and violence.

In spite of the growing literature on food pedagogies and families, there is little written on race, and in particular, mixed-race families. This is perhaps not surprising, for as several authors note; race and racialisation are under-researched and under-theorised in mainstream food studies (Williams-Forson 2006 and 2013; Slocum 2011; Guthman 2008a/b; Freedman 2011; Pandoongpatt 2011; Flowers and Swan 2012a/b). Yet as Darcy Freedman notes: the quotidian question 'What should we have for dinner?' is not so simple and innocent. Now subject to food pedagogy and research, what should we have for dinner, and its varied answers point to how gender, race and class are made and consumed through the everyday meals. Hence, when we eat food, 'we nourish and maintain our bodies but also produce and reproduce social worlds' (2011: 81). Answering the question what should we have for dinner

> illuminates the embodiment of food and food practices. We eat because of bodies that laboured to plant, harvest, preserve, procure and prepare foods for others. And these food practices both reflect and create social hierarchies. (2011: 82)

Rachel Slocum's (2008) research on 'racial practices' in food markets is one concrete way to analyse how food and bodies produce race in situ, and provide concepts which work well in tandem with Berliner's idea of cultural transmission. She writes:

> Groupings of bodies do things and are 'done to', becoming racialized in the process (Grosz 2005). From this perspective, bodies are not only inscribed; they actively participate in the material production of themselves and other bodies. Race takes shape out of the physical gathering of bodies in which phenotype matters in its connection to material objects, practices and processes (Saldanha 2007). (Slocum 2008: 854)

Racial practices are embodied and material and therefore help us to consider the cultural transmission of race in relation to food. In the context of the market, racial difference constitutes a 'corporeal relationship to growing, selling and eating food' (Slocum 2008: 856). Racial practices in the market include:

> the production and marketing of certain plants, the location and quality of someone's land, ideas about 'good' food and the gathering of racially identified people around some vendors and vegetables but not others. (Slocum 2008: 856)

Bodies 'are materially produced through what people buy, who they talk to, where they grow vegetables, as well as through phenotypic differences' (Slocum 2008: 857). In other words, it is not just skin colour that shapes racial food practices, it is how people inhabit and move in spaces, the knowledges they share, and the types of food they buy, sell and talk about. In this chapter, we take the idea of racial practices but in contrast to Slocum's concern with strangers in the public sphere of food markets, we examine family members in the private sphere of the kitchen, with a particular focus on gender. We also prise open the sensory, visceral and non-verbal dimensions of these practices which Berliner, Law, Highmore and others highlight and examine how these operate pedagogically. First, we turn to feminist literature on family feeding work to understand the 'making' of families through gender.

Making Families, Making Gender

Feminist authors (DeVault 1991, 1999; Hollows 2008; Valentine 1999; Charles 1995) emphasise how families are suffused with, and constitutive of, social and power relations including the gendered division of domestic labour. Thus, feminist writers caution us not to romanticise the food and family. For example, Gill Valentine argues that:

> within families it is usually women who shoulder the responsibility for choosing, shopping, preparing and cooking 'proper meals' for the 'proper family. (1999: 493)

This is the case, even when men may 'get involved' in domestic labour. Nicky Charles writes 'sharing food is an important part of family life and a symbol of community' but, 'this sharing, although symbolizing a community, is not necessarily equal' (1995: 101). Furthermore, meal-times can be a site of male aggression and domestic violence (1996; Charles 1995).

De-romanticising the family entails de-naturalising it. Hence, the idea of the family as a monolithic, non-changing institution – what David Morgan (2011) refers to as 'The Family' – is inaccurate due to socio-demographic changes such as same-sex relationships, divorce, and co-habitation which are creating new family forms (Stapleton and Keenan 2009). This call to diversify understandings of contemporary families, however, does not extend to research on race.

The idea of 'the' family as a pre-existing reified structure is replaced in recent family studies with the notion of 'family practices': everyday comings and goings, events and rituals which constitute the 'making' of families (Morgan 2011; Hollows 2008; DeVault 1991). Marjorie DeVault argues that 'a family' 'is not a naturally occurring collection of individuals; its reality is constructed from day to day, through activities like eating together' (1991: 15). Practices such as shopping, cooking and feeding work do not 'take place within a pre-given entity such as the "family" … but instead the meanings of home and family are produced, reproduced and negotiated through domestic practices' (Hollows 2008: 60). As a result, food practices become performative resources through which people learn about how to 'do' family, gender, and enact specific roles such as being a good mother or grateful child.

Nowhere are struggle and inequality more apparent than in what has been termed 'feeding work': the gendered tasks of shopping, preparing, cooking, serving and washing up (DeVault 1991). Feeding work is also caring and emotional labour: women organise their own and family schedules, choose and prepare food that are not their preferences, and do this in order to provide comfort for their children, partners and families. An integral part of feeding work in Anglo cultures is the provision of the so-called 'proper meal' (Murcott 1995). A proper meal is defined by a number of rules: first around food and the type and combination of ingredients; secondly, the use of specific types of labour and cooking techniques; and thirdly, gendered roles, affecting eating arrangements, organising who serves what and who gets served and women being 'proper' wives and carers.

The family table is a space where women provide material and emotional care, including 'interpersonal support work ... through talk' (DeVault 1991: 55). But it is also a site of accommodation, compromise and conflict (Lupton 1996): there can be 'tension and friction rather than peace and harmony at mealtimes' (Charles 1995: 109). Food can be used to 'punish, cajole, or reinforce hegemonic or patriarchal structures' (Roth 2005: 182). Conflict can arise when parents view the table as a pedagogical site to insist on their children performing good table manners and eating habits but it can also extend to men using domestic violence (Lupton 1996). Proper family meal-times are not always the site of a happy family.

Family food practices entail the cultural transmission of who does what in the kitchen, what foods mean, how power operates, how gender, class and ethnicity is done, what being a child means, and how to be a certain kind of family. In Berliner's terms, cultural transmission in families happens through a medley of mediators – objects, knowledges, smells, sounds and talk. In this next section, we develop this theme in more detail, turning to recent scholarship on family pedagogies and their interactional properties.

Family Pedagogies

In an early edited volume entitled *Feminisms and Everyday Pedagogies*, Carmen Luke (1996) argues that families reproduce 'pedagogical regimes of subject formation', exploring how she learned femininity as a girl through the 'everyday pedagogies' of her family, friends, and teachers. She outlines how popular culture in the home – texts, imagery and commodities – acts as a pedagogy in the production of the social identities of children, teaching socio-cultural and political lessons about class, gender, ethnicity, family and social power.

Although she doesn't write much about food, unusually for a pedagogy studies writer, she writes about pedagogy in mixed-race families, albeit briefly. Luke was a German migrant to Canada in the early 50s, and married an American-Chinese man and is parent to a mixed-race child, writes that popular culture:

> can be particularly complex for children from dual-culture households who can experience diverse and often ideologically conflicting sources of formal and informal pedagogies that often add a special burden and a unique complexion to identity formation. (1996: 9)

Echoing DeVault's (1999) reference to the pedagogical labour of anti-racism that racially minoritised families perform, Luke writes that she had to 'counter-teach' the racism and sexism that came home from her child's teachers and friends.

Since this early work of Luke's, there has been a burgeoning in what we might call 'pedagogy studies' (for example, Sandlin, Schultz and Burdick 2010; Hickey-Moody, Savage, and Windle 2010; Burdick, Sandlin and O'Malley 2014), part of which includes an incipient literature on family food pedagogies (Quarmby and Dagkas 2012; 2013; Ochs and Shohet 2006). But most of the latter focuses on interactions at meal-times between parents and children which, whilst useful, ignores other modes of cultural transmission. For example, Thomas Quarmby and Symeon Dagkas, sports-studies academics, argue that families are informal sites of learning where parents use their authority over children to teach 'healthy eating' (2013, 2012). Drawing on Pierre Bourdieu, they suggest the family is where taste, behaviours and attitudes are 'embedded' in young people. Parents teach their children through mobilising certain health food discourses, saying things directly or indirectly and habituating the family in eating certain kinds of food and meals. Through what they call 'pedagogic encounters', parents 'transfer' values and act in a 'correctional capacity' (Quarmby and Dagkas 2013: 14).

But family meal-time pedagogies are not simply correctional. For Ochs and Shohet 'meals are cultural sites for socializing children into commensality, communicative expectations, and the symbolic, moral and sentimental meanings of food and eating' (2006: 35). This involves parents, and particularly mothers, in teaching children a whole range of skills: how to converse at the dinner table, serve and eat food. Children learn about taste, appetite, pleasure and satiation. Furthermore, they are taught how food is used as a reward. This is done through explicit meal-time communication such as directives, error corrections, assessments and less direct strategies such as irony, inference, metaphor and noticeable silences (Ochs and Shohet 2006). Thus, children learn how food is used as a symbol to affirm or diminish affection and social bonds. Through food pedagogies, children are taught the hierarchy of the family, its social roles, how adults treat each other, the status of foods, and whose preferences count (Gallegos et al. 2011).

Making Mixed-race Families

Overall though, the family literature neglects race. Peter Jackson (2009) and Gill Valentine (1999) in their respective research show us that racially minoritised families in the UK have a range of feeding work practices including eating globally universal foods such as pizzas alongside more 'culturally specific' foods. But this work has not really focused on family food and meals as racial practices; nor has there been much focus on mixed-race families. As Ien Ang (2001) notes, in spite of the cultural 'celebration' of hybrid ethnic identities, the domestic dynamics of mixed-raced families are under-researched and theorised. In similar vein,

David Gilbert argues that researching the specificities of families is critical for understanding experiences and identifications of mixed-race individuals.

It should be acknowledged, however, that the term 'mixed-race' is a contentious term firstly because it is based on an essentialist idea of two 'pure' races co-mingling in equal proportions to make a new 'mix' (Tyler 2005; Gilbert 2005). Secondly, race may not be the most significant identification for mixed-race individuals and certainly should not be seen as 'always core or static' (Gilbert 2005: 65; Ali 2003). Whilst problematic, the term, however, is used to categorise individuals born with parents from different ethnic backgrounds. For Gilbert, there are indeed 'explicitly racialised contexts and experiences of members of such a group' but ones which do not have to be understood through a prominent notion of race (2005: 71).

Although there are few studies on mixed-race families, research was undertaken by Carmen Luke and Vicki Carrington on 50 mixed-race families in Australia in the late 1990s (2000). Arguing that race organises family and social life, and experiences of discrimination and alienation, their focus is family as an important site of racialisation. In more recent work, Luke writes that the idea of racial diversity should be extended from the workplace to the mixed-race family: what she calls, 'difference within difference' (2003: 8). Furthermore, differences within the family may be cultural, linguistic, religious, ethnic or racial (Luke 2003: 380). As a result, 'othering' can take place within mixed-race families rather than simply something white people 'do' to black people. In sum, this research shows that families provide sites for racial identity formation beyond dominant racial classifications. This means that new theoretical models and vocabularies are needed beyond those offered by the post-war literature and policy frameworks on immigration and multiculturalism (Luke and Luke 1998: 748).

The work of Suki Ali (2003) on British mixed-race families is important here as she too highlights that terms such as race, ethnicity and culture vary in their significance for mixed-race families in constructing individual and collective familial identities. In thinking about cultural transmission within mixed-race families, she notes that food is often understood as connected to ethnic and cultural identity and can be used as an 'ethnic resource' (Anthias and Yuval Davies 1993). Ali argues that too much emphasis has been placed on 'ethnic resources' in the public domain and that it is an oversight to ignore the mundane cultural practices of 'cooking, cleaning and shopping' in family settings when studying ethnic identifications (2003: 107). Overall, she is critical of widespread tendencies to essentialise race and ethnicity and argues that they should not be understood as fixed and homogeneous identities. Mixed-race is fluid and mixedness is a process of negotiation (2003: 18).

Her main argument about food is that although women have been seen as the 'transmitters' of cultural heritage in the home, their children may identify in multiple ways. There are no singular or fixed meanings for such 'mundane' family food practices. Indeed, Ali observes that mixed-race families eat 'traditional' and 'contemporary' food, highlighting that 'culture' is not 'static or enclosed' (2003: 107). Inter-generational relationships too are seen as important in mixed-race families.

Thus she challenges the idea that cultural knowledge is passed on only through the family: children identify with gender and class as well as race inside and outside the family. As she puts it, there is a not a 'simple relationship between proximity to a parent and racial identity' (Ali 2003: 91). Ali's work then points to wider cultural transmission processes and dynamic, temporal identificatory practices in ways which are important for our analysis. But at the same time, Ali's methodological focus on 'stories' told by children and parents means that there is less attention paid to senses – for example, smell and taste – and their pedagogical effects (Hayes-Conroy 2010).

Family Context

It is against this intellectual background we discuss food pedagogies in a mixed-race, step-family living in Australia in the 1970s. The family was remade in several ways during these years, reinforcing David Morgan's argument that there is not a single form of 'the family' (1996). In terms of mixed-race configuration, the family comprised of Anglo- and Chinese- and Filipino- Australians at different times. In this chapter, we focus on data drawn from the two sons, Steven and Oscar who are now men in their fifties. Their father, Ron is Anglo-Australian and their mother, Margaret was a Chinese nurse from Singapore who moved to Australia to undertake postgraduate study. Margaret and Ron married and lived in Melbourne for a number of years and then moved to Sydney because of Ron's work. Margaret worked as a nurse at a local hospital. She died when Steven was 9 years old and Oscar was 6. Three years later after her death, Ron's parents moved from their home in Melbourne to Sydney to live with their son and grandchildren. Ron's mother stayed at home and undertook the domestic labour in the family and Ron's father worked as a skilled tradesperson.

Four years later Ron married Angela, a recently arrived migrant from the Philippines, a medical technologist in her late 20s. Oscar was 10 and Steven 13 years old when Angela became part of an extended family living in the same house which included her Anglo-Australian husband, his parents and the two sons in a suburb 20 km from the city centre.

National Imaginary

The experiences of Margaret and Angela as professionals, wives, mothers and unpaid domestic labourers needs to be understood against a backdrop of Australian racisms, racist state policies, and national 'territorial and racial anxieties' (Anderson 2012). As Catriona Elder writes: 'The idea of a "white Australia" has been a key aspect of discourses of Australian national identity for most of the twentieth century. (2003, 2007). At its centre, was a territorial and racist belief encapsulated by statements made in Parliament in 1901 about restricting non-white immigration: '[the Australian people] are determined that Australia shall be kept free from alien invasion and contamination' (Commonwealth of Australia 1901c: 4631–3, cited in Elder 2007: 263). The 'White Australia Policy' was officially legislated in the *Immigration Restriction Act* which formed part of the creation of the Federation of Australia (Elder 2003). The colonial governments already had laws and policies from the mid nineteenth century to keep Chinese migrants and non-white contract workers out of the country (Markus 1994: 112–14 cited Elder 2003). The new legislation extended to labourers from the Pacific Islands and Japan (Elder 2003). As Zoe Anderson writes: the intensification and coming together of a territorial and racial anxiety further affected Aboriginal and Asian peoples in Australia: becoming 'suspended subjects' and 'outsiders within' the Australian nation state (Stephenson 2007: 502, cited in Anderson 2012). Indigenous people, non-white migrants and British were positioned in highly distinct ways:

> The discourse of white Australia was always produced in relation to ... two groups of non-white peoples [Indigenous and immigrants]. In addition to stories of white Australia being produced in relation to others represented as undesirable, both governmental and popular discourses of white Australia were produced in relation to a desirable Other – the British peoples, who were represented as the same 'type' as white Australians. (Elder 2007: 263)

As Elder argues, the meaning of white Australia shifted from 1901 to the end of the twentieth century. Margaret, who was Oscar and Steven's Chinese mother arrived in Australia in the 1950s. This was after the atrocities of the Holocaust and the Second World War and there was a searching reflexivity, and 'blatant and crude racism was difficult to present as good government policy' nationally and internationally (Elder 2003: 235). There was increasing embarrassment with the continuation of a White Australia immigration policy and slow but growing opposition within Australia (Ang 2000; Jayasuriya and Pookong 1999; Sheridan 2000b). Attempts were made at this time to 'turn to Asia' politically, economically and culturally: examples include initiatives such the Colombo Plan which offered scholarships to students from Asian countries. There was also increasing cultural promotion of cosmopolitanism through food as seen in the widely selling Women's Weekly magazine and government sanctioned pride in 'ethnic' food diversity at the 1956 Olympics (Sheridan 2000b). In the 1970s the restrictions on immigration criteria were lifted and large numbers of non-Europeans entered Australia (Anderson 2012). Between 1947 and 1973 the population of Australia nearly doubled (from 7.5 million) and more than half of the population increase was due to immigration (Castles et al. 1988: 25). But as Anderson (2012) notes, this was marked by ambivalence within 'white' Australia over the settlement and integration of non-white migrants into Australian society. The reception of Asian migrants was affected by a differentiated racialisation of Asian nationalities and this was highly gendered, with Japanese and Vietnamese women being orientalised into ideals of 'feminine Asianness' (Elder 2003: 241). Elder underlines how in the late 1970s, 'acceptability' was partially defined by white patriarchy:

> the fear felt by many Australians about the arrival of the Vietnamese women in Australia was assuaged through representations of them as unthreatening – at home, at the hairdressers – and also in the care of (and in many ways monitored by) (white) Australian men and families. (Elder, 2003: 241)

One of the women we discuss in this chapter is Angela, a Filipino migrant. The formal dismantling of the 'White Australia Policy' and Marcos's imposition of martial law in the Philippines in 1972 led to a rapid increase in migration, largely feminised and due to intercultural marriages (Saroca 2006). In the media, Filipino women were constructed predominantly as 'mail-order brides', as 'sexually dangerous,' a threat to white marriages and less 'passive' than other Asian femininities (Saroca 2006).

Immigration and multiculturalism were refracted through specific ideals of the 'white family' (Anderson 2012). This was a 'particular formation based upon specifically-gendered heteronormativity and held up as a filter through which Australian belonging was regulated and contested in the late 1970s' (Anderson 2012). As Elder writes:

> White Australia was about the production of a white nation (al family). The family was often imagined as a metonym for the nation. The domestic sphere and the family was a central site for the production of a 'white' Australia. (2007: 264)

In sum, Margaret and Angela, Chinese and Filipino women respectively, moved to a country where The White Australia policy embodied the idea that 'the very presence of Asians was considered a blemish on the ideal image of the white island continent' (Ang 2000: xiii). Asian people were constructed as profoundly other in a tradition of Orientalist thinking but inflected in particularly Australian and settler-colonialist ways (Anderson 2012). At the time Margaret and Angela arrived in Australia, a dominant view in the White Imaginary was of an 'obvious and threatening otherness of Asians' (Perera 1999: 189) combined with a deep-rooted fear of the Asianisation of Australia (Ang 2000).

This racialised history and context affected Margaret and Angela in various complex and often unspoken ways. Both had university qualifications and worked outside of the home in paid employment. They experienced various forms of racism; felt socially isolated and 'othered' in suburban Sydney. Both had grown up in large metropolitan Asian cities and were comfortable with, and used to, high-density living with members of their extended family close by. In contrast, in suburban Sydney many houses that were built in the 1930s were single-storey bungalows on quarter-acre blocks. The low density living exacerbated Margaret and Angela's experiences of exclusion, racism and isolation: as Asian women it was difficult to make friends and build support networks; it took extra labour to find the Asian food ingredients locally they needed; and there were very few Asian neighbours and families. Families can provide vital support in sharing experiences of racism, giving support and advice, discussing individual and collective readings of discrimination and developing survival skills (DeVault 1999, Ali 2003). But this kind of 'family work' would not have happened in Margaret and Angela's family for a number of reasons (DeVault 1999). At a cultural level, there was widespread collective and individual ignorance of racism, a belief that Australia was tolerant and migrants should be grateful for coming to the 'lucky' country; and at a family level, a type of inexpressive masculinity prevailed in which overt communication of emotions and experiences of racism was avoided.

White Food

Having provided general background to the family and wider racialised context, in this section we turn to interviews with Oscar and Steven and start with their memories of the food practices in their family after their mother's death. This was the time when the grandparents came to live with them and there was a traditional division of gendered labour in the household with both men being seen as 'breadwinners' and the grandmother responsible for the domestic labour in the home, including feeding work. For DeVault, 'feeding work' covers many different kinds of gendered labour: thus the grandmother would have been planning menus with budget and preferences in mind, shopping, preparing meals, cooking, facilitating meal-time conversations, and cleaning up after eating. Feeding work often 'goes without saying;' being routine, naturalised and invisible as labour, and of course, unpaid. As with many white Australian families at this time, the 'proper meal' was dominated by traditional lower middle-class Anglo-Celtic food: meat and two vegetables. Examples include roast chicken with a cornflake coating, tripe, ox tongue, lamb and mint sauce, roast beef and mashed potatoes, corned beef with horseradish sauce, and also children's favourites like fish fingers and spaghetti bolognese. Typical desserts included rice pudding, baked apples, blancmange and custard. Drinks included cider and lemonade with the meal, and a glass of cold milk after.

The home was a typical Australian lower middle-class bungalow in a suburban street. The creation of suburbs was a defining preoccupation of Australian society in the twentieth century, during which time, the suburban population increased from less than 1 to more than 11 million in the capital cities alone (Davison 2006: 203). Australia has been seen as the 'first suburban nation' and suburban aspirations were the butt of middle-class derision, being associated with conservative values, conformity and 'mindless banality' (ibid.: 206–7). Of course, suburban life was much more complex than this.

Suburban living was a geographical rendering of the notion of separate spheres, with public and private life detached, and with lower- and middle-class women associated with the suburban home and their role in the domestic sphere (ibid.). The younger son, Oscar recounts that they ate breakfast and lunch in the kitchen at a blue laminex table on a lino floor. Dinner was in a separate carpeted dining room which looked out onto the street through venetian blinds, and had a fireplace converted into a gas heater and a small glass chandelier over the table hanging from the ceiling. In patriarchal style, grandfather sat at one end of the table, Ron at the other and grandmother cooked food which was served in bowls or casserole dishes in the middle of the table to enable people to have second helpings. Oscar helped his grandmother prepare food in the kitchen; and Ron, grandfather and Steven with washing up. But these acts of shared domestic labour were in the masculinist mode of 'helping out' rather than taking any responsibility for feeding work. As has been noted, the symbolism of meals extends beyond the food eaten:

> Who prepares the food, serves it, and cleans up; where people take their meals; the shape of a table; and who sits where and talks about what. All these convey roles, values, and ideas about gender, hierarchy, and power. (Jones 2007: 131)

And everything about the organisation of meal-times signified traditional gendered roles and power relations.

The literature on meal-times (Quarmby and Dagkas 2013; Ochs and Shohet 2006) has emphasised the pedagogical importance of conversations and the choices of foods but does not attend, however, to sensory and embodied aspects of cooking and eating. Yet, these are crucial for cultural transmission and racial practices. Oscar remembers the smells, textures, flavours of foods as they were being cooked, served and eaten at this time. The rice of his mother's cooking was replaced by potatoes, pork belly by roast chicken, and soya sauce by mustard. There were smells of boiled vegetables and grilled, fried or roasted meat; they were not spicy or flavoured with garlic. The grandmother's use of lard and butter in savoury dishes, and the inclusion of milky, sugary sweet puddings at meal-times, presented contrasting textures to a largely dairy-free Chinese diet.

In pedagogical terms, new habits were being formed in the shift from the production and consumption of Chinese food to Anglo-Celtic food and meal-times. As Ben Highmore has written:

> changes in the smells, tastes and flavours of a social environment would be of crucial import. But perhaps more important still would be the routines and habits that would accompany them. The habit of savouring or turning your nose up, the practices of eating and cooking, the routines of what is eaten and what is not eaten. We tend to take routine and habit for granted, forgetting the massive achievement of something 'becoming habitual'. (2008: 398)

One way to understand the changing habituation of cooking, eating, bodies and senses in the family is through the notion of a pedagogy of whiteness. As Alan Han (2007) writes, all too often food consumption in Australia is presented as if white people are non-raced eaters but clearly food practices are racialised (Pandoongpatt 2011; Perera 1999; Slocum 2008, 2011; Guthman 2008b). White food practices in this family include the preparation and choice of ingredients; for example, the use of potatoes as the staple in the meal; the adoption of cooking techniques such as rapid boiling; the lack of spices, herbs, garlic and rich sauces; and the use of lard and butter as opposed to sesame seed or peanut oil. But there are clearly bodily and sensory practices: such as the ingesting and digesting of Anglo-Celtic food and smells and the performance of white masculine lower middle-class 'bodily styles' including emotional expressivities, ways of talking, sitting, eating etc. (Ahmed 2010). All in all, what we see is an Anglo-centric conception of a 'proper meal' and its cultural and emotional images of home and family (Hollows 2008: 62).

Of course, whiteness is not monolithic but variegated and structured by history, context, gender and class. At this time in the 1970s, specific forms of Australian whiteness were constructed from 'ethnic resources' such as sport, popular culture and importantly for this chapter, the consumption and production of food, its rituals and ideologies (Perera 1999; Han 2007).

For Oscar and Steven, the privileging of white food and habits constituted a considerable change from the meal-times with their Chinese mother. Her legacy and Chinese heritage were not completely erased as some of her belongings were in the house, her Chinese music albums were played, and connections to her family in Singapore were maintained through correspondence. Furthermore, their father had taken them to eat on many trips to Chinatown. Nevertheless, the change to white food racial practices became so embedded through everyday mundane pedagogies: some sensory and embodied, others produced through explicit talk about what constituted 'ethnic' or special food, and several to use Berliner's phrase, based on practices and ideas that 'go without saying'.

Potatoes in Rice Cooker

Three years later, Angela a Filipino woman married Ron and moved in to the extended family home and the family's configuration, food racial practices and identity resources changed. With Angela's arrival, not only was there a new member of the family – a young woman – but she was Filipino. Filipino women were racialised and feminised in particular ways at this time in Australia which would have affected her reception in the family however unconsciously. The introduction of a new member challenges the whole definition of the family group, its boundaries and its identity, meaning that it has to be re-defined and modified (Quarmby and Dagkas 2013). Family reconfigurations have an effect on the pedagogical practices in the family (Quarmby and Dagkas 2013). For Angela, there were issues of how to perform being a wife, stepmother, daughter-in-law and how to 'settle' into her new home. One of Angela's strategies was to cook 'Filipino' foods as a form of 'home-making,' albeit within a number of constraints – for example, access to Filipino foodways, and having to negotiate family food preferences (Law 2001; Hage 1997).

Oscar and Steven remember that at first, Angela and the grandmother were jointly responsible for the preparing and cooking of meals. This cannot have been easy emotionally or practically but the women learned to inhabit the same kitchen space, and organise their bodies, rhythms, and cooking around each other. They grew accustomed to the different smells of the food they each prepared, the look of unfamiliar ingredients, and the way each of them used particular preparation, cooking and presentation techniques. Thus, there were gendered pedagogical encounters between the women, their bodies and senses, objects and food in the kitchen.

An important change was the introduction of the Asian staple food – rice. As Oscar recounts:

> When my stepmother came to live with us, we started eating more rice for the evening meal. But I distinctly remember my [Anglo-Australian] grandmother putting potatoes alongside rice, in our rice cooker for my grandfather.

Pedagogically, enabling this culinary compromise would have entailed Angela and the grandmother in working out whether to respond to the grandfather's preference, trialling the cooking of rice and potatoes together, timing the cooking of these staples and learning which main meat course could go with both rice and potatoes. In so doing, Angela and the grandmother would have undertaken mental and manual work, deploying memory and intelligence: as Luce Giard writes of 'doing-cooking', 'one has to organize, decide and anticipate. One must memorize, adapt, modify, invent, combine and take into consideration … likes and … dislikes' (1998: 131).

In the 1970s rice in savoury dishes was an 'exotic' ingredient for many Anglo-Australians and culturally associated with 'Asians' (Ohnuki-Tierney 1994; Ang 2004). As Emiko Ohnuki-Tierney (1994) argues, staple foods such as rice have profound symbolic meaning, in particular for distinguishing 'us' from 'them', with them being 'rice-eating Asians'. Analysing the popular magazine *Women's Weekly*, Susan Sheridan (2000a) writes that wider consumption of rice among non-Asian Australian families was promoted extensively in the 1960s through adverts, recipes and magazine supplements. It took a little over a decade, however, before rice was no longer seen by white Australian families as either a poor substitute for potatoes or as a side dish, but as a possible main staple (Sheridan 2000a). Although there are many different ways in which Asian people prepare, cook and eat rice, it is still seen as a marker of a pan-Asian identity (Ang 2004).

Angela introduced an electric rice cooker. Invented in Japan in the 1950s, they were taken up enthusiastically across Asia (Nakano 2009). The title of Yoshiko Nakano's book captures this: *Where there are Asians, there are Rice Cookers*. But even today, rice cookers are not a common piece of kitchen equipment for non-Asian Australian families. Back in the 1970s they were even less so. The family as a whole would have adapted to the sight of the rice cooker as a large machine on the table, taking up considerable room, and causing bodies to move in new ways in the kitchen and the dining room to produce the rice-potato combination. For the rest of the family it may have at first seemed strange, but for Angela it created ‘homely feelings of familiarity’, an important component of home-building (Hage 1997). Feeling at home comes from knowing how to use particular objects in a home. For Angela, it was one less thing to learn.

Over time, Angela and the family extended the food accommodations. As Steven recounts:

> they [grandmother and stepmother] reached a compromise where they would both cook meals. And so then it became even more astonishing because we’d have Filipino meals with the old, you know, Australian Anglo meals; so we’d have both together.

Viscerally and bodily, the family learned to enjoy new combinations of smells, tastes, textures, flavours, and aesthetics. Their taste buds attuned to the more sweet, salty and sour flavours of Filipino dishes. Spices such as star anise, cardamom and the generous use of garlic created pungent and aromatic smells that at first arrested their noses but over time became aromas of comfort. The rooves of their mouths and tongues experienced textures that were more syrupy, glutinous and viscous. And the family members’ sense of sight learnt to appreciate the brighter and darker colours of Filipino dishes side by side with Anglo-foods on the table, and often on the same plate. Bodily responses within the family at the table included pleasurable sniffing, salivating mouths, a wrinkling of the nose and the odd screwing up of the face. These responses are not simply individual and ‘natural’ but socio-culturally located against a backdrop of expectations about food, gender and race.

The grandfather wanted to continue his cultural habit of eating Anglo cuisine; Angela and Ron wanted to instantiate new family traditions of eating Filipino food. Rice was typically eaten by Filipino people at every meal (Law 2001). For all involved, this was a symbolic issue about power and identities, individually and collectively. Everyday staples eaten as habits at home – like rice – take on a symbolic and nostalgic hue in a new context (Magno 2011). But it was also a material issue about what kinds of foods bodies can learn to eat. Bodies take time to learn. Groups acculturate around certain flavour combinations and ‘taste perception’ involves physiology: biochemical processes on the tongue and nasal sensory cells but also the interpretation of symbolism and social meaning (Lalonde 1992). The family learned to modify their ‘bodily memories’, and ‘temper their sense of taste formed from repeated exposure … to repertoires of preferred foods’ (Lee 2000: 217).

Through their cooking and accommodations to each other, the women helped remake the ‘proper’ meal and forms of commensality in which everyone ate together in spite of cultural and bodily differences in food preferences. New rituals were being created, learned and practised. These taught the family how the women would accommodate to their gendered domestic labour in the kitchen, how the men's preferences would be serviced, what and how it was acceptable to eat in the family, and how cooking and eating were to be organised in the new family structure. Mary Douglas (1984) has suggested meals are patterned culturally and ethnically; ordered like a grammar, marking social relations within and without the family. Thus, the proper meal stands for 'the home itself, a man's relation to that home and a woman's place in it' (Murcott 1982: 693). Angela rewrites the grammar and in a small way, insists that her ethnic and cultural food practices will have a place in the home, at the same time expressing independence and negotiating with family and social constraints. Using skills, learning and negotiations in a highly constrained family and national context, she changes the feeding work expectations meaning the family adapted on several fronts (DeVault 1991: 43). The term adaptation is critical here. As Amanda Wise (2007) and Greg Noble (2013) emphasise, living with difference requires more than propinquity: it needs new habits and capacities, which in this family were facilitated through food pedagogies.

The mixing of food as a practice that shaped their collective identity has now become a 'well-worn story' for members of the family (Kehily 1995). But Oscar emphasises that this was not necessarily an entirely happy arrangement. The grandfather expressed disappointment and frustration at rice being served for every evening meal, and placing potatoes in the rice cooker was seen as a grudging compromise. Nonetheless, Oscar and Steven, now middle-aged men, present this memory of mixing foods as a feel-good story of a family narrative about 'what it is like to be in our family across cultures and generations' (Curtis, James and Ellis 2009: 83). As Oscar said: 'We are a family that mixed things up.' Our next section though shows, however, that there were limits to mixing and food pedagogy in the family.

Blood Stew

After a short time, Angela took responsibility for the feeding work in the family as the grandmother developed a long-term illness. As Angela's role for feeding work became more prominent, more Filipino dishes were cooked. Filipino food, its preparation, flavours and styles is hybrid, and influenced by pre-colonial histories of trade with China and Malaysia, and by Spain through colonisation (Magno 2011). Chinese influences include the use of tofu, soya and noodles; Malay influences, certain meat and the simmering of food in vinegar; and Spain, the use of sautéing, tomato sauce and the use of garlic. Angela cooked dishes such as: Filipino sausage (longganisa); chicken and pork adobo braised in garlic, vinegar, oil and soy sauce; meat and vegetables in peanut sauce; pork and boiled eggs in soya sauce; sweet and sour fish; and used Asian cabbage, coconut, Asian fruits when she could obtain them. Angela kept ducks in the garden so she could have a Filipino favourite of duck eggs. The meals were inspired by memories of her mother's cooking when she was growing up in Cebu. Ron and the two sons ate most of the food with relish. But Steven discusses some of his limits:

> But when my stepmother came, then it was a bit awkward. Because there were foods that we obviously, not obviously, but there were foods that some people didn't like. Some of the Filipino dishes were quite standard like barbequed meat and stuff. But some of the dishes were a bit different and there was a lot of – I caused problems because when I was a teenager, when I got to about 14 or 15. Sometimes a 14 year old can get a bit surly and I turned my nose up at a few dishes.

The literature on proper family meals shows us that when a child rejects food, s/he is refusing to play happy families as imagined in the ideal of 'the proper meal' and in so doing challenges the social order (O'Connell 2010). In this example, we have an added, racialised dimension. Steven presents himself rejecting food that he regards as 'intensely' Filipino, drawing on the phrase 'turned my nose up at' connoting disgust (Highmore 2008).

He continues to recount an incident from this period when Angela served a pig's blood stew, otherwise known as 'dugo dugo' on Cebu, the island on which Angela grew up:

> Particularly there was a pig's blood soup [*sic*] and I just couldn't bring myself to say I like it. I had to say: 'Look this is just not good.' It was very awkward for my father because he wanted to make our stepmother happy … I got sent from the table a few times. That was kind of punishment to be sent from the table and not have your meal because I'd made a bit of a comment that had probably hurt our stepmother. I don't know if she was hurt but I guess she was. I didn't ask her. My father said she was.

The pig's blood stew (recte) failed pedagogically. It did so symbolically and materially. It failed to produce the ideal of the warm loving mother and the grateful son of the happy family. It failed as a proper meal, bringing about disgust and separation rather than care and connection. Steven's abjection of the pig's blood stew should be understood as deriving partly from a male sense of entitlement that the food he is served did not meet his expectations about what is acceptable. Its failure meant that a gendered pedagogy of manners ensued in which Ron used his patriarchal power to reinforce stepmother-son relations.

Steven, even in the face of reprobation from his father, regarded the pig's blood stew as too 'Other.' The pig's blood soup aroused disgust in Steven. Disgust is a highly specific form of food rejection (Rozin, Haidt and McCauley 2008). It can be the idea, smell, taste or even texture of some foods that can prompt feelings of disgust (Donovan 2007, cited in Longhurst, Ho and Johnston 2008). Examples include seaweed, insects, tapioca, cow tongue, testicles, octopus, gizzards, sheep brains, pig trotters, chicken feet, necks and giblets (Donovan 2007, cited in Longhurst, Ho and Johnston 2008).

For Steven, the disgust arose from the stew's material properties, and their gendered and racialised symbolism. Steven's response should be seen against a background where Filipino food has not been taken up like other Asian foods in Australia such as Thai, Japanese and Chinese; and where Filipino femininity has been stereotyped in racist ways. This hierarchy reflects the racialised and cultural politics in which food is always located (Magno 2011). Symbolically pigs have been seen in Western culture as dirty and unrefined. Blood is imagined as unclean and abject. Both are seen as polluting. Julia Kristeva (1982) has written about how bodily fluids such as blood come to symbolise a danger to identity because of its links with life, death, and taboos associated with women's bodies. Blood has particular resonance as it is slimy, having a half-life between solid and fluid. Such fluids are imagined to engulf, defile, seep and infiltrate (Lupton 1996: 114). In this way, blood connotes threats to boundaries. Of course, blood is also central to biological understandings of race.

Disgust at food is fundamentally about expressing individuation (Rozin et al. 2008). Steven is distancing himself from the food and its provider. Disgust 'works to push away others, and in the process, establish one's own identity as non-disgusting' (Lawler 2008: 141). As William Miller writes:

> Disgust … recognizes and maintains difference. Disgust helps define boundaries between us and them, me and you. It helps prevent *our* way from being subsumed into *their* way. (2009: 50 cited in Lawler 2008: 140)

In summary then we can see that food pedagogy in families can be about exclusion as much as about belonging and communitas (Roth 2005). Whilst the blood stew failed pedagogically on a number of counts, it was one of the lessons that taught Steven his distancing to any Filipino ethnic identification.

Pork Belly

To date, we have discussed Oscar and Steven's memories of family meal-times when they were children but our final vignette recalls Oscar's life when he is at university in London where he has to shop and cook for himself. His mixed-race identity became a prominent issue for him at this time as it was widely called into question. As a result of his mixed-race appearance, people would ask him in the classic question asked of mixed-race people, where he came from. They expressed surprise that he was Australian. This was because the prevailing dominant image of an Australian was that they were white. Oscar had various non-white, visual racial markers including his skin colour, eye-shape and hair colour. At the same time, people in London rarely read these racial markers as Chinese as Oscar had white cultural and social capital, education, style and manner. But as a result of the attempts to pin down his identity, Oscar described a variety of strategies he mobilised to sustain comfort and pride in his mixed-race identity. One was to be mischievous and say to people that he was an Eskimo [*sic*]. (In London in the 1980s, the term Eskimo was widely understood but is now regarded as derogatory; the term Inuit being preferred.) Oscar commented that it was easier and quicker to present a single-race identity. He added that it amused him to hear people say he was the first 'Eskimo' they had met. Usually he would disclose that he was half Chinese and white Australian.

Against this identity when Oscar remembers this being a time when he set out to learn more about his Chinese heritage, in particular through his food practices. His Chinese mother had died when he was 6 years old but Ron, his father had occasionally cooked Chinese food and taken the sons to Chinatown. Oscar had been cooking rice, the Asian staple from childhood for some time and had cooked a few Chinese dishes when he was younger at school, including sweet and sour pork. He recounts experimenting with various soya sauces to conjure up the salty rich flavour of his childhood. Sometime he ate with chopsticks in his student accommodation. He recounts buying Chinese Communist Party posters and a Mao style jacket, but food was the main source for his identificatory practices. He bought a Chinese cookbook, a wok and cooking implements from Chinatown and taught himself how to cook various recipes. Sometimes this was for him alone or for his brother and girlfriend. As well as the cookbook he bought, he would read Chinese cookbooks in bookshops and from the library. Several authors have noted how cookbooks can be an important pedagogy of ethnic heritage-making for migrant women providing techniques, recipes and know-how not learned in the more traditional embodied apprenticeship with an older woman (Sutton 2001; Holtzman 2006). As pedagogical devices, the cookbooks were one element that enabled Oscar to learn how to do Chinese cooking but it was memory and embodiment that changed his material and visceral habits in relation to food as a mode of identification.

Oscar visited Chinatown, a sensory space of race-making (Knowles 2003) and food racial practices (Slocum 2008). Oscar found himself in streets lined with Chinese food shops, and restaurants with formal and informal signs in Chinese script. He smelled Chinese fruit, vegetables, and cooked food. He walked past Chinese people moving through the shops, streets and alleys, talking Cantonese and Mandarin, playing Chinese radio and songs. These had visceral effects on Oscar, eliciting feelings of nostalgia, curiosity and excitement. In terms of pedagogy, as Alison Hayes-Conroy writes bodies are attentive and active (Hayes-Conroy 2010) and can learn through movements, sounds and aromas in ways which are outside consciousness and cognition (Sutton 2001).

In particular Oscar learned to cook pork belly, a Chinese comfort food but also a Filipino dish from his childhood. As Gilbert and Ali suggest, Oscar did not have a static notion of his ethnicity. He yearned after Asian flavours that he associated with his mother, father, and stepmother and was less concerned with reproducing 'authentic' culinary traditions – be they Chinese, Filipino or Anglo-Australian – and cared more about drawing on bodily memories of Chinese foods to express a connection to a Chinese part of his mixed-race identity. Oscar, like respondents in Ali's research, was keen to stress that Chineseness was not the core of his identification, and was mobilised through food but not other cultural practices. It was produced through a sensory need for connection not simply a cognitive one.

Learning to cook food from one's ethnic heritage has been described as a form of food-centred nostalgia (Holtzman 2006). Food can be used to recollect family and childhood. It can be more commemorative, so partaking of a collective past – 'the long roots of wisdom of our ancestors' (Bardenstein 2002: 356). Food works so well mnemonically because it has material and symbolic properties which evoke cognitive, emotional and physical recollecting (Holtzman 2006). Comfort foods such as pork belly with its soft, fatty and slippy texture are particularly catalytic because of its soothing material properties. But comfort foods are affective, often being nostalgic and remind us of being cared for; we eat them to connect us to others (Locher, Yoels, Maurer and Van Ells 2005).

Importantly food nostalgia need not be linked to actual memories of happy childhoods but post-hoc fantasies of them (Lupton 1996; Duruz 1999). This was the case for Oscar. Materially, learning to prepare and cook Chinese food would have re-created smells and tastes from his past but also from an imagined world in which his mother was still alive. Fenella Cannell (2011) argues that we try to 'remake kinship relations' through caring for the dead, 'enlivening our sense of the dead as persons', and 'activating relatedness' (2011: 463–5). In learning how to mobilise his hankering for Asian flavours, to cook Chinese foods and in particular, pork belly, Oscar uses food and feeding work to animate connections to his mother. Feeding work is often understood as a kind of care associated with femininity. Here it is a form of care Oscar as a young man directs at reanimating connections with his Chinese mother and his Chinese heritage as part of building his mixed-race identity, and produced through a range of food pedagogies involving memory, yearning, imagined pasts, racialised spaces, objects, embodiment and senses.

Conclusion

In this chapter, we argue that food practices in families work pedagogically in dynamic and heterogenous ways. This can be at the level of how to 'behave' at dinner in our family: how to eat, how to talk, how to be grateful. It can be cultural and identitarian: this is what our food means, this is how men and women act and this is what we do in our family. Influenced by Berliner's conceptualisation of cultural transmission as a way to prise open what Tony Bennett, Greg Noble and Megan Watkins (2012) have called the 'black box of pedagogy', we show that family food pedagogies operate through a congeries of modes, objects and media to reproduce skills, knowledge, ideologies, emotions and identifications. Importantly, his definition brings in the significance of sensory and embodied learning and 'ways that go without saying' which we connect with the recent so-called sensory and material turns in food studies (although the 'newness' of these turns can been debated). In this regard, we moved beyond seeing family meal-times as simply 'conversationally pedagogic'. As Highmore writes, the body is a learned form and one which is:

> constantly in the process of learning: of learning to accept new flavours, tastes … In this way we need to see ourselves as unfinished and in process and that our most intimate teacher is the material world around us. (2008: 393–4)

Our chapter emphasises, like Ali and Gilbert who theorise about mixed race, how individual and family mixed-race identifications are also unfinished.

Highmore highlights how foods work on us as 'agents of transformation' or what we might think of as pedagogues. And here we have focused on the way foods – their material properties, their smell, texture, and taste, who prepared them and to whom they were served – worked in the making of mixed-race identities. Berliner emphasises the congeries of modes and mechanisms of learning. In the chapter, we see bodies learning to eat new flavours and some bodies refusing to learn. In families; tongues, noses, stomachs, eyes, and hands, all play a role in teaching and learning. In the family that we discuss in this chapter, women from different racial backgrounds and ages learned to work together to produce new 'proper meals'. But some meals failed to work pedagogically: for example, the blood stew. And bodily memories teach care and connections to the dead.

In drawing on a wider repertoire of pedagogical mechanisms, our chapter expands beyond much recent scholarship on food pedagogies which remain stubbornly Foucauldian. In particular, we show food as a multifaceted object which smells, tastes, satiates, repulses, and comforts, and has situated racialised, gendered and classed social and symbolic meanings. Our contribution is to suggest that food in its varied manifestations – material, symbolic, sensory, political – needs to be placed at the centre of debates on food pedagogies. This would not mean privileging a narrow view of the material or the sensory but would mean attending to what food is taken to be and what it does in food pedagogies. In focusing more closely on food in food pedagogies, we can also redefine what we understand by pedagogy.

We began the chapter with Freedman's argument that the question 'what's for dinner' is important for examining racial and gendered politics. We show how the answers it inspires are forms of home- and identity-building. As Hage argues ethnic home-building through food is about settling, helping you make a life in a new country. But home-building through food also entails processes of making families and identities, skilled and complex learning of bodies, senses and cognition; and negotiation in the face of gendered, racialised and classed constraints. In mixed-race and step-families, homes and identities are not settled. The memories of Oscar and Steven reveal how the question 'what's for dinner' was repeatedly asked and to answer it involved a congeries of pedagogical politics, modes and practices.

References

Ahmed, S. (2010). Orientations matter. In D. Coole and S. Frost (eds), *New Materialisms: Ontology, Agency and Politics*. Durham: Duke University Press, 234–57.

Ali, S. (2003). *Mixed-race, Post Race: Gender, New Ethnicities and Cultural Practices*. Oxford: Berg.

Anderson, Z. (2012). Borders, babies, and 'good refugees': Australian representations of 'illegal' immigration. *Journal of Australian Studies*, 36:4, 499–514.

Ang, I. (2000). Introduction: Alter/Asian cultural interventions for 21st century Australia. In I. Ang, S. Chalmers, L. Law and M. Thomas (eds), (2000). *Alter/Asians: Asian-Australian Identities in Art, Media and Popular Culture*. Annandale: Pluto Press.

——— (2001). *On Not Speaking Chinese: Living between Asia and the West*. Routledge, London: Routledge.

——— (2004). Between Asia and the West: The cultural politics of food. *Life Writing*, 1/(1):, 147–54.

Anthias, F. and Yuval-Davis, N. (1993). *Racialized Boundaries: Race, Nation, Gender, Colour and Class and the Anti-racist Struggle*. New York: Psychology Press.

Bajic-Hajdukovic, I. (2013). Food, family, and memory: Belgrade mothers and their migrant children. *Food and Foodways*, 21(1), 46–65.

Bardenstein, C. (2002). Reconfiguring food, memory, and gender in the cookbook-memoirs of middle eastern exiles. *Signs: Journal of Women in Culture and Society*, 28(1), 353–87.

Bennett, T., Noble, G. and Watkins, M. (2012). Cultural Pedagogies: An International Workshop (brochure cover note), University of Western Sydney, August 2012 http://www.uws.edu.au/ics/events/cultural_pedagogies.

Berliner, D. (2013). New directions in the study of cultural transmission. In L. Arizpe and C. Amescua (eds), *Anthropological Perspectives on Intangible Cultural Heritage*. New York: Springer International, 71–7.

Burdick, J., Sandlin, J. and O'Malley, M. (eds). (2014). *Problematizing Public Pedagogy*. London and New York: Routledge.

Cannell, F. (2011). English ancestors: The moral possibilities of popular genealogy. *Journal of the Royal Anthropological Institute*, 17(3), 462–80.

Charles, N. (1995). Food and family ideology. In S. Jackson and S. Moore (eds), *The Politics of Domestic Consumption*. Hemel Hempstead: Harvester Wheatsheaf.

Castles S., Kalantzis, M., Cope, B. and Morrissey, M. (1988). *Mistaken Identity: Multiculturalism and the Demise of Nationalism in Australia*. Sydney: Pluto.

Chen, T.G. (2013). Homemade: An exploratory study on the impact of cooking on family relationships and cultural identity development. Master's degree dissertation in Smith College School for Social Work, Northampton, Massachusetts.

Curtis, P., James, A. and Ellis, K. (2009). 'She's got a really good attitude to healthy food … Nannan's drilled it into her': Inter-generational relations within families. In P. Jackson (ed.), *Changing Families, Changing Food.* Basingstoke: Palgrave, 77–92.

Dagkas, S. and Quarmby, T. (2012). Young people's embodiment of physical activity: The role of the 'pedagogized' family. *Sociology of Sport Journal*, 29(2), 210–26.

Davison, A. (2006). Stuck in a cul-de-sac? Suburban history and urban sustainability in Australia. *Urban Policy and Research*, 24(2), 201–16.

DeVault, M. (1991). *Feeding the Family: The Social Organisation of Caring as Gendered Work.* Chicago: University of Chicago Press.

——— (1999). Comfort and struggle: Emotion work in family life. *The Annals of the American Academy of Political and Social Science*, 561, 52–63.

Donovan, A.M. (2007). Tentacles? Testicles! A sampling of perceptions on uneatable food items among undergraduate students. Paper presented at *The Association of American Geographers Meeting*, 17–21 April, San Francisco, California.

Douglas, M. (ed.). (1984). *Food in the Social Order: Studies of Food and Festivities in Three American Communities.* New York: Russell Sage.

Duruz, J. (1999). Food as nostalgia: Eating the fifties and sixties. *Australian Historical Studies*, 30(113), 231–50.

Elder, C. (2003). Invaders, illegals and aliens: Imagining exclusion in a white Australia. *Law, Text and Culture*, 7(1), 221–50.

——— (2007). 'Diggers' Waifs': Desire, anxiety and immigration in post-1945 Australia. *Australian Historical Studies*, 38(130), 261–78.

Flowers, R. and Swan, S.E. (2012a). Eating the Asian Other? Pedagogies of food multiculturalism in Australia. *Portal Journal of Multidisciplinary International Studies*, 9(2), 1–30.

——— (2012b). Why food? Why pedagogy? Why adult education? *Australian Journal of Adult Learning*, 52(3), 419–33.

Freedman, D. (2011). Embodying food studies: Unpacking the ways we become what we eat. In M.J. Casper and P. Currah (eds), *Corpus: An Interdisciplinary Reader on Bodies and Knowledge*. Basingstoke: Palgrave Macmillan.

Gallegos, D., Dziurawiec, S., Fozdar, F. and Abernethie, L. (2011). Adolescent experiences of 'family meals' in Australia. *Journal of Sociology*, 47(3), 243–60.

Giard, L. (1998). Doing cooking. In M. De Certeau (ed.), *The Practice of Everyday Life: Living and Cooking,* vol. 2. Minneapolis: University of Minnesota Press, 149–247.

Gilbert, D. (2005). Interrogating mixed-race: A crisis of ambiguity? *Social Identities*, 11(1), 55–74.

Guthman, J. (2008a). Bringing good food to others: Investigating the subjects of alternative food practice. *Cultural Geographies*, 15(4), 431–47.

——— (2008b). 'If they only knew': Color blindness and universalism in California alternative food institutions. *The Professional Geographer*, 60(3), 387–97.

Hage, G. (1997). At home in the entrails of the west: Multiculturalism, ethnic food and migrant home-building. In G. Hage, L. Johnson, J. Langsworth, and M. Symonds (eds), *Home/World: space, Community and Marginality in Sydney's West*, Sydney: Pluto Press, 99–153.

Han, A. (2007). 'Can I tell you what we have to put up with?': Stinky fish and offensive durian. *Continuum: Journal of Media & Cultural Studies*, 21(3), 361–77.

Hayes-Conroy, A. (2010). Feeling slow food: Visceral fieldwork and empathetic research relations in the alternative food movement. *Geoforum*, 41(5), 734–42.

——— and Hayes-Conroy, J. (2008). Taking back taste: Feminism, food and visceral politics. *Gender, Place and Culture*, 15(5), 461–73.

Hayes-Conroy, J. and Hayes-Conroy, A. (2010). Visceral geographies: Mattering, relating, and defying. *Geography Compass*, 4(9), 1273–83.

Hickey-Moody, A., G.C. Savage and Windle, J. (2010). Pedagogy writ large: Public, popular and cultural pedagogies in motion. *Critical Studies in Education,* 51(3), 227–36.

Highmore, B. (2008). Alimentary agents: Food, cultural theory and multiculturalism. *Journal of Intercultural Studies*, 29(4) 381–98.

Hollows, J. (2008). *Domestic Cultures*. Maidenhead: McGraw-Hill.

Holtzman, J. (2006). Food and memory. *Annual Review Anthropology*, 35, 361–78.

Jackson, P. (2009). Introduction. In P. Jackson (ed.), *Changing Families, Changing Food.* London: Palgrave Macmillan.

Jayasuriya, L. and Pookong, K. (1999). *The Asianisation of Australia?: Some Facts about the Myths*. Melbourne: Melbourne University Press.

Jones, M.O. (2007). Food choice, symbolism, and identity: Bread and butter issues for folkloristics and nutrition studies. *Journal of American Folklore*, 120(476), 129–77.

Kehily, M. (1995). Self narration: Autobiography and identity construction. *Gender and Education*, 7(1), 23–31.

Knowles, C. (2003). *Race and Social Analysis*. London: Sage.

Kristeva, J. (1982). *Powers of Horror: An Essay on Abjection*, trans. Leon S. Roudiez. New York: Columbia University Press.

Lalonde, M.P. (1992). Deciphering a meal again, or the anthropology of taste. *Social Science Information*, 31(1), 69–86.

Laurier, E. and Wiggins, S. (2011). Finishing the family meal: The interactional organisation of satiety. *Appetite*, 56, 53–64.

Law, L. (2001). Home cooking: Filipina women and geography of the senses in Hong Kong. *Ecumene*, 8(3), 264–83.

Lawler, S. (2008). *Identity: Sociological Perspectives*. Cambridge: Polity.

Lee, S.S.J. (2000). Dys-appearing tongues and bodily memories: The aging of first-generation resident Koreans in Japan. *Ethos*, 28(2), 198–223.

Locher, J.L., Yoels, W.C., Maurer, D. and Van Ells, J. (2005). Comfort foods: An exploratory journey into the social and emotional significance of food. *Food & Foodways*, 13(4), 273–97.

Longhurst, R., Ho, E. and Johnston, L. (2008). Using 'the body' as an 'instrument of research'. Kimch'i and pavlova. *Area*, 40, 208–17.
Luke, C. (2003). Glocal mobilities: Crafting identities in interracial families. *International Journal of Cultural Studies*, 6, 379–401.
——— (ed.) (1996). *Feminisms and Pedagogies of Everyday Life*. New York: SUNY Press.
——— and Carrington, V. (2000). Race matters. *Journal of Intercultural Studies*, 21(1) 5–2.
——— and Luke, A. (1998). Interracial families: Difference within difference. *Ethnic and Racial Studies*, 21(4), 728–54.
Lupton, D. (1996). *Food, the Body and the Self*. London: Sage.
Magno, N.F. (2011). Filipino food ways in Japan: A case of Filipino migrant women married to Japanese men in Tokyo. *Philippine Sociological Review*, 48, 52–71.
Miller, W. (2009). *The Anatomy of Disgust*. Boston: Harvard University Press.
Morgan, D. (1996). *Family Connections: An Introduction to Family Studies*. Cambridge: Polity.
——— (2011). *Rethinking Family Practices*. Basingstoke: Palgrave Macmillan.
Murcott, A. (1982). On the social significance of the 'cooked dinner' in South Wales. *Social Science Information/sur les sciences sociales*, 21(4/5), 677–96.
——— (1995). 'It's a pleasure to cook for him': Food, mealtimes and gender in some South Wales Households.' In S. Jackson and S. Moores (eds), *The Politics of Domestic Consumption*. Critical Readings. London: Prentice Hall.
Nakano, Y. (2009). *Where There are Asians, there are Rice Cookers: How 'National' Went Global via Hong Kong*. Hong Kong University Press: Hong Kong.
Noble, G. (2013). Cosmopolitan habits: The capacities and habitats of intercultural conviviality. *Body & Society*, 19(2/3), 162–85.
Ochs, E. and Shohet, M. (2006). The cultural structuring of mealtime socialization. *New Directions for Child and Adolescent Development*, 111, 35–49.
O'Connell, R. (2010). (How) is childminding family like? Family day care, food and the reproduction of identity at the public/private interface. *The Sociological Review*, 58(4), 563–86.
Ohnuki-Tierney, E. (1994). *Rice as Self: Japanese Identities through Time*. Princeton: Princeton University Press.
Pandoongpatt, T.M. (2011). Too hot to handle: Food, empire and race in Thai Los Angeles. *Radical History Review*, 110, 83–108.
Perera, S. (1999). Whiteness and its discontents: Notes on politics, gender, sex and food in the year of Hanson 1. *Journal of Intercultural Studies*, 20(2), 183–98.
Quarmby, T. and Dagkas, S. (2013). Informal mealtime pedagogies: Exploring the influence of family structure on young people's healthy eating dispositions. *Sport, Education and Society*, 20(3), 1–17.
Roth, L.A.K. (2005). 'Beef. It's what's for dinner': Vegetarians, meat-eaters and the negotiation of familial relationships. *Food, Culture and Society: An International Journal of Multidisciplinary Research*, 8(2), 181–200.

Rozin, P. (1996). Towards a psychology of food and eating: From motivation to module to model to marker, morality, meaning, and metaphor. *Current Directions in Psychological Science*, 5(1), 18–24.

———, Haidt, J. and McCauley, C.R. (2008). Disgust. In M. Lewis, J. Haviland-Jones and L. Feldman Barrett (eds), *Handbook of Emotions,* 3rd edn. New York: Guilford Press, 757–76.

Sandlin, J., Schultz, B. and Burdick, J. (eds) 2010, *Handbook of Public Pedagogy: Education and Learning Beyond Schooling*. Routledge, London and New York.

Saroca, N. (2006). Woman in danger or dangerous woman? Contesting images of Filipina victims of domestic homicide in Australia. *Asian Journal of Women's Studies*, 12(3), 35–74.

Sheridan, S. (2000a). Eating the other: Food and cultural difference in the *Australian Women's Weekly* in the 1960s. *Journal of Intercultural Studies*, 21(3), 319–29.

——— (2000b). The 'Australian Woman' and her migrant others in the postwar *Australian Women's Weekly*. *Continuum: Journal of Media & Cultural Studies*, 14(2), 121–32.

Slocum, R. (2008). Thinking race through corporeal feminist theory: Divisions and intimacies at the Minneapolis Farmers' Market. *Social & Cultural Geography*, 9(8), 849–69.

——— (2011). Race in the study of food. *Progress in Human Geography*, 35(3), 303–27.

Stapleton, H. and Keenan, J. (2009). (New) family formation and the organisation of food in households: Who does what and why? In P. Jackson (ed.), *Changing Families, Changing Food*. Basingstoke: Palgrave.

Sutton, D. (2001). *Remembrance of Repasts: An Anthropology of Food and Memory*. Oxford: Berg.

Tyler, K. (2005). The genealogical imagination: The inheritance of interracial identities. *The Sociological Review*, 53(3), 476–94.

Valentine, G. (1999). Eating in home, consumption and identity. *The Sociological Review*, 47, *492–524.*

Williams-Forson, P.A. (2006). *Building Houses out of Chicken Legs: Black Women, Food, and Power*. Chapel Hill: University of North Carolina Press.

——— and Walker, J. (2013). Food and race: An overview. In K. Albala (ed.), *Routledge International Handbook of Food Studies*. London and New York: Routledge.

Wise, A. (2007). Multiculturalism from below: Transversal crossings and working class cosmopolitans. In A. Wise and S. Velayutham (eds.) *Everyday Multiculturalism*. Basingstoke: Palgrave Macmillan.

Xu, W. (2008). *Eating Identities: Reading Food in Asian American Literature*. Honolulu: University of Hawaii Press.

Chapter 4
'You Are What You Eat!'?: Crafting the (Food) Consuming Subject through Cooking Shows

Seline Szkupinski-Quiroga, Jennifer A. Sandlin, and Robin Redmon Wright

In this chapter, we explore cooking shows as a form of food pedagogy, and examine how they attempt to shape postmodern subjectivities characterised by a preoccupation with lifestyle practices and the 'self–referential concern with style and image' (Usher, Bryant and Johnston 1997: 18). Using a Foucauldian framework (Rose 1996), we sought to understand how different genres of cooking shows enacted, embodied and/or produced particular food pedagogies. We pay attention to how these food pedagogies problematise particular issues, to what kinds of authorities they invoke, to what technologies they employ and to what kinds of subjectivities they seek to create in learners/viewers (see Flowers and Swan 2012 for an earlier application of this framework). We focus on the multiple pathways – to employ a term from Nikolas Rose (1996) – used by celebrity chef cooking shows to facilitate their promotion of consumerist lifestyles. We also discuss the pathways of two alternative cooking shows that offer different aesthetics of consumption while also propagating subjectivities linked more to a particular form of conviviality than consumerism. As envisioned by the alternative cooking shows we analyse here, conviviality is a result of gathering together around food and induces the positive affective qualities of harmonious, joyful feasting with good company[1] that then serves as a precursor to opening up sometimes difficult and challenging dialogues about the ethical and cultural politics of food.[2]

1 Gathering together around food is a potent cultural indicator of belonging, of identity and of social structure (Sobal 2000). Ignored in the idealised views of alternative cooking shows are the conflicts and tensions around who does and does not belong, who is excluded and why, who is privileged to be served and who is relegated to serving, and so on.

2 Unlike the conviviality characterised by habitual interactions put forth by Gilroy (2004) and Noble (2013), the alternative cooking shows we analyse promote a conviviality linked to the transient nature of communitas (Turner 2012).

Exploring the Pedagogical Pathways of Cooking Shows

We draw from a Foucauldian analytical framework originally proposed by Rose (1996) and utilised by other scholars examining adult education and food pedagogies (Flowers and Swan 2012). In this framework, there are four linked 'pathways' to explore, each of which yield insights about the pedagogical aspects of cooking shows: problematisations, authorities, technologies and subjectivities (Rose 1996). Analytically, *problematisation* involves paying attention to the processes through which certain phenomena and the individuals associated with the phenomena become 'problems' that then require resources, interventions, policies and solutions. Key to the process of problematisation is the knowledge mobilised to support particular definitions, moral judgements and subject positions.

The end goal of the interventions suggested by problematisations is the production of particular *subjectivities*/subject positions. The self is always the target of these interventions/projects, and technologies are deployed to guide, direct, encourage and compel the self to engage in a constant process of improvement and adherence to an ideal put forth by authorities and bolstered by knowledge (Rose 1996). Individuals are not governed by unidirectional, top-down power relationships, but rather participate in their own self-government through 'capacitisation' rather than 'constraint' – that is, individuals participate in their own self-disciplining through the productive practices and experiences of enacting their 'freedom' and 'desire' rather than through 'prohibition, coercion and punishment' (Flowers and Swan 2012: 535). Capacitisation and self-government thus work 'in quite unsystematic, dispersed, contradictory and localised ways across innumerable and unexpected sites' (Flowers and Swan 2012: 535). Furthermore, subject positions are not singular entities; rather, individuals targeted by multiple interventions simultaneously can take up multiple positions that can be complementary or contradictory (Madden and Chamberlain 2010).

The nature, form and source of the knowledges that are mobilised to suggest particular problematisations and subsequent interventions fall under the analytical purview of *authorities*. Here we investigate which knowledges are authorised or privileged and held forth as credible, truthful and authoritative by chef-pedagogues.

Subjectivities are created through the mobilisation of particular *technologies*, which Rick Flowers and Elaine Swan define as 'hybrid assemblages of diverse forms of knowledge such as advice, techniques, judgements, experts, texts and sanctions' (2012: 535). Technologies are those physical and material practices with transformative functions used to shape the bodies, minds, conduct and lifestyle of both others and one's self with the aim of producing certain desired effects and avoiding other undesired ones (Foucault 1988, Rose 1999). For example, some types of television shows can be considered a cultural technology and lifestyle education that teach viewers how to 'better' themselves. A reality television show like *The Biggest Loser*, which showcases efforts to lose weight, exercise, eat well and change unhealthy behaviours, models to viewers how to self-monitor their own daily lives and make changes guided by the discourses of responsibility, choice and empowerment prevalent in the show (Ouellette and Hay 2008). However, the effect on viewers is not a given, as the individual viewer can choose a variety of responses, including to follow these models, mock them, or ignore them.

Analysing Food Pedagogies

Richard Johnson and colleagues (2004) argue that while there are a variety of specific methods used in the study of popular culture, in general there are two broad methodological approaches: *readings*, which focus on understanding culture through textual means, and *meetings*, which focus on direct encounters with other humans, via ethnographic methods. We were concerned with *reading*, via qualitative textual analysis, the meanings of cooking shows.

Our research is located in the United States and we take up US-based shows in our analysis. We welcome comparisons of our findings with cooking shows in other countries and contexts; however, a comparative analysis was beyond the scope of our current research. As representative of US shows featuring celebrity chefs, we conducted a textual analysis of the *Food Network*'s instructional[3] cooking shows (for example, *Emeril Live* and *30 Minute Meals with Rachael Ray*). The *Food Network* (hereafter *FN*) currently airs over 200 shows, the majority showcasing the personality and showmanship of celebrity chefs. As counterpoint, we also analysed two 'alternative' (that is, non-corporate-sponsored, non-celebrity-chef-based) cooking shows: the *Post Punk Kitchen* (hereafter *PPK*), a public-access television cooking show, and *The Cooking Show con Karimi & Comrades* (hereafter *TCS*), an interactive cooking show hosted live by a performance artist/cook. Data included episodes and performances of the shows; websites, blogs and videos sponsored by the shows; and written statements by chefs (cookbooks, interviews and so on).

Consuming Lifestyles: The Celebrity Chef Genre

The rise of the celebrity chef genre parallels the rise in popularity of television food programming. While several countries now have entire channels devoted to food programming, *FN*, founded in 1993, was the first channel completely dedicated to food and entertaining (Adema 2000). While the individual personalities and cooking style of each chef differs, there are some common elements that characterise the celebrity chef genre. Kathleen Collins (2009) describes celebrity chefs as chefs who are represented by entertainment management agencies, whose celebrity has

3 In general, the instructional shows we analyse air in the daytime and are known collectively as *Food Network in the Kitchen*. While fascinating and relevant, we will not analyse the food pedagogies of entertainment shows (comprising the cooking competitions, reality shows and travelogue style shows airing in primetime).

been created and/or bolstered by broadcast media. Celebrity chefs promoted by *FN* – examples include Emeril Lagasse, Nigella Lawson, Anthony Bourdain and Rachael Ray – value entertainment as much as and sometimes over instruction, often performing in front of a live audience that allows direct interaction, and comprise 'sparkly personality-centric programming' (Collins 2009: 180). In addition to their own shows, celebrity chefs become media personalities and regularly appear on television and in other media in order to maintain a high profile. As the reality/competition show *The Next Food Network Star* makes clear, individuals who aspire to be the next celebrity chef on the *FN* are judged on much more than their ability to cook or instruct an audience. Celebrity chefs must have a unique identity, a visual performance style suited for television, a marketable personality and the ability to sell a variety of products – the food being prepared, the expertise and credibility of the celebrity chef and ultimately their persona – as their task is to market culinary and consumption experiences on television. When potential celebrity chefs are judged on their presentations – which focus on the explanation of the dish they have prepared – mentors tell them they must be able to 'reel in' the audience with their descriptions. Ideally, the description should not just focus on the food but should reveal something personal about the celebrity chef because, ultimately, the chefs are selling themselves. As mentors on *The Next Food Network Star* frequently intone, 'the product is yourself'. The celebrity chef can then equal a brand and the marketable personality created can be used to sell other products.

The manufacturing of a celebrity chef with the aforementioned qualities lays the groundwork for diversification into related areas of entertainment and (cultural) consumption. This diversification is known as synergy, part of a strategy to create a 'lifestyle' package that includes branding, endorsements and influence (Negus 1997). As a whole, the products promoted by celebrity chefs present a context of consumption, a lifestyle that becomes an element of the brand associated with the chef (Arvidsson 2005). Thus the exemplar *FN* celebrity chef with an established persona, culinary point of view and credibility with an audience becomes a marketing tool, and their show within the celebrity chef cooking show genre becomes 'a type of commercial – for food, for lifestyles, and for the celebrity chef who represents and promotes both' (Ketchum 2007: 171). The power and influence of the chef's persona to provoke consumption is dependent on how the credibility, attractiveness and expertise of the celebrity chef are experienced by consumers (Byrne, Whitehead and Breen 2003).

A Taste of Something Different?: Alternatives to the Celebrity Chef Genre

Below, we examine two 'alternative' cooking shows. By 'alternative' we mean that they are not sponsored by or hosted on commercial television networks such as the *FN*, and they are not driven by the commercial and consumerist ethos of the celebrity chef genre we discussed above. That is, both Isa Chandra Moskowitz of

PPK and Robert Karimi/*El Mero Cocinero* of *TCS* position themselves as different from and often in opposition to the celebrity chefs on mainstream cooking shows.

PPK was a public-access television cooking show hosted by vegan cookbook author Isa Chandra Moskowitz and her co-host Terry Hope Romero that aired between 2003 and 2005 on Brooklyn and Manhattan, New York public-access television. Six shows were produced during that time period and were available on DVD as well as posted on the Internet. During this time period, Moskowitz also created a blog and website as a way to create a vegan cooking community online, where people could 'submit recipes, share ideas, and maybe gossip a bit' (www.thePPK.com). A self-professed cooking show fan, in 2003 she became disillusioned with the cooking shows on commercial TV because they lacked any connection to the politics of food. While the show no longer airs, the website continues to flourish, and the message boards especially have become a 'bustling metropolis' where vegetarians can interact with each other. In addition to maintaining an active community-focused website and authoring cookbooks, Moskowitz also regularly speaks and provides cooking demonstrations at vegetarian conferences and festivals all over the world.

El Mero Cocinero aka The People's Cook is the alter ego of Robert Karimi, a Minneapolis/St. Paul-based performance artist. Mero has hosted an interactive cooking show – *TCS* – for 16 years. *TCS* is not televised regularly,[4] but, rather, is performed in unlikely spaces in cities where Karimi has formed partnerships with local activists, educators, artists and arts organisations. For example, an art gallery is turned into a pop-up restaurant or a community centre meeting room into a kitchen stage.

TCS is modelled after the Public Broadcasting System (PBS) cooking show format which Karimi remembers watching growing up with his immigrant mother as she adapted to life in the United States. In addition to live cooking instruction and demonstration, Mero adds music, storytelling, humour and audience participation. These additions are not just to entertain, but to jump start one of the principles of *TCS*: to create community through cooking and eating together. For every gastronomic creation Mero cooks, he also tells a story, often one that highlights his upbringing in an Iranian–Guatemalan household where culinary traditions were remixed and reinvented. He prompts audience members to become storytellers as well, as in a recent dinner/performance in which one course was designated as time to 'feed each other stories'.

Karimi (2007) aims for the audience of *TCS* to learn 'revolutionary recipes in order to cook as a community and dialogue about the issues important to our stomachs and hearts'. The use of the term 'revolutionary' is fitting as the persona of Mero Cocinero is that of a 1960s-style leftist revolutionary. He addresses his kitchen helpers as 'comrade' during the show, and his chef's hat and coat

4 Performances of *TCS* featuring the character of *El Mero Cocinero* are available on *The People's Cook* website (http://thepeoplescook.com) and on vimeo (http://vimeo.com/channels/thepeoplescook).

are emblazoned with a power fist holding a cooking spoon. The motto of *TCS* is 'Revolution begins in the kitchen!' and Mero echoes this credo through his persona, recipes, patter and explicit inclusion of socio-political commentary and cultural pride into his cooking instruction. The names of the dishes and recipes he shares with the audience are infused with political significance and humour. The food he cooks and the recipes he shares emphasise foods that are easily securable, affordable and less detrimental to a chronic-disease prone multicultural audience (Etheridge Woodson et al. 2015) in an acknowledgement of health disparities and urban food justice issues.

Unlike celebrity chefs and similar to the ethic of *PPK*, Mero positions himself as explicitly anti-consumerism and anti-corporate, often starting a performance of *TCS* with a hand washing ritual which fulfils kitchen sanitation guidelines, but also washes away the 'germs of capitalism.' His patter while cooking references topics as varied as grocery store redlining in Baltimore, the historical amnesia of America towards Native Americans, the dangers of mono-crop agriculture and the expense of eating organic. While *TCS* has aprons for sale (the only nod to commercialism), Mero counts it as a point of pride that he gives away food he has prepared in every city where *TCS* has been staged.

Crafting the Subject of (Food) Consumption through Food Pedagogies

In this section we use the framework of problematisation, subjectivities, authorities and technologies to explore the ways in which these various chefs, through their food pedagogies, offer potential subject positions from which audience members can draw as they craft their identities. Within each 'category', we briefly discuss the celebrity chef genre before discussing in more detail the two alternative chefs.

Problematisation

The problems celebrity chef cooking shows purport to solve are ostensibly cooking-related: how to be efficient with time so as to 'still have time to enjoy your family' (*30 Minute Meals with Rachael Ray*); how to make dishes using store-bought ingredients (another time–saver) that 'taste like they were made from scratch' (*Sandra Lee Semi-Homemade*); how to entertain with elegance and ease (*Barefoot Contessa*); or how to liven up bland cookery with spice (*The Essence of Emeril*). The framing of these problems assumes the subject positions of the viewing audience; for example, that the home cook/viewer is a family member (implicitly female) in charge of meals, who is pressed for time or who aspires to the easy elegance associated with the upper class.

The problematics of food preparation are narrowly defined as occurring in an individual household. Larger economic, social, and cultural issues that affect the household – such as pesticide use, food safety and the US industrial food system – are systematically ignored (Ketchum 2007). There is no mention of global hunger, no discussion of genetically altered food and no discussion of the recent increase in food-borne disease. The celebrity chef genre also ignores issues of cheap labour, human exploitation and environmental damage in global food production.

Since the celebrity chef genre focuses its problematisations on individual consumers in discrete households, the main solutions its shows offer comprise various configurations of consumption. For example, the tips celebrity chefs on *FN* shows propose to make life easier often require or encourage, through product placement, the use of branded kitchen equipment and food ingredients or, through the highlighting of various corporate sponsorships, the purchase of packaged consumer goods or specialised and celebrity-chef-themed equipment. In contrast, the alternative chefs we examined problematise contemporary American eating habits and contemporary American food production and processing systems, policies and practices. Karimi and Moskowitz critique Americans' reliance on processed and pre-packaged foods, the neglect of cultural and social aspects of food, and the disconnects between the sensual experiences of food and its preparation.

For Isa Moskowitz of *PPK*, the problem is the ways in which American food production and processing systems harm both humans and non-human animals. She firmly holds to the principle that food and politics are inextricably linked. A solution she offers in her cookbook, *Vegan with a Vengeance*, is for her audience to avoid convenience foods because relying on such foods 'makes us vegans dependent on huge corporations with shady policies' (Moskowitz 2005: 1). Avoiding such foods 'will help wean you from the corporate teat while at the same time saving you money and encouraging you to support local growers' (2005: xiii). For Moskowitz, cooking and eating a vegan meal with whole, non-processed ingredients is itself a political act – a move away from corporate agribusiness and towards more sustainable and ethical ways of living and being. She states, 'Eating is a moral act or a political statement, depending on whom you ask. When you choose to stop eating animal products and supporting big business, you prove both statements to be correct' (2005: xiv).

Moskowitz also problematises the ways in which some vegans engage with the moral and political aspects of food – arguing that while corporate food production and processing systems are part of the problem, so are self-righteous vegans who criticise and harshly judge non-vegans because of their cooking and eating habits, or who engage in vegan foods and cooking that are alienating to non-vegans. Moskowitz argues that many people do not want to engage in the ethics of veganism because they are turned off by its aesthetics, and by the shame and blame they receive from many vegans. Instead of shame and blame, Moskowitz encourages fellow vegans to aestheticise and pleasurise the vegan experience and thus make it more inviting to non-vegans or those who might not know about or actively reflect upon the politics of factory farming and corporate food production. Moskowitz encourages vegans to make and share delicious, pleasurable, comforting vegan foods with others as a way to reach them and share veganism with them in an open and non-judgemental way. She seeks to create connections among those cooking and eating together by promoting dialogue between vegetarians and omnivores, to encourage them in 'understanding each other and listening to each other.' The opening to this dialogue, however, is the sharing of delicious vegan food. Moskowitz encourages viewers/readers of her blog to find ways to get vegan food into the hands and mouths of omnivores – through hosting dinners for friends and family, neighbourhood brunches and bake sales, for example – and in her own community hosts vegan dinners to raise funds for various human and non-human animal rights causes and organisations.

Karimi also focuses on how American food practices are detrimental to one's health. Specifically, in *TCS* episodes entitled *Diabetes of Democracy*, Karimi borrows from health authorities the idea that diabetes is a problem that can be ameliorated by changing one's eating patterns. For Karimi, however, health is conceptualised more holistically than just physical health, but also encompasses emotional health and one's relation to others. Karimi problematises how diabetics (and other modern populations) eat, and more significantly, how diabetics are told to eat by health professionals: without a deep consideration of culture and the accompanying social context.

In *TCS*, Karimi presents a variety of inter-related solutions to this complex of problems. Primary is the directive to appreciate and actively engage in the communal aspects of food. Captured in his mantra of 'Cook. Eat. Together.', which appears on the top of his webpage and as a tagline on blog posts, like Moskowitz, he exalts the bonds formed when people create something together – in this case preparing food – and the social exchanges facilitated by eating and sharing a meal together. A related corollary is that cooking a meal from scratch is valuable and, when done in community, can be fun rather than a chore. Karimi's concept of community – one shared with Moskowitz – is not one that is geographically bounded or held together by attributes of ethnicity, culture, or class. Rather it is an ideal configuration of communitas (Turner 2012) that comprises more than the discrete households where meals are commonly shared and is temporarily formed through the sharing of an intense culinary experience.

The valorisation of food made with fresh ingredients over pre-packaged and processed ones is based on health concerns: processed foods usually contain high amounts of sodium, fat and sugar. As part of his attention to diabetes and other dietary-related diseases that disproportionately affect communities of colour, Karimi actively promotes eating more vegetables and less meat and carbohydrates. Like Moskowitz, who relishes the smells of ingredients she works with, proclaiming how delicious the cocoa powder and homemade curry blend she's cooking with are, when showing ingredients to his audience, Karimi rhapsodises over the colour of mango flesh, the fragrance of mint, the bite of chilli. This is both congruent with and demonstrative of the solution of respecting/loving your food and delighting in the sensory and sensual aspects of food. This emphasis on pleasure is an antidote to the food-related proscriptions of health authorities whose rhetoric of self-discipline and control usually ignores the sensual. As well – and here is where the 'alternative' chefs move beyond the embracing of pleasure and sensuality that some celebrity chefs also engage in – the alternative chefs attempt to explicitly wed sensory pleasures of consumption to ethics and politics, in what Kate Soper (2007) calls an alternative hedonism.

Subjectivities

The celebrity chef cooking shows we analysed on the *FN* seem to seek to produce viewers who, to at least some degree, will begin adopting the particular lifestyle of consumption on offer, and who are receptive to the influence of celebrity chef recommendations – in short, a consuming subject who actively engages with a discourse of the self that is to a large extent defined by certain kinds of consumption-based lifestyle practices (Voight 1997). This consuming subject was originally assumed to be middle-class, white and female, as cooking shows traditionally targeted those viewers. However, *FN* has actively sought to capture a male demographic as they have developed more shows, such as *BBQ with Bobby Flay* and *Boy Meets Grill*, featuring 'masculine' cooking techniques. They have also increased the number of shows focusing on ethnic cooking such as *Big Daddy's House* and *East Meets West with Ming Tsai*, although these shows do not appear to target a different demographic but rather a non–ethnic (read white) audience who want to spice up their culinary repertoires. When celebrity chefs present ethnic food, it is often stripped of its context and symbolic of a sophisticated cosmopolitanism (Heldke 2001).

The subject positions that Moskowitz and Karimi aim to produce in their audiences are similar to their own – progressive, politically aware, individuals who are respectful of other cultures, enjoy food and value community and who are thus willing to make changes compatible with this stance and to share knowledge and delicious food with others, to encourage them to move in similar directions. A critical element of the desired subject position is that one both recognises the need for making changes – be it in the interest of physical or emotional health or human/animal ethics – and also feels inspired to and capable of making these changes. The changes in eating and food preparation habits Moskowitz and Karimi propose are linked to what they see as the areas that would benefit from improvement.

Lifestyle, as applicable to the alternative cooking shows exemplified by *PPK* and *TCS*, encompasses the modifiable choices about daily habits and the implied responsibility to make the 'right' choices to live well, that is, ethically and with lower disease risk (Coreil and Levin 1984: 105). This is in contrast to lifestyle as employed by the celebrity chef genre in which living well is associated with increased consumption of consumer goods.

Authorities

As the genre of cooking shows feature different kinds of celebrity chefs, the authorities they draw on vary. Signe Rousseau (2012) categorises celebrity chefs as either the professional (for example, Emeril Lagasse and Bobby Flay) or the amateur (for example, Rachael Ray and Paula Deen). The authority of the former is grounded in the codified formal knowledge of culinary school, bolstered by the experiential knowledge of working as a professional chef. The latter privilege experiential knowledge, as these celebrity chefs have no formal culinary training but have worked in the food industry as caterer and restaurateur. These chefs also draw upon the additional constructed authority of celebrityhood, as being a celebrity is in and of itself sufficient to grant authority in contemporary media worlds, since many people pay attention to what celebrities advise and recommend (Rousseau 2012). We recognise, of course, that not all people heed the advice of celebrities and some, in fact, mock celebrities, hold them in disdain, or simply pay them no attention.

Like amateur celebrity chefs, both Moskowitz and Karimi draw on experiential knowledge in order to be seen as a credible food instructor. However, while Rachael Ray and Paula Deen's expertise was acquired in the commercial food industry, Moskowitz and Karimi turn to quite different domains for their authorisation. Moskowitz draws upon her own Jewish heritage in her cooking as well as the experiential authority of having grown up in a racially and ethnically diverse neighbourhood, being invited to dinners at friends' houses and learning from their parents. She describes herself as 'technically self-taught' – but explains that she was really taught by

> the 'awesome and skilled' people she worked beside throughout her life – 'from the guy at *Food Not Bombs* who showed me how to slice 10 pounds of broccoli in under 10 minutes, to the prep cook at a Brooklyn restaurant where I was a waitress who taught me to slice onions – the world has been my cooking school'. (www.thePPK.com)

Moskowitz also draws upon her experiences as a teenager participating in the New York City punk scene, helping to turn abandoned buildings into homes, to create community gardens, and to create news, music and entertainment, including 'zines (do-it-yourself magazines). Also during this time, Moskowitz was introduced to vegetarianism, became involved with social justice groups such as *Food Not Bombs*, and began connecting food to politics and health. *PPK* embraces the punk idea of 'Do It Yourself', or DIY, wherein 'the unpolished, improvised nature of DIY projects results in something much more interesting than most overtly commercial efforts' (Moskowitz 2005: xiii). Within this ethic, Moskowitz explains, 'we can create our own forms of entertainment. We don't have to sit back idly and wait for something to happen – we can make it happen' (2005: 3). These experiences help shape her DIY approach to cooking and instruction as well as provide a platform from which she educates people about veganism. Moskowitz became vegan at the age of 16 and began 'cooking breakfast for everyone before a demonstration, making snacks as we silk-screened or made banners' (Moskowitz 2005: 3). Drawing upon the DIY punk aesthetic, she decided she could create her own show, cooking in her own kitchen and producing the show with her friends.

With this ethic in mind she took classes at Brooklyn Community Access TV and learned the basics of editing, camera work and lighting so that she could start producing *PPK*. While drawing upon this authority, she also strives to share it with her audience, encouraging them to explore vegan cooking, to share recipes and to experiment with her recipes as well as their own.

Like Moskowitz, Karimi privileges the knowledge imparted by mothers and grandmothers from the home kitchen, a location 'identified with reproduction of family and gender as non-commodified caring' (Walter 2009: 2). The food he cooks and teaches others to cook is grounded in recipes handed down by his own mother, other mothers he knew growing up and the mothers of his community partners. In this practice, his knowledge claim is implicitly gendered in that he invokes the emotional appeal of maternal care (albeit romanticised and curiously uncritical of the gendered division of domestic labour). The knowledge claim is also classed, as what is served in the home and prepared by mothers has less cultural cachet than that prepared in the kitchens of high-end restaurants by credentialed [male] chefs.

Karimi's ethnic-racial subject position affects both the body of knowledge he draws on and the authority he possesses. When he highlights an Iranian dish his Guatemalan mother learned to cook – *ghormeh sabzi*[5] – he also tells the story of the colonial enterprises and US interventions in Latin America and the Middle East that shaped his parents' histories, experiences and food practices. Karimi's insistence of the importance of history to food runs counter to the prevailing trends of food consumerism which 'ignores history and context in favour of fashion and corporate concerns' (Rousseau 2012: 10) and to the constraints of television cooking shows where food, in the interest of palatability, is usually 'de-fused of its political bite' (Pearson and Kothari 2007 quoted in Cook et al. 2008: 825). Dominant audiences may see Karimi's privileging of 'ethnic' food without the accompanying exotification as undermining his authority. Yet, this is a specific technology, which he (and to a lesser extent, Moskowitz) employs: a conscious and subversive de-authorisation.

Technologies

As pedagogues, all these chefs deploy a variety of technologies – that is, material practices with transformative functions used to shape the bodies, minds, conduct and lifestyle of others. Here we will specifically focus on three technologies of celebrity chef and alternative cooking shows: staging, content and host persona.

The staging of celebrity chef cooking shows – the pedagogical arena if you will – relies on well-appointed kitchens equipped with the latest luxury gadgets and tools that aim to incite envy and desire in the eyes of their viewers and appeal to a consumer fantasy of 'vicarious consumption' (Adema 2000). The display kitchen/set thus becomes a highly tuned merchandising system with the branded tools available for purchase on celebrity chef websites and in other retail outlets

5 *Ghormeh sabzi* is a stew of beans and greens known as the Iranian national dish.

(Ray 2007). The filming of the shows are slick and calculatingly produced, with a three-camera set-up, allowing for dynamic shots, flashy editing and lingering shots on the final dish which have been likened to the 'money shots' of pornography (Chan 2003).

Karimi's inspirations, in contrast, are the PBS cooking shows of a generation ago with their decidedly low-budget sets and earnest presentations broadcast uncut and unedited. Karimi stages *TCS* in unconventional spaces such as art galleries, public school classrooms and community centres. The colours of the set, the accompanying music (often hip hop), the props used and the recipes presented are all decidedly déclassé from the perspective of those for whom food is cultural capital, a presentation of taste and class (Ketchum 2005). With these deliberate choices, he adheres to a Chicano rasquache[6] aesthetic in which the non-mainstream is privileged.

Moskowitz, too, consciously works against the ideal of the typical *FN* production. Friends filmed *PPK* in the cramped kitchen of Moskowitz's tiny Brooklyn apartment while local punk rock bands played in her living room. Unlike the celebrity chefs featured on the *FN*, who cook with new, top-of-the-line equipment in fancy staged kitchens, Moskowitz cooks with the worn hand-me-down pots and pans that she already owns or borrows from friends or family, and provides tips about how to improvise with ingredients and tools that most home cooks would already have in their kitchens, actively discouraging people from buying new equipment. In some episodes, the stove malfunctions, Moskowitz and her co-host Terry Hope Romero appear nervous and get tongue-tied as they stumble over each other, make mistakes and jokingly ask the camera person to edit out mistakes – an acknowledgement of how celebrity chef shows' mistakes are typically erased from the final broadcast. In these ways, *PPK* embodies the idea of DIY, wherein 'the unpolished, improvised nature of DIY projects results in something much more interesting than most overtly commercial efforts' (Moskowitz 2005: xiii). The informality of Moskowitz's production and the transitory nature of Karimi's sets also signal to viewers that the kitchen is potentially a space for play.

Celebrity chef cooking shows purport to 'teach' audience members to be 'better' and to cultivate 'more refined' tastes than they currently have. Most implicitly offer the identity of *connoisseur*, as they promote the appreciation of gourmet ingredients, hard-to-find organic foods and specialty items – even if such items are beyond the financial or time expenditures of a working parent. For example, with her catch phrase EVOO, Rachael Ray consistently communicates that only extra virgin olive oil is appropriate to use in her recipes, rather than cheaper olive oil or vegetable oil. Phebe Shih Chao critiques television cooking shows for offering

6 Rasquachismo has been defined as 'an outsider viewpoint [that] stems from a funky, irreverent stance that debunks convention and spoofs protocol' (Ybarra-Frausto 1991: 155) … which often features an impulse of political resistance, one which plays with appropriation, reversal and inversion as artistic strategies (Ybarra-Frausto 2003).

'visions of food and lifestyle of and for the middle class, especially that sector aspiring to rise higher' while ignoring 'the lower or blue-collar class' (1998: 19).

The food that is prepared on *PPK* and *TCS* is not aspirational but rather is rooted in personal classed and ethnic experiences of 'home.' Moskowitz, drawing on her own Jewish heritage and working class background, demonstrates how to make matzoh ball soup and coconut cream pie, declaring that 'those tastes and flavours are a part of who I am' (Moskowitz 2005: 2). Karimi makes a dish – '*Lumpia Campesina*' (farmworker *lumpia*), a variation on a traditional Filipino eggroll that substitutes vegetables for pork in acknowledgement of his Muslim background – while singing a politically infused ditty. In his teaching and in the space Karimi creates, he generates a discussion with audience members on ethnic food, cultural diversities, colonial and multicultural encounters, political activism and how all these factors affect one's choice of food consumption.

Cooking, by its very nature, involves the sensory aspects of food. Chefs working both within the celebrity chef genre and alternative cooking shows highlight the pleasurable qualities of food – colour, smell, taste – but to different ends. Celebrity chefs, like Nigella Lawson, embrace the pleasures of food and the gratification of the senses but seemingly as ends in themselves, and with a focus on the pleasures of the individual self. Moskowitz and Karimi, while extolling gustatory delights, both maintain that pleasure comes with responsibility for a larger social good. They ask viewers to consider the ethical and political meanings of food via the cultivation of pleasure in consumption (Sassatelli 2010). Alongside the sensory celebration of Moskowitz and Karimi is an explicit acknowledgement of cost and accessibility, as they communicate to viewers that critical consumption is not just an activity of the elite and perhaps also attempt to counter the critiques made of other alternative food movements as being paternalistic and imperialist (Donati 2005). Through their shows' content, Moskowitz and Karimi emphasise supplying their audiences with the tools to change their behaviour and ethos associated with food. Moskowitz provides practical information regarding how to create vegan baked goods and main dishes without the ingredients cooks usually rely on – butter, eggs, milk and so on – as well as how to cook with meat substitutes without having to rely on such foods created by multinational food corporations and their 'shady politics' (Moskowitz 2005: 1). Additionally, she gives audience members ideas about how to host vegan community breakfasts and potlucks, thus encouraging the communal cooking and eating of food. Both Moskowitz and Karimi reframe the meaning of food through their focus on the importance and desirability of cooking and eating in community, and by their attempts to awaken the audience's consciousness through an overt politicisation of food and eating.

Celebrity chefs use the technique of captivation through which they hope to seduce and charm the audience by the charismatic force of their personality. A charismatic yet approachable persona is integral to the definition of the celebrity chef and something that the *FN* requires of its food 'ambassadors.' Celebrity chefs must be approachable to construct an immediate faux familiarity with the audience. If celebrity chefs are judged to be likeable and approachable, they are more likely to gain the trust of their audience, an important property that can be leveraged to encourage consumption.

While Moskowitz and Karimi also employ pedagogical techniques associated with captivation that increase their relatability, they both approach the instructional format in more playful and tongue-in-cheek ways bordering on parody. Moskowitz, with her cutesy aprons, Bettie Page haircut and punk band and/or political t-shirts, is charmingly irreverent and sarcastic. Between instructing her viewers where to buy different ingredients locally and cheaply, she talks about local punk bands, tells corny jokes, laughs at herself and declares how happy she was when she found out she could curse on public-access TV. When hosting *TCS*, Karimi strategically performs the persona of *Mero Cocinero*. The Spanish word *cocinero* translates to 'cook', a designation Karimi embraces, rather than the more lofty (in the hierarchy of professional kitchens) title of chef. Like Moskowitz, Mero is somewhat of a buffoon (something anathema to the celebrity chef genre). He regularly dances goofily to rap music, and exchanges his squashed white toque, symbolic of mastering a body of codified knowledge (Shepard 1995), for a Che Guevara style black beret. He engages his audience through presenting recipes as history and storytelling, rather than using the more masculine style of relaying recipes as scientific formulas (Swenson 2009).

In a further technique of de-authorisation, Moskowitz and Mero both acknowledge and undermine bodies of knowledge considered to be authoritative. Moskowitz strays from standard culinary authority by privileging her audience's instincts and whims, rather than the codified and tested knowledge found in cookbooks. She writes:

> I remember once reading a Betty Crocker cookbook that asked readers not to deviate from a recipe – well I say no such thing. Deviate all you want, recipes are mere guidelines and everyone has different tastes. If the final dish tastes good to you, then it's a success. (Moskowitz 2005: 5)

Mero also defers to the expertise of his audience members while downplaying his own, still portraying 'enlightened' eating as something everyone can and should do. In Karimi's words, Mero 'is the fool, and this brings his message, if the fool can do it so can you' (Karimi 2013).

Through a subversive de-authorisation accomplished through the staging, content and host personas of *PPK* and *TCS,* Moskowitz and Karimi work with/in the cultural phenomenon of cooking shows but invest them with a meaning and purpose that differs from the interests of the economically and ideologically dominant (Fiske 1989). The active de-authorisation that Karimi and Moskowitz deploy can create a path for people to craft their own subject positions with more fluidity than that offered by the celebrity chef genre. The technologies for change Moskowitz and Karimi use and impart to their audiences in a classic technology-of-the-self-move can be selectively taken up, rejected or combined with other techniques from other sources. While this is true for how viewers might receive the techniques from celebrity chefs as well, the subversive de-authorisation deployed by Karimi and Moskowitz is an open invitation to play with multiple subject positions, rather than just the unitary consumer subjectivity privileged by the celebrity chef genre. Karimi and Moskowitz aim to inspire change – be it in eating habits, opinions, or just openness to an ephemeral experience of trying something new.

Conclusion: Consumerism and/or Conviviality?

While we believe it is impossible to escape being a consuming subject, our analysis raises questions about the possibilities of cooking show food pedagogies to shape subjects that problematise, navigate around, or operate outside the frames of consumerism. *PPK* and *TCS*'s emphasis on conviviality as a pre-condition to dialogue about social change suggests a fruitful line for further inquiry into these questions. We do not mean to suggest that conviviality is an antidote to consumerism, for the promotion of conviviality is present in the celebrity chef cooking show genre as well, though less explicitly than in the alternative cooking shows and to a different purpose. An assumption of the celebrity chef cooking show genre is that the viewer will often be cooking for others – family members or one's social circle – a nod to conviviality. But the shows model that the best way to impress one's guests is through the cook presenting her/his most idealised complete self as defined by consumer purchases. Conviviality, as practised in the celebrity chef genre sponsored by corporate interests, is achieved through meeting a standard of culinary entertaining which demonstrates that one has learned *style*, that most 'important and purchasable commodity … at the heart of successful sociability' (Julier 2002: 76). Conviviality here is thus a culmination of consumerist lifestyle and consumption-focused learning practices. The food pedagogies of the celebrity chef cooking show genre are potentially self-perpetuating, as viewers may learn that consumption is a way to define themselves, and re-define themselves as new products and culinary styles are presented. There is thus a kind of bounded flexibility in the subject position presented as ideal by the food pedagogies of the celebrity chef cooking show genre, as the viewer's identity is restricted to being able to reinvent oneself within the confines of consumerism. This style of food pedagogy is constantly reinforced through the ubiquitous corporate support it enjoys.

Within *PPK* and *TCS*, however, conviviality plays a different role, as it is the foundation for the process of forming new bonds, even if only temporarily, within the 'ritual parenthesis of a meal' (Grignon 2001: 30). Karimi and Moskowitz are interested in this aspect of conviviality, and the exchange of ideas across difference it may facilitate. Sincere discussion in an environment of conviviality about the responsibilities that come with pleasure is the beginning of creating a conscientious subject willing to make changes. The conviviality espoused by their alternative cooking shows, rather than a culmination, is, rather, a starting point for other lifestyle projects. The ideal subject positions presented by the alternative cooking shows' pedagogies are more flexible in that they can be selectively incorporated into viewers' practices. In other words, you don't need to embrace veganism to appreciate and desire to bake a delicious vegan cupcake.

While these alternative food pedagogies offer greater flexibility and perhaps point towards a way to craft identities and lifestyle practices that are less dependent on commercial and corporate culture, they are limited in that they are not widely supported, as they are contrary to the prevailing consumer ethos of modern society. In addition, alternative cooking shows are not as widely available to a viewing/learning public as celebrity chef cooking shows, which enjoy ubiquitous corporate support.

Despite the different visions espoused by cooking shows, there are also limits to thinking of cooking shows as food pedagogies as we do not know if the celebrity chef genre's attempts to encourage consumerism or Moskowitz's and Karimi's efforts, fostered by conviviality, to create community dialogue around the politics of food, are then translated into everyday consumption practices by their audiences. Most likely there are attempts by audiences, as suggested by Adams and Raisborough (2010), to negotiate and re-articulate suggested practices to fit into the contours of their lived realities.

References

Adams, M. and Raisborough, J. 2010. Making a difference: Ethical consumption and the everyday. *The British Journal of Sociology*, 61(2), 256–74.

Adema, P. 2000. Vicarious consumption: Food, television and the ambiguity of modernity. *Journal of American & Comparative Cultures*, 23(3), 113–23.

Arvidsson, A. 2005. Brands: A critical perspective. *Journal of Consumer Culture*, 5(2), 235–58.

Byrne, A., Whitehead, M. and Breen, S. 2003. The naked truth of celebrity endorsement. *British Food Journal*, 105(4/5), 288–96.

Chan, A. 2003. 'La grande bouffe:' Cooking shows as pornography. *Gastronomica: The Journal of Food and Culture*, 3(4), 46–53.

Chao, P.S. 1998. TV cook shows, gendered cooking. *Jump Cut*, 42, 19–27.

Collins, K. 2009. *Watching What We Eat: The Evolution of Television Cooking Shows*. New York: Continuum Publishing.

Cook, I. et al. 2008. Geographies of food: Mixing. *Progress in Human Geography*, 32(6), 821–33.

Coreil, J., and Levin, J.S. 1984. A critique of the life style concept in public health education. *International Quarterly of Community Health Education*, 5(2), 104–14.

Donati, K. 2005. The pleasure of diversity in slow food ethics of taste. *Food, Culture and Society*, 8(2), 227–42.

Etheridge Woodson, S., Underiner, T., Szkupinski Quiroga, S., Winham, D. and Todd, M. 2015. Moveable feasts and immoveable paradigms: Can theatre

artists and health scientists cook, aat, and play well together? In *Food and Theatre on the World Stage*, edited by D. Chansky and A. White. New York: Routledge Press, 189–206.
Fiske, J. 1989. *Reading the Popular*. Winchester, MA: Unwin Hyman.
Flowers, R. and Swan, E. 2012. Pedagogies of doing good: Problematisations, authorities, technologies and teleologies in food activism. *Australian Journal of Adult Learning*, 52(3), 532–72.
Foucault, M. 1988. *The History of Sexuality*, vol. 3. New York: Penguin.
Gilroy, P. 2004. *Postcolonial Melancholia*. New York: Columbia University Press.
Grignon, C. 2001. Commensality and social morphology: An essay of typology, in *Food, Drink and Identity: Cooking, Eating and Drinking in Europe since the Middle Ages*, edited by P. Scholliers. New York: Berg, 23–33.
Heldke, L. 2001. Let's cook Thai: Recipes for colonialism, in *Pilaf, Pozole, and Pad Thai: American Women and Ethnic Food*, edited by S.A. Inness. Amherst, MA: University of Massachusetts Press, 175–98.
Johnson, R., Chambers, D., Raghuram, P. and Tincknell, E. 2004. *The Practice of Cultural Studies*. London: Sage.
Julier, A. 2002. Feeding Friends and Others: Boundaries of Intimacy and Distance in Sociable Meals. Dissertation, University of Massachusetts Amherst.
Karimi, R. 2007. Feed art, not war. *My power fist holds a cooking spoon*. http://www.kaoticgood.com/merococinero/http://www.kaoticgood.com/merococinero/.
———. 2013. Personal communication.
Ketchum, C. 2005. The essence of cooking shows: How the *Food Network* constructs consumer fantasies. *Journal of Communication Inquiry*, 29(3), 217–34.
———. 2007. Tunnel vision and food: A political-economic analysis of the *Food Network*, in *Cable Visions: Television Beyond Broadcasting*, edited by S. Barnet-Weiser, C. Chris and A. Freitas. New York: NYU Press, 158–76.
Madden, H. and Chamberlain, K. 2010. Nutritional health, subjectivity and resistance: Women's accounts of dietary practices. *Health*, 14(3), 292–309.
Moskowitz, I.C. 2005. *Vegan with a Vengeance*. Cambridge, MA: Da Capo Press.
Negus, K. 1997. The production of culture, in *Production of Culture/Cultures of Production*, edited by P. duGay. Thousand Oaks: Sage, 67–118.
Noble, G. 2013. Cosmopolitan habits: The capacities and habitats of intercultural conviviality. *Body & Society*, 19(2/3), 162–85.
Ouellette, L. and Hay, J. 2008. *Better Living through Reality TV: Television and Post-Welfare Citizenship*. Oxford: Blackwell Publishing.
Rose, N. 1996. *Inventing Our Selves: Psychology, Power, and Personhood*. Cambridge: Cambridge University Press.
———. 1999. *Powers of Freedom*. Cambridge: Cambridge University Press.
Rousseau, S. 2012. *Food Media: Celebrity Chefs and the Politics of Everyday Interference*. New York: Berg.
Ray, K. 2007. Domesticating cuisine: Food and aesthetics on American television. *Gastronomica: The Journal of Food and Culture*, 7(1), 50–63.

Sassatelli, R. and Davolio, F. 2010. Consumption, pleasure and politics: Slow food and the politico-aesthetic problematization of food. *Journal of Consumer Culture*, 10(2), 202–32.

Shepard, R. 1995. For caring chefs, headgear is their crowning glory, in *Dress and Identity*, edited by M.E. Roach-Higgins, J.B. Eicher and K.K. Johnson. New York: Fairchild Books, 193–4.

Sobal, J. 2000. Sociability and meals: Facilitation, commensality, and interaction, in *Dimensions of the Meal: The Science, Culture, Business, and Art of Eating*, edited by H.L. Meiselman. Gaithersburg, MD: Aspen, 119–33.

Soper, K. 2007. Re-thinking the good life: The citizenship dimension of consumer disaffection with consumerism. *Journal of Consumer Culture*, 7(2), 205–29.

Swenson, R. 2009. Domestic divo? Televised treatments of masculinity, femininity and food. *Critical Studies in Media Communication*, 26(1): 36–53.

Turner, E. 2012. *Communitas: The Anthropology of Collective Joy*. New York: Palgrave Macmillan.

Usher, R., Bryant, I. and Johnston, R. 1997. *Adult Education and the Postmodern Challenge*. London: Routledge.

Voight, C. 1997. *You are What You Eat: Contemplations on Civilizing the Palate with 'Gourmet'* (magazine). Master's thesis, McGill University.

Walter, L. 2009. Slow food and home cooking: Toward a relational aesthetic of food and relational ethic of home. *Provisions: The Journal of the Center for Food in Community and Culture*, 1, 1–23.

Ybarra-Frausto, T. 1991. Rasquachismo: A Chicano sensibility, in *Chicano Art: Resistance and Affirmation, 1965–1985*, edited by R. Griswold del Castillo, T. McKenna and Y. Yarbro–Bejarano. Los Angeles: Wight Art Gallery and University of California Press, 155–62.

———. 2003. Rasquachismo: An aesthetic of the underclass, in *Puro Border: Dispatches, Snapshots and Graffiti from La Frontera*, edited by L. Humberto Crosthwaite et al. El Paso, TX: Cinco Puntos Press, 191–3.

PART II
Transformation and Affect

Chapter 5
Food and Passion: Technologies of Self-transformation in *Jamie's Kitchen*

Lyn Harrison, Peter Kelly and Perri Campbell

Introduction

Since the 1990s there has been a surge of televisual dramatisations of real-life cooking shows in industrialised countries (Versteegan 2010: 447). Through reality television cooking shows such as, *MasterChef*, *Jamie's Kitchen*, *Hell's Kitchen*, viewers have encountered celebrity chefs, 'foodies', hospitality trainees, contestants, cooking competitions and customers. These shows have been understood as an indication of – and intervention into – contemporary consumption trends and as vehicles for social change. Many reality-based cooking shows have been regarded as educational, pedagogical sites that 'encourage populations to undertake surveillance of their own and others' bodies' and eating habits with messages like: 'You are what you eat!' or 'Organic is better' (Rich 2011: 3; see also Lewis 2007 and Chapter 4 in this book by Szkupinski-Quiroga, Sandlin and Redmon Wright).

In this chapter we explore the reality television programme *Jamie's Kitchen* as a pedagogical site which seeks to transform young people's understandings about food, work and ultimately themselves. In 2002 the high-profile celebrity chef Jamie Oliver set out to transform a group of unemployed young Londoners into the enterprising, *ideal* workers of twenty-first century, flexible capitalism.[1] This process of transformation was represented in the enormously successful Channel 4 TV series *Jamie's Kitchen*.[2] In Australia, we viewed the series, as it was screened on Channel 10 over five weeks during July and August 2003. In the series Jamie Oliver

1 As a social enterprise the Foundation claims that it 'exists to inspire disadvantaged young people to believe that they can create for themselves great careers in the restaurant industry' (Fifteen 2005).

2 Jamie Oliver's biographer Gilly Smith (2006) points out the series was one of Channel 4's top two shows in 2002 with an average weekly audience of over five million. It would go on to be televised in a further 34 countries. The original series was followed by *Jamie's Kitchen Australia* – a successful, high-rating 13-part series that was screened on Channel 10 (Australia) during September–November 2006.

took 15 unemployed young Londoners and tried to turn them into trainee chefs who had the capacity to work in his new London restaurant called, Fifteen.[3]

Like many reality television shows, *Jamie's Kitchen* brings the once private transformations of the self into the public sphere. We watched as young people were encouraged to develop skills and to go on a journey of – partially scripted, usually prescribed – self-transformation and self-discovery.[4]

Jamie's Kitchen encourages particular relationships with, and attitudes towards food, food consumption and production. In particular, passion plays a central role in the drama of the show. Passion itself among the participants is not a problem – many display passion for fast food or junk food. It is the particular type of passion that Jamie Oliver supports and seeks to develop that challenges the trainees and informs this pedagogical space: a passion for slow food, organic food, sustainable foods, local foods and home grown food. Throughout the series, food is used to engender passion and becomes a pedagogical tool supporting self-transformation. The *Jamie's Kitchen* series, and the figure of the entrepreneurial, passionate, risk-taking, small businessman (who in this instance is also a global celebrity brand) seeks to develop similar dispositions and behaviours in a workforce that initially does not display these.

We suggest that *Jamie's Kitchen* provides a vehicle to explore food pedagogies: how knowledge, behaviour and selves are shaped in relation to certain uses of, and ideas about food.[5] We argue that Michel Foucault's (1988) concept of technologies of the self enables us to analyse particular understandings of food and passion – and the manifestations of these in *Jamie's Kitchen* and in the training of marginalised young people – as powerful technologies of self-transformation. Technologies of the self refer to those 'procedures, which no doubt exist in every civilization, suggested or prescribed to individuals in order to determine their identity, maintain it, or transform it in terms of a certain number of ends, through relations of mastery or self knowledge' (Foucault 1988: 18; see also Flowers and Swan 2012).

---

3 The Melbourne franchise closed at the end of 2010; however, other community projects have been initiated by Oliver in Australia. The Fifteen Foundation is now called the Jamie Oliver Foundation.

4 We understand self-transformation as a process of ethical reflection and practice. This denotes a particular attitude towards the self: 'self-knowledge in the service of a transformative effort' (Nehamas 1998: 179; see also Foucault 1987: 6). This is an attitude that involves questioning one's own views and those of others, critiquing and reflecting upon preferred ways of being or codes of conduct. This is a self-shaping exercise or practice of the self. A reflexive, critical mode of engagement with societal norms. For more on the different uses of terms 'self-discovery' and 'self-transformation' see Swan (2010: 209).

5 The account of food pedagogies and trainee transformations we provide in this chapter can be situated in a larger and more detailed discussion of work related identity (work ethics), enterprise culture, and the possible education, training, management and policy implications related to young people's transitions. These areas are examined in detail in Kelly and Harrison's (2009) book *Working in Jamie's Kitchen: Salvation, Passion and Young Workers*.

It is our claim that food, passion, enterprise and work – bundled together and understood in certain ways in these training environments – promise to produce, in these young people, new understandings of themselves and others, their choices, responsibilities and opportunities. As the Fifteen Foundation (2005) claim:

> This involves a unique encounter with food and Jamie's inspiring approach to cooking and service. But Fifteen is so much more than a chef-training project. Food and cooking are the means to the end. The purpose is personal transformation for each young person.

Oliver himself plays a vital role in the narrative of *entrepreneurial, hospitality oriented self-development* that pervades the show. In the first section of this chapter we provide a glimpse of this narrative with reference to Jamie Oliver: celebrity chef, global brand, author and social entrepreneur. We build a picture of Jamie Oliver as a product of time and place, a moment in history in which food is understood in particular ways.

We then present a narrative about one young male trainee named Dovid, from the Australian Fifteen programme (*Jamie's Kitchen Australia*). Dovid struggles to adopt Oliver's preferred attitudes towards food and in doing so is seen to be impeding his own personal development, transformation and progress in the programme. We have chosen to present Dovid's story here because the types of challenges he faces in becoming passionate can be recognised in the stories of other trainees. His story also enables us to unpack the problematic dimensions of passion in *Jamie's Kitchen*. Drawing on Foucault's concepts of the self we discuss Dovid's transformation and examine the ways in which accounts of food, passion, and the training of marginalised young people expose some of the challenges and opportunities faced by them, as they seek to transition into the uncertain and risky labour markets of twenty-first century capitalism. The drama of *Jamie's Kitchen* suggests that as a technology of the self, passion for food promises to provide precarious, possibly temporary, forms of salvation, meaning and purpose for the young people engaged in the Fifteen Foundation's social enterprise transitional labour market programme. The young people involved in the programme, of course, construct their identities in other ways, and in other social spaces. However, our intention in this chapter is to focus on the ways in which they are represented as shaping a passionate self in the limited field of *Jamie's Kitchen*.

Jamie's Passion: Celebrity Teachers and Globalised Foods

Part of the work of this section is to profile Jamie Oliver and his somewhat chequered history as a high-profile celebrity chef who has taken on a variety of social causes and continues to position himself in a pedagogical role in relation to particular understandings of food. Through this brief introduction to Jamie Oliver we will map the types of experiences that shape his attitudes and philosophies towards food and thus his plan for the Fifteen Foundation training programme and his expectations for participants.

Throughout his television career we have seen many different sides of Jamie Oliver: the celebrity chef, the transformative and/or charismatic leader, the social entrepreneur, the food revolutionary, the lad, the respectful son, the husband, the father. Who or what is the *real* Jamie Oliver? All of these figures are representations produced in a range of media texts. In one sense they are all fictions (can we know the *real* Jamie Oliver?), but they all have effects in the everyday (Couldry 2006; Hage 2003). What is important for our argument is not whether the representations of Jamie Oliver and his trainees that we see across a range of media are *real*, but that these representations come to signify certain aspects of contemporary forms of the self.

Jamie Oliver is presented to us as the amiable, likeable, energetic, cool country boy made good through hard work, determination and a prodigious talent. Born in Essex, England in 1975, Jamie arrived in London in 1991 at the beginning of a 'new exciting food scene' and the advent of a 'new breed of superstar chef' (Smith 2006: 55). We now recognise him through his numerous television series in the UK, USA and Australia including: *The Naked Chef* (renamed *Oliver's Twist* in the US), *Jamie's Italy* (2005) *Jamie's Kitchen, Jamie's School Dinners, Jamie's Kitchen Australia, Jamie at Home* (2007), *Jamie's 30 minute meals* (2010) and *15 minute meals* (2012).

In the way of the modern entrepreneur and media personality, Oliver has a proliferation of websites (some devoted to him and others against him), and an unauthorised biography, *Turning up the Heat*, written by journalist Gilly Smith (2006). Smith charts Jamie's career from growing up in the village of Clavering in Essex and learning to love food and food preparation in *The Cricketers*, his parent's pub, through to his television series *Jamie's School Dinners* and then *Jamie's Italy*.[6]

One of Oliver's main aims has been to change attitudes towards food, food consumption practices and healthy eating. Oliver's social change agenda is evidenced, in part by his focus on fresh, locally sourced ingredients; a celebration and promotion of what has become known as *slow food*; and an associated campaign against processed, industrialised, *fast food*. In addition he is renowned for his mission to change the eating patterns of UK school children. This particular, ongoing campaign, was promoted and popularised in yet another television series, *Jamie's School Dinners*. *School Dinners* documented his attempts to change the eating habits of school children in schools in the UK, and was perhaps the most controversial of his initiatives. The parents of the targeted children resisted being

6 After his initial period of significant success in the UK, US and Australia sections of the British press began to suspect that he 'was becoming too big for his boots'. In response he was quoted as saying: 'I have done more for English food throughout the world in the past two years than anyone else has done in the past 100. I have put it on the map, for Chrissakes' (Connolly 2003; see also Lyall 2003).

told what to feed their children; school dinner ladies rebelled against the extra work involved in *preparing* meals rather than *opening* packets of pre-prepared and processed food; and the children themselves were resistant to change. Some commentators likened the battle to class wars as the *darling of the middle classes* attempted to tell mainly working-class women what they should be doing. His actions also included petitioning then British Prime Minister Tony Blair to increase budget allocations for school dinners.

Oliver's efforts to change the lives of a select group of marginalised young people through his *Jamie's Kitchen* television series, facilitated through the philanthropic Fifteen Foundation, is another example of his social entrepreneurship which engages ideals of social justice and responsibility.[7] In many respects Oliver is a man of a particular time, reflecting as he does the focus on corporate social responsibility that was a significant element of the New Labour's Third Way political agenda/manifesto in the UK for the 15 years prior to 2010.

Oliver himself argued that he was forced to develop his approach to training marginalised young people because governments (in the UK, Europe, Australia and the US) are increasingly withdrawing from such social responsibilities; or else were insisting that the responsibility should be shared with the private sector.[8] All of this social entrepreneurship on Oliver's part is underpinned by contemporary preoccupations with food: food is too fast, too processed, it is making us fat, or unhealthy or ill, we are eating too much of it, some of us are not eating enough, it causes cancer, it prevents cancer.

So, is Jamie Oliver a middle-class *tosser* telling the working classes what they should be eating (see Rich 2011: 17)? Possibly. But, we would argue, this sort of characterisation is, in many respects, unsophisticated and not one that sits well with the analysis we want to develop. It is more interesting, and possibly provocative, to think about a range of issues to do with the *Naked Chef* phenomenon, Oliver's social entrepreneurship, and the meanings associated with food, the way that Jamie (and others) think about it, by providing a snapshot of Oliver's engagement with ideas regarding: the industrialisation and rationalisation of food; globalisation and the aestheticisation of food (food porn); celebrity culture and social enterprise.

Food used to be something that people grew, hunted, caught, fished for. Many around the world still do. We should not romanticise this past with this statement. Pre-industrialised food supplies, quantity and quality were heavily dependent on climate, luck (good and bad) and skills as hunter/gatherer, farmer, trader. Industrialisation in this sense is also rationalisation. The industrialisation

7 Social entrepreneurship, the social impact of activities and corporate social responsibility are emphasised as key elements of social enterprise. Social entrepreneurship denotes an innovative approach towards social needs and problems 'taken by individuals in fostering business … mainly through non-profit organisations, but also in the for-profit sector' (Defourny and Nyssens 2006: 4–5).

8 For more on social enterprise in Australia and the UK see: Campbell, Kelly and Harrison (2011a) and (2011b).

and rationalisation of food removes, largely, the matter/question of fate from food production, processing, distribution. We need no longer learn, develop, or pass on a variety of skills, knowledges related to food production, preparation, cooking, and presentation in order to feed ourselves (Lyon et al. 2003: 167–8; see also Jaffe and Gertler 2006: 143).

In many respects we have been de-skilled in terms of food, or at the very least food preparation skills and the ways in which we understand cooking has changed significantly (Short 2003: 177). There now exist different 'creative' modes of food preparation shaped by fast-paced contemporary lifestyles. As Lyon et al. suggest:

> While questioning the past distribution of good cooking skills, we can acknowledge changed skill acquisition and application in recent years. The interaction of social and technological factors has meant that modern products demand less in response to the reduced consumer time allocation for food preparation and cooking. (2003: 171–2)

At a time when different food preparation skills are emerging, Lyon et al. (2003: 167) note that 'domestic interest in preparation of food has probably never attracted greater public interest', sparked by cookery programmes, celebrity chefs and magazines. This is one of the key elements or features of much of what Jamie Oliver has attempted throughout the various phases and manifestations of his TV career as celebrity chef. Through training and television programmes he has sought to inspire and educate people about ways of understanding food as slow, organic, local, personal rather than as pre-packaged, processed, fast, and imported.

These matters of education, skilling, training are key points because all of these, in different ways, involve processes that seek *transformations of the self*, the development of different sorts of self-understandings that can be located in the physical, visceral, embodied process of eating food. And the myriad processes that can be involved in the production, processing, preparation and presentation of the food we consume (Rich 2011; Wood and Skeggs 2008: 179). These relationships between eating, food preparation and self-development are depicted (and encouraged) in *Jamie's Italy* where consumption of food is a family activity, and consumers are part of its production in a working-class, local context.[9]

Against this complex background Jamie Oliver has appropriated, translated and transformed elements of these processes in his version of what food production, preparation, presentation and consumption should involve. The way in which food

---

9 Of interest here is the circulation, translation and transformation of foodstuffs on a global scale (New Zealand lamb in the UK, Californian oranges in Australia, etc.). This element has much to do with industrialisation and rationalisation of food. But alongside these processes we witness the transformation of the understandings and meanings associated with food within increasingly mediated and globalised settings (Kuehn 2009: 473; see also Lyon et al. 2003).

is understood by Oliver gives shape to the field in which Oliver's trainees find themselves. This is Oliver's world, where passion for food can be life changing.

His food philosophy emerges in different contexts, for example through his exploration of regional food variations in his journey through Italy (see Oliver 2005). The 'journey' operates as a pedagogical tool, a vehicle through which the viewer is taught about food production, preparation, presentation and consumption, based in peasant or working-class, rural and urban contexts: contexts in which knowledge about these elements is fiercely, proudly, and loudly articulated and defended. For instance, Hollows and Jones refer to Oliver as a 'moral entrepreneur' – 'able to give focus and leadership to debates about the place of cuisine within national life ... the moral entrepreneur makes explicit the relationship between consumption and morality' (2010: 309). This knowledge locates food – understood in these ways – at the centre of collective, social, familial, village, and neighbourhood life. These understandings of food are applauded, respected, honoured, sometimes romanticised by Oliver as expressions of what ought to be in terms of food. Yet, in these spaces the middle-class Essex boy – in the globalised/regionalised/localised spaces of twenty-first century food – was often represented as being out of his depth, and seen by many of the people he encounters as unskilled in the ways that *they* understand food.

Celebrity Culture and Social Entrepreneurship is also a complex field in which Oliver is positioned as a brand and as a particular type of pedagogue: someone involved in trying to (re)educate large populations about food, and as a charismatic and 'laddish' individual who provokes diverse, often passionate, forms and levels of attachment and antagonism (Hollows 2010: 308). In the globalised, mass mediated spaces that characterise the start of the twenty-first century we *consume* celebrity, and develop relationships and attachments to celebrities. The concept of *para-social* interaction or relationship highlights the ways in which we locate ourselves in what is, essentially, a one-way relationship with a celebrity. To illustrate: we know that Jamie Oliver exists. We form a sense of who he is. As a consequence of his media presence, profile, personae, we develop an orientation towards him. We *know* Jamie Oliver. Yet, importantly, he does not need to know that we exist for him to continue to be a celebrity, or to involve himself in media, educational, and political processes. This educative capacity can be understood and critiqued in various ways (see for instance Kelly and Harrison, 2009: 39–41). But the power of this capacity is enhanced within a context that is also shaped by the idea, practice and products of social entrepreneurship.

In the section that follows we present a glimpse of one young trainee from the Fifteen programme – Dovid. We provide a short account of his experiences in the programme, the challenges and expectations he faced, and the ways in which he responded to incentives to relate to food and to himself in particular ways. We then unpack Dovid's story using Foucault's ideas of technologies and practices of the self to show the ways in which *passion* pervades the philosophy of the moral entrepreneur and the training environment of *Jamie's Kitchen*.

Dovid's Story

> Dovid: My dad left when I was younger and stuff. Don't know what happened there you know. Like before mum passed away I spent a little bit of time with her and stuff like that and knowing her really well, but as you get older you realise how you haven't got a mum, haven't got a dad. What's going on? On days I cry and stuff you know because I miss her. (*Jamie's Kitchen Australia*, Episode Seven, Broadcast in Australia on Channel 10, 26 October 2006)

Dovid was a homeless 20 year old when he applied to be a Fifteen trainee, and during the series lived in a Melbourne refuge. He had not had parental support since he was 11. His mother is deceased. He did not know his father and was unsure why he left the family home. At his initial interview Dovid stated that he 'didn't really pass school'. He confessed to having a nervous disposition and said that he did not usually follow through with things and would often take the easy way out.

Dovid struggled for most of this series. In particular, it was thought that he showed a lack of confidence, skill, ability and to some extent passion – passion the way in which Oliver understands it. Jamie's Australian friend/fellow chef/ programme manager Toby Puttock had this to say about Dovid:

> Toby: Dovid is incredibly quiet and I don't know where his self-confidence is at. Like he always hesitates about doing things. He's really smart so I am sure if he just jumped in he'd nail it and it would be fine but he thinks 'What if I'm doing it wrong?' and he's kind of looking around at what everyone else is doing and I think he just needs to trust himself and just go with it and I've said that to him. (*Jamie's Kitchen Australia*, Episode Four, Broadcast in Australia on Channel 10, 5 October 2006)

Fellow trainees and others believed in Dovid and tried to help him along the way. At one point early on in the series another trainee Erin, a young mother on methadone treatment for a drug addiction, tried to help him out by swapping her successful rice dish for one that he had made a mess of. Dovid did the swap but confessed to Toby that he 'had help' when Toby asked him: 'Where did you pull this one from?' Toby took a measured approach to the situation and was supportive and encouraging. Despite Erin's concerns that no one was noticing it was obvious that they were. Eventually, Andrew Sankey (a trainer from Box Hill TAFE in Victoria, Australia) put Dovid on notice that he may fail the course.

Despite the willingness of chefs and trainers to support them, the trainees still had to pass the theory and training hurdles put in front of them – and in a short period of time. Episode Five saw Dovid in further difficulty when he studied recipes for the wrong day and quickly became overwhelmed.

> Andrew Sankey: He can't organise himself. He did work for the wrong day. He had it all wrong.

Voice Over: After a slow start it's an apprehensive Dovid serving up his first dish. The clock's ticking. Despite having three dishes still to cook Dovid's been sprung by Training and Development Chef Glenn taking a break.

Dovid: I don't want to say I don't want to do it and stuff but it's confusing.

Glenn: Look you're going okay. You're giving it something but you are not giving it enough. Do you think you've got what it takes to make it in the kitchen?

Dovid: No.

Glenn: See you've already quit before you've even started. If you think like that you'll never get anywhere.

Dovid: Yeah.

Glenn: You're like 45 minutes before your exams due and you've got something boiling there on the stove and you're not even a quarter of the way into what you need to be done. You're down here having a cigarette. To me that's not commitment. That's running away. That's not stepping up to the plate and getting back in the kitchen and putting it out.

Dovid: It's not running away … It's saying … I'm sorry that you see it that way and stuff.

Glenn: I'm just saying it the way I see it. I've got all you guys. I'm here to help. Don't get me wrong mate, I'm on your side 100% but if you don't pass this

TAFE … If Andrew doesn't give you a pass through you're not going to make it into the restaurant and we want all you guys to go through cos that's why you're here. Okay so you need to really put your head down. Alright? And get into it. Keep focussed and make it happen.

Dovid to camera: It just seems that they can see more in me than I can actually see in myself. You know they can see that I can do this but really … you know what I mean? Like put yourself in my shoes. I don't think I'm doing a real perfect job. (*Jamie's Kitchen Australia*, Episode Five, Broadcast in Australia on Channel 10, 12 October 2006)

Dovid, here, displays a particularly limited sense of self, of the possibilities and choices that he imagines are open to him, of the skills and capacities that he thinks he brings to the training and work environment. Throughout the Fifteen series we develop a sense of a lifecourse characterised by loneliness and ongoing failure, marginalisation and exclusion from mainstream institutions and relationships.

Dovid eventually observes that 'If I didn't pass it then I guess there's no more chances from this point on', and with this realisation he put in the extra effort. Despite Andrew Sankey's predictions, Dovid managed to pass his theory and practical tests. His success seemed to mark a turning point in his progress.

> Dovid: That just shows I am learning a lot of things out of this. I was impressed with myself but at the same time I was like confident about what I had done as well. I didn't want to get the perfect score I just wanted to get a little bit of good feedback you know, on what I'd actually done. (*Jamie's Kitchen Australia*, Episode Six: Broadcast in Australia on Channel 10, 19 October 2006)

Even though Dovid appeared more confident in the training environment where he was well supported, this confidence was very fragile and work experience at La Luna restaurant in Melbourne saw him struggling again. Adrian Richardson, the head chef at La Luna, decided to work with Dovid one to one and slowly his confidence in the kitchen grew. Despite some further setbacks Dovid seemed to find his feet amid the heat and noise of the kitchen.

In the final episode the trainees cooked and played host to the chefs that welcomed them into their restaurant kitchens for their work experience. Dovid was selected to stand up in front of everyone and thank the chefs on behalf of the rest of the trainees.

In many respects the processes of self-transformation that we witness with Dovid exemplifies the sorts of outcomes Fifteen aims for: 'We want to provide skills and experience in food preparation and service at the same time as helping our people to believe in themselves, to know that they can achieve anything they want in their lives despite what setbacks they may already have experienced' (Fifteen 2005). In the section that follows we unpack Dovid's story to show how processes, systems, support structures and rationalities come together to facilitate Dovid developing new forms of self-understanding, that promise, as the programme hopes, to create new options and choices, new fields of possibilities in which Dovid might imagine and fashion a future; a future where there are still no certainties or guarantees.

Food, Passion and the Transformation of the Self

> Jamie: None are formally trained as far as we know. They are all unemployed and not in education. So all we can look for really is a bit of passion with food.
>
> *The trainees file in one at a time for the taste test.*
>
> Jamie: What are you tasting? What do you like about it? What does it make you feel?

They have trouble expressing themselves.

> Jamie: Would you say you are not good at expressing yourself? (Pause) … with regard to flavours? (Young man agrees) If you want to be a chef it comes from the palate really, and from the heart. (*Jamie's Kitchen*, Episode One, Broadcast in Australia on Channel 10, 21 July 2003)

Although Dovid managed to transform himself and his attitudes towards food throughout the programme, his initial lack of 'Oliver style' passion was a concern for trainers.[10] This *lack of passion* is situated against the expectations of Oliver: '*I wasn't expecting loads, only inspiration.*' Efforts to overcome this problem, drive the anxieties, uncertainties, confrontations and collaborations that manufacture the drama we witness in *Jamie's Kitchen*. Against this dramatic backdrop the idea that trainees need to develop passion – to *be* or *become* passionate – is made concrete.

In the selection and training of young people Oliver and his staff indicate that *being* passionate about food is a desirable and positive attribute that will make trainees more effective, more productive, more creative. Passion underlies motivation and enhances performance. In this section we will turn to a more detailed analysis of the role of passion in *Jamie's Kitchen* framed by Foucault's *technologies of the self*. This analytic enables us to understand passion, and its particular manifestations in *Jamie's Kitchen*, as a powerful technology of self-transformation. We understand passion as emerging in three ways in the discursive field of Jamie's Kitchen:

- It emerges from particular forms of knowledge and ways of knowing the self, vocational training, paid work, the restaurant industry, food.
- It is produced, regulated and managed within relations of power – sovereignty, discipline and government – that emerge from and give structure/shape to particular fields of possibilities.
- It seeks to provoke and produce certain practices of the self – understood in terms of the development and performance of an entrepreneurial, passionate self.

Passion becomes a pedagogical device or framework for self-transformation, and food is the vehicle which is used to engender that passion and disposition. That is, the philosophical approach of *Jamie's Kitchen* is that passion can help you turn your life around, and food is a way of getting in touch with, awakening and operationalising that passion.

---

10 This lack of passion is a trait shared by other potential Fifteen candidates. Although some appeared more passionate, articulate and convincing than others, it was clear from the beginning that their food repertoires were limited in terms of the variety of food available to them, their food preferences and their previous cooking experience.

In his later work Foucault developed and introduced certain concepts to open up the field of historical analysis of the forms that the self, power and knowledge assumed at particular moments. In this section we want to think about passion by using a number of these tools. In analysing the forms that the self, that self-knowledge, and the incitements and encouragements to know the self in certain ways have taken at different times, Foucault argued that; 'neither a recourse to an original experience nor the study of the philosophical theories of the soul, the passions, or the body' (2000b: 87–8) could be the principal interest. Rather, the sorts of studies that he undertook were guided by the concept of *technologies of the self* – encouragement or incitements to behave in one way or another encountered by the individual. The self, in this frame, has no originary or ultimate essence, but takes, instead, a number of forms that emerge in particular ways, in particular contexts, in relation to particular purposes.

In this sense, argued Foucault (2000b: 88), histories of the care of the self would be histories of subjectivity – that is, histories of the way in which subjects are formed and give themselves meaning in any given time/place. Such histories would be concerned with the 'putting in place, and the transformations in our culture, of 'relations with oneself', with their technical armature and their knowledge effects' (Foucault 2000b: 88). Within this sort of analytical project the question of governmentality would become one in which the central concern would be; 'the government of the self by oneself in its articulation with relations with others (such as one finds in pedagogy, behaviour counselling, spiritual direction, the prescription for models of living and so on)' (Foucault 2000b: 88). From this perspective we can analyse passion, and the characteristics it assumes in *Jamie's Kitchen* and in the training of marginalised young people, as a powerful technology of self-transformation.

First, passion is represented as emerging from, and framing, particular forms of *knowledge and ways of knowing* – the self, vocational training, paid work, the restaurant industry, and food. So, marginalised young people are understood in certain ways and as requiring certain processes and practices to be put in place to enable a passion to emerge or develop from an initial sense of self that is anything but passionate. Dovid's interactions with Glen demonstrate the attitudes that are encouraged. Glen says: 'When you're down here having a cigarette. To me that's not commitment. That's running away. That's not stepping up to the plate and getting back in the kitchen and putting it out'. This type of regular training aims to connect young people like Dovid with the preferred work ethic and attitude towards food and food preparation.

In the time and spaces spanned by the original series, the emergence of a vision to develop Fifteen as a global social enterprise brand, and the Australian series, knowledges (*truths*) about how to achieve this vision have been reflexively reformulated. The aim has been to produce, for example, different ways of understanding the entering behaviours of these young people, and of the practices, processes and relationships that might facilitate processes of self-transformation – with lower attrition rates and less focus on individual failings/lacks.

The sorts of understandings of food that Jamie Oliver is famous for are produced as *truths* about food. Food, understood in these ways, is something to get passionate about. It can excite the passions. It can be produced, prepared, presented and consumed with passion. Because food is understood in these ways the work that goes on in a restaurant kitchen is also something to be passionate about (Palmer et al. 2010: 311). Through the two series, we see that for many trainees, not all the training and regimentation, the rule learning and obeying, and the skill development that is a necessary precursor to becoming a cook or a chef is all that passion provoking. Indeed, the menial and mundane nature of many of these practices of the self can dampen passion, can make you bored (for more see Kelly and Harrison 2009: 109). For instance, even when Dovid wants a cigarette break he is encouraged to stay in the kitchen and continue his work, whether he wants to or not.

Second, passion is produced, regulated and managed within relations of power – *sovereignty, discipline and government* – that emerge from and give structure/shape to particular fields of possibilities (Foucault 1991). In the context of this training programme – undertaken in various spaces including training colleges and restaurant kitchens – sovereignty represents the relationship of power which locates authority in the hierarchy of chefs, cooks, assistants that characterise the restaurant kitchen. An example of technologies of the self that explicitly seek to discipline, can be seen in the use of military metaphors to identify *command and control* structures that are understood as being vital to the task of preparing and presenting substantial amounts of food, *to order*, and on time – 'Yes Chef' and 'Right away Chef!'. Throughout both series, in kitchens, in off-the-job training spaces, we witness the exercise of sovereignty by head chefs, trainers and teachers, at the same time as we witness trainees resisting, or choosing to conform, to these demands. The aim of the exercise of sovereignty is to establish the field, and its limits, in which appropriate forms of passion might emerge. This type of discipline is however exercised with caution; this is not a regular apprenticeship course. Apart from the trainees' journey being televised and monitored by outsiders, their development is monitored by a number of trainers with particular goals in mind. For these trainees discipline is balanced with behind-the-scenes moral guidance from Oliver and the training chefs, with the aim of seeing the trainees complete the programme.

In this training environment disciplinary power takes a form that requires trainees to submit to the often menial, mundane tasks of cleaning, of maintaining a work place/space and utensils such as pots, pans, knives. It also involves learning, repeating, and mastering the mechanics of food preparation. At one level this cleaning, sweeping, tidying, dicing, slicing treadmill seeks to develop essential skills. At another level, it promises to develop new forms of self-awareness and self-knowledge: as someone who can discipline themselves: can conform to the demands of rationalised clock time, workplace practices and behaviours: can situate and understand their membership of a crew or team which is more than the sum of its individual parts: can become passionate about doing these things well through a sense that they have a purpose, and that this purpose contributes to a larger project which can deliver feelings and understandings of self-worth, competence, ability. Discipline cannot *will* passion into existence, but these forms and relations of power promise to produce a skill, knowledge, attitude base from which passion might be uncovered or emerge.

Third, passion seeks to produce certain entrepreneurial *practices of the self*. These practices take their shape from the field of possibilities structured by the relationships between knowledge and relations of power outlined above. In *Jamie's Kitchen* and in the Fifteen programme these practices of the self include attendance requirements at both college and in work placements; the mundane, menial tasks of cleaning work benches, ovens, grills and hotplates, floors and utensils; learning how to correctly dice, slice and generally prepare and present ingredients so that dishes can be cooked, assembled and presented for consumption – the seemingly endless practice of diverse skills and techniques that are vital to food preparation in the hectic, frenzied, chaotic context of commercial kitchens; tasting and testing of foods in ways that develop new vocabularies, understandings and orientations to food and its possibilities; shopping and sourcing expeditions to develop and practice skills necessary to knowing food as having different origins, different qualities, different possibilities in terms of preparation and as ingredients for particular dishes; team-building excursions to test the limits of the self, to locate the self in different fields where different understandings of the self, and of others, and of a team might be encouraged to form. This training and knowledge – these practices that become fragments of the trainees themselves – is the basis from which it is hoped entrepreneurial young people/futures will emerge. This development can be seen in Dovid, towards the end of his time in Jamie's kitchen. Dovid develops a way of knowing himself that is different from the ways in which he understood and critiqued himself at the beginning of the course. From a lack of confidence and replacing his meals with those of other students during assessments, to the reflection: 'I am learning a lot of things out of this. I was impressed with myself but at the same time I was like confident about what I had done as well.' Dovid also becomes aware of the greater purpose of the programme – the particular type of education and employment opportunity that has been offered. An opportunity that means seeing the self as entrepreneurial: 'If I didn't pass it then I guess there's no more chances from this point on.'

Conclusions

The television series *Jamie's Kitchen* provides a glimpse into the ways in which popular, public and personal understandings of food are shaped and deployed as knowledge, practice and passion (Luke and Luke 1997). In this context, food is not only to be consumed and enjoyed; it is a vehicle for the communication of preferred ways of knowing and understanding the self, and preferred ways acting – on ourselves, and in relation to others. These technologies of the self-structure and emerge from a variety of fields in which social class, gender, ethnicity, age and a number of other relations shape our understandings of ourselves and others.

The evidence from *Jamie's Kitchen* and from the Fifteen programme is that passion has the capacity to transform the self, to be a vital ingredient in processes of salvation – however precarious these processes may be – promoting performance, productivity, and motivation. Passion can energise the self, can give direction or purpose or meaning to a life. It can be creative, it can be a skill.

But this reading of passion should be approached and analysed as being problematic – as a particular truth that in certain contexts seek to produce particular outcomes. Marginalised young people, may not appear as passionate, may not approach a variety of tasks, activities and skill development processes with much passion – at least not initially (and in a sense this is tied to the valorisation of affective labour). They may be passionate, but just not about the things that work organisations and labour markets demand, or not in ways that their trainers, mentors, supervisors and bosses imagine as appropriate. Passion, as a vital ingredient in processes of self-transformation in Jamie's Kitchen, is disciplined and exercised by a self capable of practising well regulated, self-governing autonomy. The self here needs to be *made* passionate via a variety of pre-approved practices of the self.

These pre-approved or socially acceptable practices of the self are given shape within a much wider social context. As Bauman (2004: 6) argues the 'totality of human production and consumption has become money and market mediated, and the processes of the commodification, commercialization and monetarization of human livelihoods have penetrated every nook and cranny of the globe.' In these spaces – where salvation is precarious and uncertain, where trimming the fat and rationalisation, re-organisation, and re-engineering conspire to produce human waste, and where marginalised young people may, indeed, be condemned to material and social oblivion – then the training and development processes of social enterprises such as the Fifteen Foundation offer possibilities for young people to develop and practise forms of selfhood that might enable them to imagine and secure a different future (that is something no one can be sure of). For someone like Dovid this training and transformation of the self enabled him to imagine a future that was not characterised by homelessness, failure, loneliness, lack of a sense of worth. It enabled him to imagine a different Dovid: a Dovid that didn't sleep rough, a Dovid that was employed at something that he wanted to do, something that he could be passionate about, something that gave him different possibilities for understanding himself and his life.

As a pedagogue, as a moral entrepreneur, and as a lad, Jamie Oliver himself is an artefact of a particular moment in history. Oliver embodies a time when innovation and passion, willingness to learn new skills, and meet the demands of industries that hold out no promise of job security – are dispositions not only relevant to the lives of young trainees in *Jamie's Kitchen*. Young people like Dovid who are part of the Fifteen programme, are encouraged by Oliver's understanding of food to know themselves as capable of the transformation necessary to survive in a commodified, commercialised world. Those viewers who tune in to watch the trials, challenges and success of the trainees, can perhaps relate to the lessons taught in Oliver's kitchen and how passion can be practised in their own lives towards different ends.

References

Bauman, Z. 2004. *Wasted Lives: Modernity and its Outcasts*. Cambridge: Polity Press.

Campbell, P., Kelly, P. and Harrison, L. 2011. The Problem of Aboriginal Marginalisation: Education, Labour Markets and Social and Emotional Wellbeing. [Online: Alfred Deakin Research Institute Working Series No.20, Alfred Deakin Research Institute, Deakin University, Geelong]. Available at: http://www.deakin.edu.au/research-services/forms/v/3280/wps-31w.pdf [accessed: 10 March 2012].

———, Kelly, P. and Harrison, L. 2011. Social Enterprise: Challenges and Opportunities. [Online: Alfred Deakin Research Institute Working Series No.20, Alfred Deakin Research Institute, Deakin University, Geelong]. Available at: http://www.deakin.edu.au/alfred-deakin-research-institute/publications/workingpapers.php#working_paper_no_19_%27social_enterprise:_challenges_and_opportunities%27_48_55 [accessed: 10 March 2012].

Couldry, N. 2006. *Listening Beyond the Echoes: Media, Ethics, and Agency in an Uncertain World*. Boulder: Paradigm.

Defourny, J. and Nyssens, M. 2007. Defining Social Enterprise, in *Social Enterprise: At the Crossroads of Market, Public Policy and Civil Society*, edited by M. Nyssens, S. Adam, and T. Johnson. London: Routledge, 1–26.

Fifteen Foundation.2005. What's right with these young people. London: Fifteen Foundation.

Flowers, R. and Swan, E. 2012. Pedagogies of doing good: Problematisations, authorities, technologies and teleologies in food activism. *Australian Journal of Adult Learning*, 52(3), 532–72.

Foucault, M. 1987. *The History of Sexuality*, vol. 2. New York: Vintage.

———. 1988. Technologies of the Self, in *Technologies of the Self: A Seminar with Michel Foucault*, edited by L.H. Martin, H. Gutman and P.H. Hutton. London: Tavistock, 16–49.

———. 1991.Governmentality, in *The Foucault Effect: Studies in Governmental Rationality*, edited by G. Burchell, C. Gordon and P. Miller. Hemel Hempstead: Harvester Wheatsheaf, 87–104.

———. 2000b. Technologies of the Self, in *Michel Foucault Ethics, Subjectivity and Truth*, edited by Paul Rabinow. London: Penguin, 223–52.

Hage, G. 2003. A Viable Ethics: Journalists and the 'Ethnic Question', in *Remote Control: New Media, New Ethics*, edited by C. Lumby and E. Probyn. Cambridge: Cambridge University Press, 74–86.

Hollows, J. and Jones, S. 2010. 'At least he's doing something': Moral entrepreneurship and individual responsibility in Jamie's Ministry of Food. *European Journal of Cultural Studies*, 13(3), 307–22.

Jaffe, J. and Gertler, M. 2006. Victual vicissitudes: Consumer deskilling and the (gendered) transformation of food systems. *Agriculture and Human Values*, 23(2), 143–62.

Kelly, P. and Harrison, L. 2009. *Working in Jamie's Kitchen: Salvation, Passion and Young Workers*. Victoria: Palgrave Macmillan.

Kuehn, B.M. 2009. Melamine scandals highlight hazards of increasingly globalized food chain. *JAMA: The Journal of the American Medical Association*, 301(5), 473–5.

Lewis. T. 2007. He needs to face his fears with these five queers!: Queer eye for the straight guy, makeover TV and the lifestyle expert. *Television and New Media*, 8(4), 285–311.

Luke, C. and Luke, H. 1997.Techno-Textuality: Representations of Femininity and Sexuality. *Media International Australia* 84(May): 46–58. Available at: http://www.razonypalabra.org.mx/ anteriores/n9/techno.htm.

Lyall, S. 2003.The Naked Chef's Wicked Act. [Online: *New York Times*, 29 January. Available at:http://query.nytimes.com/gst/fullpage.html?sec=travel&res=9B0 7EFDC1039F93AA15752C0A9659C8B63 [accessed: 14 March 2007].

Lyon, P., Colquolhoun, A. and Alexander, E. 2003. Deskilling the domestic kitchen: National tragedy or the making of a modern myth? *Food Service Technology*, 3(3/4), 167–75.

Nehamas, A. 1998. *The Art of Living: Socratic Reflections from Plato to Foucault*. Berkeley: University of California Press.

Oliver, J. 2005. *Jamie Oliver: Jamie's Italy*. London: Penguin.

Palmer, C., Cooper, J. and Burns, P. 2010. Culture, identity and belonging in the culinary underbelly. *International Journal of Culture, Tourism and Hospitality Research*, 4(4), 311–26.

Rich, E. 2011. 'I see her being obesed!': Public pedagogy, reality media and the obesity crisis. *Health*, 15(1), 3–21.

Short, F. 2003. 'Domestic cooking practices and cooking skills: Findings from an English study. *Food Service Technology*, 3(3/4), 177–85.

Smith, G. 2006. *Jamie Oliver: Turning up the Heat*. Sydney: Pan Macmillan.

Versteegan, H. 2010. Armchair Epicures: The Proliferation of Food Programs on British TV, in M. Gymnich and N. Lennartz (eds), *The Pleasures and Horrors of Eating* (Representations and Relections 1). Bonn: Bonn University Press, 447–64.

Wood, H. and Skeggs B. 2008. Spectacular Morality: Reality Television, Individualisation and the Remaking of the Working Class, in *The Media and Social Theory*, edited by D. Hesmondhalgh and J. Toynbee. London: Routledge, 177–93.

Chapter 6

The *Loi Evin*: A Pedagogical Experiment in Responsible Drinking

Julie Robert

Introduction

Amid concerns about health and other social costs, a large number of countries have adopted strategies (such as social marketing, formal education initiatives, regulation of the industry and criminalisation of behaviours associated with overconsumption) to promote drinking in morally, socially and physically 'responsible' ways.[1] This chapter examines how efforts to promote 'responsible drinking' in late twentieth century France proceeded via stringent regulation of advertisements for alcohol. The French government's approach, encapsulated in the 1991 *Loi Evin*, is predicated on a number of assumptions about the power of advertising, namely that it succeeds in selling products, promoting consumption, creating brand loyalty and manipulating consumers by enticing them to act in ways that may contradict their own volition. Anne Cronin (2004) has dubbed these perceived effects 'advertising myths', owing to their relatively unquestioned status as truths about advertising's efficacy.

The law's framers have taken up these myths in relation to alcohol advertising and have construed them as pedagogies of alcohol consumption. The *Loi Evin* was accordingly formulated as a way of countering and blocking the advertisers' pedagogies with ones that put public health interests first. Conceived as a tough measure to limit the influence of advertising and its effects on consumption patterns, the law's basis on suppositions about how alcohol advertisements and public health messages educate consumers about drinking might more realistically be seen as an experiment in which hypotheses about how advertising and public health messaging 'work' are tested. This experiment consisted of both blocking 'bad' or 'dangerous' but effective pedagogies and countering these messages with 'good' pedagogies more consistent with the goals of government and the public health sector. This chapter examines the hypotheses or 'imagined pedagogies' underpinning this experiment and considers the outcomes in terms of what

1 What constitutes responsibility has been a contentious issue, for as Adam Barry and Patricia Goodson (2010) note, industry definitions (which tend to be centred on social dimensions) vary significantly from those in public health (which focus more on moderation).

impact the law had (more symbolically than epidemiologically) in relation to its understanding of how pedagogies of alcohol consumption operate.

The *Loi Evin* presupposes three imagined pedagogies, or assumptions about how people come to learn about alcohol consumption. In the first instance, there is the belief, founded mostly on hypodermic models of mass communication and public health research (Tulloch and Lupton 1997), that advertising (especially for products like alcohol) constitutes a dangerous pedagogy. The imagined pedagogies, however, also extend to presumptions about *how* alcohol advertising influences choices.

What kinds of pedagogies are most effective in teaching people about consumption? How are they communicated? What is communicated that makes a given pedagogy more or less effective? How are consumers connecting with messages? These questions lead to the second imagined pedagogy, which is that affective identification with drinkers portrayed in advertisements is a key facet of alcohol advertising. The law thus blocks so-called lifestyle advertising and mandates 'information only' advertisements that ostensibly appeal only to rational judgements about a product. This prohibition posits affect as a key pedagogical process, insofar as 'aspects of embodiment and desire are already and always sources of action in pedagogical relationships' (Evans et al. 2008: 111).

The third imagined pedagogy tested by the law is a corollary of the second, namely that positive affect about drinking can be countered by an affect of fear of its consequences. The dissemination of knowledge about moderate drinking and warnings about the health risks of immoderation were thus put forth as a means to motivate rational choices about alcohol consumption.

For all its attention to how advertisements function as pedagogies, the *Loi Evin* – among the world's strictest codes of its kind – has not generated the results anticipated. Using a visual and discursive analysis of a post-Evin advertising campaign and a close reading of its mandatory health message as a case study, this chapter shows how the legislation has not blocked the more influential aspects of affect-driven pedagogies of drinking promoted by the industry. Moreover, it has failed to produce successful counter-pedagogies of responsible drinking, which is to say messages about health and moderation that would subvert or undermine the 'unhealthy' or 'irresponsible' pedagogical effect of the advertisements the among the target population. These shortcomings owe to a variety of factors: a hollow distinction between objective information and affect-generating narrative, an over-investment in the interpellative pedagogical capacity of health warning messages and a disregard for the way in which pedagogies are received by learners. These failures suggest that those looking to mitigate or otherwise influence the circulation and reception of public pedagogies ought to pay careful attention to not only the way in which they are produced, but also the ways how they may be taken up and transformed by learners.

Before proceeding, a quick note on terminology might be helpful. This study uses the terms 'public pedagogy' and 'pedagogy' interchangeably. This is not to deny the importance of the debates about classification of cultural, everyday and public pedagogies highlighted by Anna Hickey-Moody, Glenn Savage and Joel

Windle (2010), but simply to situate this particular study within the mass media framework. Henry Giroux's media studies work on what he has labelled 'public pedagogies' informs my terminology, but I also propose to think more broadly about the term. Hence, I take public pedagogy to mean the cultural, social and political spaces and discourses in which processes of normalisation (although also contestation and resistance) occur. At the same time, 'public pedagogy' also refers to the processes and functions that operate within these spaces and on and within learners to generate experiences and impressions from which meaning is made and through which learning happens.

The *Loi Evin*: A Plan for Public Health

The *Loi Evin*, introduced in 1991 and put into effect on 1 January 1993, restricts the ways in which alcohol can be marketed and sold.[2] In addition to tightening up loopholes in prior legislation, it aims to mitigate the impact of substances deemed harmful and addictive through controls on advertising and other forms of promotion.[3] A product of academic physicians and public health experts (Sulkunen and Ugland 2005), the law centres on a conception of public health that is less focused on changing individual behaviour, a common facet of what Alan Petersen and Deborah Lupton (1996) characterise as the neo-liberal inflected 'new public health,' than with modifying the environment that would influence health-related behaviours (Sulkunen and Ugland 2005).[4] It relies on communications strategies such as the 'effects' and 'knowledge-attitude-behaviour' models (Tulloch and Lupton 1997), which aim to 'get the message out' using health care networks, schools, community groups and the media in its 'public service', entertainment and information variants. The goal of such campaigns is to inform the public by introducing a message that counters either other discourses, like advertising, or to undermine persistent cultural beliefs, for instance that alcohol will warm you up on a cold day.[5] This environmental orientation recognises that public health is just

2 The law also contains provisions that concern the sale of alcohol to young people, the locations and hours for alcohol sales and regulations about tobacco advertising.

3 Sponsorship of sports teams, sporting and cultural events and even media coverage of alcohol-related events (such as the annual release of Beaujolais Nouveau) that are thought to err too much toward the promotion of consumption (Loi Evin/Censure: La presse du vin s'inquiète 2008; Rigaud and Craplet 2004) are among the 'promotional' aspects of alcohol that also fall under the purview of the law.

4 A school within the field of public health (Dorfman and Wallack 1993; Mosher and Wallack 1981) has argued that this global approach is preferable in that it reduces the potential for stigma and targets systemic causes of unhealthy behaviour. Critics of what they term the universalising nature of French public health (Caron 2001) have nonetheless protested that it frequently fails to target services and messaging toward those at greater risk.

5 Health education and health promotion also employ a number of other strategies, many of which rely on models other than message dissemination, to accomplish their aims.

that – public – and operating at the broad social and cultural level whereby it is society as a whole that is influenced by the national media landscape.

The *Loi Evin* states that alcoholic beverages can be marketed only on the radio (during hours when children would not reasonably expected to be listening), online (via sites that are, in theory, accessible only to adults), in print advertising and on billboards using information-based promotion relating to the product's origin, composition, production, distribution, colour, alcohol content and potential uses. All advertisements must also include a standardised warning about the (non-specific) health dangers of alcohol consumption and a reminder to drink in moderation. The provisions for the inclusions of this statement are not subject to prescriptions in terms of placement, colour or size.

Table 6.1 The *Loi Evin* in brief

Permitted	Prohibited
• Billboard and print advertisements, subject to health messaging • Radio advertisements, during certain hours only • Online content, subject to health messaging and age restriction • Content relating to a product's: – Origin (national, terroir) – Composition (ingredients, alcohol content) – Production (methods, producers) – Distribution – Colour – Uses (recipes, serving suggestions) – Logo – Packaging – Name	• Television advertisements • Sponsorship of sports teams or events • Placement of advertisements near sports facilities • Depiction of people (including body parts) so long as they cannot be readily identified as professional producers or distributors of the product (i.e. sommeliers, winemakers)* * Technically anything not explicitly authorised is prohibited, but the restriction on people has been particularly controversial

Henriette Touillier-Feyrabend (2006) notes the *Loi Evin* shifted French policy from one, common to most nations with legislation of this nature, whereby anything not prohibited is allowed, to one where anything not explicitly authorised is forbidden. The visuals of post-Evin ads therefore disproportionately feature imagery such as bottles, glassware and close-up shots of the product. With the exception of

Some of these (including having target audiences design campaigns) have been used in conjunction with the Loi Evin, but both independent scholars and health officials have been critical of the measures for being insufficient, sporadic, underfunded, embarrassing and for, therefore, failing to produce results (Direction Générale de la Direction Générale de la Santé 2001; Sulkunen and Ugland 2005; ANPAA 2003; Craplet 2001).

depicting those that can be readily associated (for instance by their uniform or the image's backdrop) with either the production or distribution of the product (i.e. a sommelier, brewer or winemaker), people have also effectively been banned from visual advertisements. These restrictions have been court tested and upheld, as recently as 2012, on the grounds that the presence of people constitutes 'lifestyle advertising', or the attempt to promote a product through the marketing of a way of living. Such tactics are deemed to foster a (false) causal relationship between drinking and conviviality or emotional states resulting from consumption (Andrieu 2012) and thus violate the spirit of the law to allow only the provision of objective product information. What is accordingly at issue is a presumption that positive, affect-driven pedagogies are more effective – and thus more dangerous from a public health point of view – than supposedly 'information-only' pedagogies.

Since its introduction, industry pressure has weakened some of the law's provisions, notably around where advertisements may appear – so much so that government reports have blamed the inconsistencies and loopholes for turning a good idea in theory into a problematic and ineffective practice (Sulkunen and Ugland 2005). Advertisers have found ways to innovatively subvert the law's intent, for even whilst working within the content restrictions, they continue to market their products and build brand recognition. Pascal Beucler and Fanny Favreau (2003) have called these restrictions 'productive constraints' in that they have pushed advertisers toward tactics that exalt the brand and its qualities and which infuse elements of surprise and creativity into advertisements in ways not typical of the pre-Evin era. Commentators associated with the wine industry in particular have nonetheless argued that advertisers are self-censoring to an extreme degree for fear of costly legal sanction (Gillis 2012). The conclusions about the law's efficacy are varied and reveal almost as much about the commentator as they do about the statute itself.[6] Despite these debatable successes and shortcomings, other nations have been looking at Evin-style measures to address the public health issues relating to alcohol, if only because France's media landscape now bears the definitive imprint of the restrictions.

Imagined Pedagogy #1: Alcohol Advertisements as Public Pedagogy

As mentioned above, pedagogical power comes from the ability to normalise attitudes and behaviours. Hickey-Moody, Savage and Windle (2010) see this normative facet of public pedagogy as crucial, for once established as a cultural norm, a practice need no longer depend on explicit (and in this case paid)

6 French wine producers, many of whom operate independently or in small collectives, have been most critical of the law because their marketing budgets are relatively small and do not allow them to do the kind of in-person marketing (hosting events, maintaining a flashy online presence) favoured by larger conglomerates for getting around the law (Georges 2013).

pedagogies to be taught, for it becomes an almost self-perpetuating cultural practice. The first hypothesis or imagined pedagogy to be tested by the *Loi Evin*, therefore, is advertising's efficacy in setting norms relating to how and why people should consume alcohol.

The notion that advertisements impact upon norms and thus constitute a form of public pedagogy has been well studied from both public health and cultural points of view. From the effect-centric perspective of traditional public health, advertising is an all too effective form of pedagogy in that it that succeeds in inculcating knowledge and changing attitudes and behaviours to products and practices deemed unhealthy (Gerbner 1990), hence the lobbying for greater regulation of the advertising industry. From the health education perspective, these three outcomes (knowledge, attitudes, behaviours) represent the trifecta of effective pedagogy (Tulloch and Lupton 1997). A host of studies link exposure to media messages and images about alcohol (alcohol advertising in particular) to attitudinal shifts and increased alcohol consumption among children, teenagers and adults (Robinson et al. 1998; Connolly et al. 2006; Martin et al. 2002; Anderson et al. 2009).[7] Although findings about the extent and nature of the correlation between exposure to advertising and consumption vary, there is broad consensus (from studies done in a number of countries with a wide variety of sample advertisements that conform to the respective laws and codes governing advertising content) that advertising increases favourable perceptions of alcohol and influences decisions about when and how much to drink. Liz Stewart and Sally Casswell (1990) have gone so far as to argue that marketing has allowed the alcohol industry to position itself as a 'drug educator', which is to say a giver of norms in relation to the ways in which alcohol is to be consumed and the responses it is meant to evoke. Indeed, alcohol companies have used advertisements and other promotional schemes to campaign aggressively around normalising alcohol as a beverage like any other or returning it to its former classification as a foodstuff, as was the case in Southern Europe (Gual and Colom 1997), and resisting the public health community's attempts to consider it a drug akin to cannabis or tobacco.

Scholars of public pedagogy such as Godfrey Hodgson (2006) and Henry Giroux (1993) have upheld advertising in general as a highly effective vector of pedagogy, which lends broader cultural credence to the more empirical public health studies. As Cronin's (2004) discussion of popular 'antidote' discourses suggests, focusing on the power of one message or another does not contest the underlying principle that advertisements are effective public pedagogies. The *Loi Evin*, therefore, accepts the fundamental premise that alcohol advertising is both effective and dangerous

7 Many of these studies were conducted in controlled settings (laboratories, classrooms) and most focused on assessing the impact of advertising on children and adolescents (for whom models of hypodermic media influence are more accurate), not adults. While the findings cannot be discounted, more nuanced results are likely to emerge from studies that give greater weight to cultural factors beyond those variables which are normally controlled (Baillie 1996).

and in doing so concedes that the battle for responsible drinking and public health will and should be fought within the field defined by advertisers.

The Association Nationale de Prévention en Alcoologie et Addictologie (ANPAA, or the National Association for the Prevention of Alcoholism and Addiciton), a public health watchdog group that lobbied heavily for the changes brought in under the *Loi Evin* and which now initiates legal proceedings against infringing advertisers, embraces this first imagined pedagogy as justification for its interventions:

> Despite their reputation, public health experts do not whish [*sic*] to regulate peoples' lives and do no [*sic*] wish to treat them solely as consumers, unlike alcohol producers whose only wish is to impose consumption levels and are paradoxically the new 'norms givers'. On the contrary, the philosophy of the associations promoting prevention is to give citizens back their freedom of choice regarding products, consumption patterns and rituals and to prevent patterns and rituals to become bounds limiting freedom. (Rigaud and Craplet 2004: 5)

Of primary importance to the ANPAA is stripping alcohol advertisers of their (perceived) capacity to set cultural norms in relation to drinking practices in France. This defence of the *Loi Evin* also implicitly highlights the attempt to restore such influence to those whose primary mission is not to encourage maximum profit through maximum consumption. At issue in this question of norms-giving is agency, namely a deep unease with the prospect of 'citizen' freedom being impinged upon by commercial, drink-promoting interests. The ANPAA's discourse draws on questions of social values, political orientation and even French tradition (in an era when most alcohol is marketed by multinational conglomerates), but the organisation's public health roots are still evident in that it does not dispute the pedagogical power of advertising (and the need to combat it). Indeed, its statements and its decades-long campaign against advertisers reifies the advertiser's role in acting as (dangerous) norms-giver and its own function as necessary opposition.

There are nonetheless valid critiques that truly test and unsettle this imagined pedagogy. Taking up the methodological underpinnings of much of the public health care literature, Richard Baillie contends that 'the influence of the media has been examined in isolation without taking into consideration other variables which contribute to changes in levels of alcohol consumption/alcohol-related problems' (1996: 240). Similar reservations have been expressed by Jeffery Bineham (1988) and Keith Tones (1996). From a media studies perspective, Cronin has questioned the 'certainty' about advertisements as public pedagogies, arguing that public and private regulators 'nowhere clarify how to recognize an advertisement engaged in these persuasive practices' (2004: 42). Across both disciplines, scholars call for greater attention to how pedagogies of advertising are actually taken up by learners who are embedded in particular contexts. As will be shown below, such oversights are at the core of the *Loi Evin*'s failings.

The law has nonetheless attempted to do what Cronin argues should be done, which is to pinpoint how an advertisement becomes a pedagogy. This has come not through the rhetoric defending and promoting the law, but rather very implicitly through its design and prohibitions. It is thus that the role of affect emerges as the second imagined pedagogy to be tested.

Imagined Pedagogy #2: Dangerous Affect

The *Loi Evin*'s most controversial dictate, that people cannot (except for in very specific circumstances) appear in advertisements, is predicated on the notion that people are particularly effective norms-givers, which is to say that they are pedagogically powerful in the context of advertising. Public health officials see the use of people and positive scenarios in advertisements as the marketing of fantasies (Stewart and Casswell 1990; Nathanson-Moog 1984). Public pedagogy scholars, for their part, recognise this effect as the impact of embodiment and affect (Mankekar 1999; Hickey-Moody et al. 2010; Sandlin and Milam 2008). Affect, defined as 'what sustains or preserves the connection between ideas, values, and objects' (Ahmed 2010: 29), pedagogically operates in a number of ways, including but not limited to aspirational emulation and modelled behaviour (Goodman 2009). Theories of affective pedagogy hold that 'learning is fundamentally affective: it always entails the embodied labour of generating particular emotional states' (Hickey-Moody et al. 2010: 230). Controlling affect is thus hypothesised as the way to control learning.

The imagined pedagogy of affect underpins many of the law's prohibitions and subtly acknowledges what Elizabeth Ellsworth (2005: 2) calls the 'impetus [of] particular … affects of bodies/mind/brains in the midst of learning', which is to say the manner in which pedagogies of alcohol consumption generate learning by producing sensations and feelings that are particular to the individual and which thus have resonance. From the simple insinuation that a product will make one feel good or provoke enjoyment (defined as the illicit solicitation of 'l'émotion gustative' [tasting emotion]) (Andrieu 2012) to obvious uses of sex appeal, the *Loi Evin* attempts to impede the association of alcohol and positive affect. This prevents advertisers from using role models, be they celebrities or seemingly ordinary people who enjoy 'a socially and sexually fulfilling, as well as an economically satisfying, lifestyle' (Mosher and Wallack 1981: 334) to incite aspiration or emulation centred on their product.[8] The law removes these figures,

8 The ban on using logos on sports jerseys, for example, definitively prohibits a link between the accomplished and fit sporting body of the athlete and alcohol. Moreover, it deprives advertisers of the potent symbolism of the logo-clad body while the wearer's body exhibiting peak physical form and whilst the viewer is most attentive to it, which is to say during play (Hill and Casswell 2004). On a more quotidian level, aspirational emulation is denied when the seemingly average fellow who is lavished with attention by women, who

those with whom the public can associate, in whose shoes they can and/or want to see themselves and proscribes even the notion of a drinking (and by extension tasting and emotive) body.

The *Loi Evin*'s imagined pedagogies accordingly subscribe to several intertwined notions about the role of affect, pedagogy and embodiment, and the presence of people in advertisements. First, there is an assumption that that learning is driven by affect. Second, is the thought that affect is generated through embodiment. Third, the law presupposes that in removing people, who can be not only models for emulation, but also catalysts for emotions (from the minute to the grandiose), the influence of embodiment, and thus affect, might be controlled, which would limit the pedagogical power of alcohol advertisements. A series of advertisements for Gordon's London Dry Gin, shows in what ways the law's identification of these imagined pedagogies about affect and learning are mostly valid but, as the following case study reveals, cannot be controlled by the law.

The Gordon's advertisements in question feature an anthropomorphised boar (the head of which is the Gordon's logo) attempting to return home from a long night of partying at a London nightclub. The advertisement's copy varies slightly, but all advertisements in the series follow the formula of 'Gordon's au Limelight Club jusqu'aux … ' [Gordons, from the Limelight Club to …] and an indication – either textual, visual or both – of a safe way to return home. The cartoonish animal permitted by the allowances for emphasis on logos and elements thereof facilitates affective association for the viewer (Beucler and Favreau 2003). Its human-like poses – feet crossed, leaning against an umbrella or perched on a bus seat with one arm draped across the back of another bench – encourage viewers to see the boar as a plausible stand-in for themselves in situations in which empathetic association is desirable. The anthropomorphism and the cartoonishness of the advertisement, nonetheless, facilitates dissociation and reminders of the situation's unreality when it comes to considering matters that would be unpleasant – a hangover, being the victim of alcohol-related violence – but which might reinforce a more precise affective pedagogy relating to responsible drinking. Showing a lone, drunken, young woman trying to hail a cab in the middle of the night, for instance, might just prompt viewers to think about those omitted consequences.

In addition to the attempts to eliminate affective identification, the law's ban on television commercials and cinema advertising is suggestive of an imagined pedagogy concerning narrative's role in producing affect. The information-only rhetoric surrounding the law implies that creating narrative within its strictures will be difficult. A storyline nevertheless emerges from our sample advertisement – albeit in elision – for the jovial boar is no less a protagonist in this snapshot of an evening than embodied human actors would be in a television commercial. That this narrative is not delivered to the audience fully constructed, but rather as a sort of puzzle that must be put together in order to fully comprehend the interplay

---

drives an expensive car and who is the life of the party because he drinks a particular kind of spirit is no longer granted a place in French ads.

of product, protagonist, visual setting and text means that it requires processing, which is to say time spent engaging with the advertisement and its message. This kind of mental engagement is what Gina Agostinelli and Joel Grube (2002) call 'issue-relevant thinking' and describe as the kind of processing most likely to lead to changes in attitudes and behaviours. Gordon's Gin is therefore likely to become associated with the allure of partying in London.

As the creative play with the law's prohibitions and allowances suggest, the *Loi Evin* as pedagogical experiment in controlling affect in favour of information-based pedagogies cannot really be considered a success. I would, nonetheless, argue that its recognition of *how* advertising influences its target audience is notable. The law's ban on people, and to a lesser extent its prohibition of narrative, arises from the requirement that advertising address only certain permissible factors deemed to constitute 'information only' advertising.[9] Information is thus positioned as antithetical to affect insofar as information-based advertising is, at least according to the law's design, not meant to elicit affect. In practice, however, advertisers have gone to great lengths to circumvent and undermine the law's intent, perhaps indicating the underlying validity of the affect hypothesis.[10] Beucler and Favreau (2003) highlight the new strategies advertisers have used post-Evin to market their products more creatively than before and conclude that what remains unsaid and invisible in contemporary advertisements invites the audience's participation in a co-construction of meaning about the product. Affective engagement is thus solicited rather than meaning imposed.

One might surmise that the *Loi Evin* was predicated upon a binary construction of two imagined pedagogical powers. On the one hand, information is seen as controllable, subject to rationality and therefore a manageable risk. This kind of thinking about the role of information in pedagogy is common in public health circles. Known as 'information transfer' pedagogies, they assume that correct information (about a product or situation) and rationality will dictate choices (Flowers et al. 2001). On the other, affect is posited as dangerous in the hands of advertisers, for it is a way of manipulating audiences into consuming in irresponsible ways. The statute presupposes that stripped of the alluring trappings of sex appeal, desirable social settings, connotations of success and sensorial pleasures, consumers will be presented information about products in a vacuum of prejudicial and biased tactics. They will then be able to make rational and informed choices about their consumption. Affect, however, is not solely dependent upon

9 The decision to ban commercials has just as much if not more to do with the exposure that people have to television advertisements and the belief that marketing done via this medium is particularly effective and, therefore, dangerous from the point of view of the law's objectives.

10 Much can also be said about the 'non-advertising' pedagogies of alcohol consumption, such as product placement (Gupta and Gould 1997) and the ubiquity of alcohol in television and music videos (Robinson et al. 1998) and movies (Cin et al. 2008).

role models or embodiment; it can be generated in myriad ways and can thus influence learning even though its most obvious pathways are legally blocked.

A further problem comes from assuming that consumers/learners will act rationally if (in theory) presented with objective information. Drinking, as Thomas Wilson (2005) attests, is a highly contingent cultural practice that is informed by a host of factors that influence, cloud and even defy logic. Our ethno-cultural background, religion, geographic setting, age, gender and situational factors (employment situation, personal experience) influence our ability to generate (or fail to generate) particular affects in response to given stimuli. Thus even if the law succeeds in having the products marketed in a vacuum of other meanings, the message will always be received by consumers who are deeply embedded in situations that influence how messages will be taken up and acted upon. In most of the commentary on the law though, matters of particularised audience or learner reception are absent. 'Society' and 'youth', its most vulnerable segment, are discussed as almost homogeneous entities despite the implicit acknowledgement of the affective and therefore individualised nature of how pedagogies of alcohol consumption operate in advertisements.

Imagined Pedagogy #3: Fear Motivates Change

So far, the *Loi Evin* has been examined as a mostly reactive measure to the imagined pedagogical power of alcohol advertising. The third imagined pedagogy can, nonetheless, be seen as part of a proactive strategy to promote more responsible drinking. As with the second pedagogy, affect is at the core of the pedagogical experiment, for the goal is to elicit certain affective responses among the population and to consequently transform them into learners. The pedagogy finds its form in the mandatory health message that must appear on all print, billboard and Internet advertising. As will be explained below, however, the success of this pedagogical experiment hinges on knowing one's audience, both in terms of being able to predict their affective response to a given pedagogy and to recognise themselves as potential learners.

The health message typically appears in all caps, in a relatively small font size (approximately one-fiftieth of a standard-sized magazine ad) in all print advertisements and on billboards. Most often, the message is in thin white script, which may or may not be the most visibly contrasting colour given the advertisement's background. The message reads: 'L'abus d'alcool est dangereux pour la santé. À consommer avec modération' [Alcohol abuse is a health hazard. Consume in moderation]. The first part of the statement is a warning that is meant to play on the viewer's assumed fear of illness and/or death and on the presumed desire to minimise health risks. The word 'dangereux' functions as a caution that must be heeded. Commonly used on signage to mark less quotidian dangers such as high voltage, it has the potential to trigger alarm. This sense of the extraordinary is necessary to achieve the desired result, for as Emma Rich

(2011) notes in her work on the panic generated by anti-obesity reality television, fostering a sense of impending disaster or urgency is central to motivating changes in line with the objectives of a given pedagogy. Linking this danger to health, a prominent social and cultural issue in a country where in 2010, public and private spending on healthcare reached 11.6 per cent of GDP (OECD 2012) – the highest percentage among OECD countries – reinforces the idea that something that is both collectively and individually valued is threatened.

Although the health message is clear in its intent of reminding consumers about the dangers of alcohol abuse and its suggestion of moderation, its effects – even the symbolic ones – are debatable. This owes both to a misalignment between the message being articulated (or rather that is thought to be articulated according to an idealised notion of what the health message will do and what affects will be elicited, pedagogically speaking) and the medium of its articulation as well as to ambiguities within the message itself.

Health warnings have become not only the tell-tale sign of government intervention in alcohol advertising in France, but also the most visible counter-pedagogy in circulation. While there is at least one such message for every alcohol advertisement, the warning has been criticised for having become mundane, an all too often seen feature that is now more frequently ignored than noticed or contemplated as a prompt for behaviour change (Direction Générale de la Direction Générale de la Santé 2001). Thus ignored, the overt pedagogical message becomes something of a mute signifier amid a landscape already declared poor in public health messages promoting responsible drinking (Direction Générale de la Santé 2001, Craplet 2001, Sulkunen and Ugland 2005). As a pedagogy that fails to perform (pedagogy being both the spaces *and* processes that effect learning), the message ceases to be pedagogical, or rather in a case such as this, is disallowed its pedagogic power by virtue of being unnoticed. In a variation of that old chestnut about a tree falling in the forest, the *Loi Evin* and similar 'ignorable' messaging pedagogies prompt us to think about whether or not pedagogy must connect with an audience, in practice and in theory, for it to have any pedagogical power.

Within the message itself, the *Loi Evin* not only meets with but also produces its own resistances to desired pedagogical outcomes. Most of these problems centre around what Charles Atkin, Sandi Smith and Hae-Kyong Bang (1994) call 'strategic ambiguity', or the leaving up to viewers what constitutes the key terms that form the basis of the warnings. Undoubtedly, any attempts to change the legal message's wording to a more prescriptive formulation would meet with the same resistance from producers and distributors that the law initially faced when it had to be passed using exceptional parliamentary procedures.[11] These key

11 Although most of the world's commercially sold alcohol is distributed by multinational corporations, production in France remains closely tied to the agricultural sector, which exerts tremendous political influence. With rural voters being over-represented in parliament, politicians are by and large opposed to measures that would cost them the support of this influential constituency.

terms, notably 'abuse' and 'moderation', are nonetheless vital to the interpellative mechanism necessary to the health pedagogy. This is to say that people must recognise themselves as the warning's audience, as those needing to heed the message's warning, in order for the message to be effective in generating affect or even logical considerations, in short, for it to have any pedagogical power. The environmental approach to public health argues that everyone, not only those exhibiting certain risks, are targeted by these sorts of health messages. In actuality, however, it is individuals who must take up the message, consider it, and ideally act in the ways suggested. The interpellative function of health messaging is therefore paramount in thinking of them as pedagogy, for if interpellation fails, the pedagogy fails to find its audience and its effects remained solely imagined.

It is for these reasons that the term 'abuse' is problematic in relation to the law's objectives, particularly insofar as one would have to recognise the stigmatised term as relating to oneself. Medical and public health messaging about what is considered safe or healthy consumption varies, therefore what will be considered abuse will vary as well. In France, current definitions place acceptable levels at three standard units per day (each unit defined as 10 grams of pure alcohol) for men and two for women, but such notions are far from universal. From one country to another, standards about safe consumption are up for debate (Furtwængler and Visser 2013). How these standards are actually taken in and applied by the public also influences their effectiveness. The translation of medical standards for a single 'drink' do not necessarily correspond to those used by bar or cafe patrons or those drinking in private spaces, where a 'drink' is most often measured by the container in which it is served, not by the volume of pure alcohol. A 2001 Ministry of Health report found that upon surveying the population, the question of what qualifies as a standard drink aside, knowledge about what constitutes acceptable levels of consumption would have had men safely consuming 3.7 drinks per day, women 3 (Direction Générale de la Direction Générale de la Santé 2001).

Medical definitions of 'abuse', especially when such definitions are not widely known, are less likely to take precedence than cultural ones, which are influenced by time, ethnicity, religion and local customs. Members of the older generations, for example, are less likely to recognise consumption in excess of 'safe' levels as abuse given previous medical and social paradigms that defined alcoholism and alcohol abuse in terms of impaired function and/or the presence of withdrawal symptoms. These older citizens were, after all, those who would also recall advertisements warning consumers about the dangers of driving after a heavy meal without first having a Cointreau (or other digestive) for the road, lest they risk sleepiness from trying to digest a sumptuous meal unassisted (Touillier-Feyrabend 2006: 59). The presence of migrants from different ethno-cultural and religious backgrounds is also likely to influence personal definitions of alcohol abuse. Even within France, regions in the North and East have a popular reputation, one backed by epidemiological data, for being harder drinking than their Parisian and Southern compatriots (Direction Générale de la Direction Générale de la Santé 2001).

The second sentence of the health message and its focus on moderation is as vague as the first, for many of the same reasons. What constitutes moderation? Whose definition should apply? To use the average figure derived from survey data about what would constitute moderate drinking for an evening of friendly festivities, three aperitifs or digestives *along with* four glasses of wine would be considered moderate (Direction Générale de la Direction Générale de la Santé 2001), a far cry from the official recommendations for low-risk drinking.

All of this is to say that abuse and moderation, although defined in medical terms also carry lay definitions that are equally if not more prevalent in the process of self-identification necessary for pedagogies to find their audiences. Discrepancies between the intended audience (everyone) and the actual audience (those who recognise the health message as being addressed to them) reveal that cultural factors are significant here as well.

Audience Reception: The Unimagined Pedagogy?

All three of the imagined pedagogies underpinning the *Loi Evin* make assumptions about the power of pedagogies to connect with learners and influence them. By far, the greatest concentration of these suppositions clusters around audience reception: whether or not a member of an audience will see themselves as a learner, how somebody will react to health-related scare-tactics, what affective responses an advertisement will generate. Given that such matters are fundamental not only to connecting with an audience, but also to having them engage with the pedagogy (much less in the ways anticipated and desired), the *Loi Evin* evinces the gaps in its own rationales about pedagogical power.

These gaps help to explain why the *Loi Evin* has been so roundly criticised and why claims of success are largely limited to those of a qualitative or symbolic order (Casswell and Maxwell 2005). The law's impact has, by admission of even its strongest proponents, been near impossible to measure with any accuracy (ANPAA 2003). If the goal was to promote more moderate drinking, crude statistics such as average annual per capita consumption of pure alcohol do not separate out abstainers (who are likely to represent a significant segment of the population in light of Maghrebian Muslims representing France's largest minority group) from heavy drinkers. Yet, the law's effect on even these gross statistics has been difficult to gauge since average per capita alcohol consumption has been steadily declining since the 1970s (Gual and Colom 1997).

The very nature of these measures of 'success' shows a concern for population-level statistics. Yet to assess what is at the basis of the pedagogical experiment requires greater attention to the questions of audience reception inherent in pedagogies reliant upon affect. This important issue has been taken up in much of the unofficial and popular discussion of the law and its effects (Andrieu 2012; Georges 2013), but audience reception ought to figure more prominently in the official discourse about a law that concerns itself with how norms about alcohol consumption are communicated, internalised, acted upon and perpetuated.

Conclusion

The scientific method involves the formulation and testing of hypotheses in carefully controlled circumstances. For the authors of France's *Loi Evin*, the hypotheses put to the test were the imagined pedagogies of alcohol advertising, namely that advertising acts as a powerful public pedagogy due largely to its ability to generate positive affective states that motivate emulative behaviours. Also tested was a counter-hypothesis concerning the efficacy of traditional health messaging in playing upon similar, albeit fear-motivated, affective responses to generate responsible drinking behaviours. The test was a law that prescribed supposedly 'information-only' advertising and health messages embedded within these advertisements. The result was a distinctly French approach to alcohol advertising that all but eschewed people and traditional forms of lifestyle advertising, but which nevertheless allowed affective identification between the viewer and the product being marketed. Another outcome was a health message that neither connected with audiences nor was specific enough in its health messaging to be pedagogically useful. The pedagogical hypotheses, while in some ways validated, were also never fully tested due to the ambiguities of the experimental process.

In scientific circles, however, failed experiments may, nonetheless, be considered successful insofar as they advance understandings about the topic being studied. In this vein, the *Loi Evin*'s partial successes serve as valuable reminders to public health officials and pedagogy scholars about the role of specificity of messages, the vagaries of pedagogical interpellation, the negotiation of 'productive constraints' (Beucler and Favreau 2003) and the importance of recognising the different ways in which audiences will engage with pedagogies.

References

Agostinelli, G. and Grube, J. 2002. Alcohol counter-advertising and the media: A review of recent research. *Alcohol Research & Health*, 26(1), 15–21.

Ahmed, S. 2010. Happy Objects, in *The Affect Theory Reader*, edited by M. Gregg and G.J. Seigworth. Durham: Duke University Press, 29–51.

Anderson, P., De Bruijn, A., Angus, K., Gordon, R. and Hastings, G. 2009. Impact of alcohol advertising and media exposure on adolescent alcohol use: A systematic review of longitudinal studies. *Alcohol and Alcoholism*, 44(3), 229–43.

Andrieu, E. 2012. La campagne des Vins de Bordeaux sanctionnée par la Cour de cassation. *Le Monde du Droit*, 5 March 2012.

ANPAA. 2003. L'abus de publicité, dangereux pour la santé? *Addictions*. Paris.

Atkin, C., Smith, S. and Bang, H.-K. 1994. How young viewers respond to televised drinking and driving messages. *Alcohol, Drugs & Driving*, 10(3–4), 263–75.

Baillie, R.K. 1996. Determining the effects of media portrayals of alcohol: Going beyond short term influence. *Alcohol and Alcoholism*, 31(3), 235–42.

Barry, A.E. and Goodson, P. 2010. Use (and misuse) of the responsible drinking message in public health and alcohol advertising: A review. *Health Education & Behavior*, 37(2), 228–303.

Beucler, P. and Favreau, F. 2003. La loi Evin dix ans après ou le paradoxe de la contrainte féconde. *Communication et langages*, 136(1), 31–42.

Bineham, J.L. 1988. A historical account of the hypodermic model in mass communication. *Communication Monographs*, 55, 230–46.

Caron, D. 2001. *AIDS in French Culture: Social Ills, Literary Cures*. Madison: University of Wisconsin Press.

Casswell, S. and Maxwell, A. 2005. Regulation of alcohol marketing: A global view. *Journal of Public Health Policy*, 26(3), 343–58.

Cin, S.D., Worth, K.A., Dalton, M.A. and Sargent, J.D. 2008. Youth exposure to alcohol use and brand appearances in popular contemporary Movies. *Addiction*, 103, 1925–32.

Connolly, G.M., Casswell, S., Zhang, J.-F. and Silva, P.A. 2006. Alcohol in the mass media and drinking by adolescents: A longitudinal study. *Addiction*, 89(10), 1255–63.

Craplet, M. 2001. Alcohol problems: Is there a specificially French view? *Addiction*, 96, 805–807.

Cronin, A.M. 2004. *Advertising Myths: The Strange Half-Lives of Images and Commodities*. London: Routledge.

Direction Générale De La Santé. 2001. Stratégie d'action alcool: Intensifier la prévention et le traitement des problèmes de santé liés à la consommation d'alcool. Paris: B.D.C.a.S.-D.S.E. Société.

Dorfman, L. and Wallack, L. 1993. Advertising health: The case for counter-ads. *Public Health Reports*, 108 (6), 716.

Ellsworth, E. 2005. *Places of Learning: Media, Architecture, Pedagogy*. New York: Routledge.

Evans, J., Rich, E., Davies, B. and Allwood, R. 2008. *Education, Disordered Eating and Obesity Discourse: Fat Fabrications*. London: Routledge.

Flowers, R., Chodkiewicz, A., Yasukawa, K., Mcewen, C., Ng, D., Stanton, N. and Johnston, B. 2001. *What Is Effective Consumer Education? A Literature Review*. Sydney: Australian Securities & Investments Commission.

Furtwængler, N.A. and Visser, R.O. 2013. Lack of international consensus in low-risk drinking guidelines. *Drug and Alcohol Review*, 32(1), 11–18.

Georges. 2013. La loi Evin: Une hypocrisie bien française. *For Georges* [Online]. Available from: http://www.forgeorges.fr/la-loi-evin-une-hypocrisie-bien-francaise/ 2013].

Gerbner, G. 1990. Stories that hurt: Tobacco, alcohol, and other drugs in the mass media. *Youth and Drugs: Society's Mixed Messages. OSAP Prevention Monograph*, 6, 53–127.

Gillis, R. 2012. Life Under Loi Evin. *Un-Official Partner: More Questions Than Answers* [Online]. Available from: http://www.unofficialpartner.co.uk/?p=785 2013].

Giroux, H.A. 1993. Consuming social change: The 'United colors of Benetton'. *Cultural Critique*, 26, 5–32.

Goodman, M.K. 2009. The mirror of consumption: Celebritization, developmental consumption and the shifting cultural politics of fair trade. *Geoforum*, 41, 104–16.

Gual, A. and Colom, J. 1997. Why has alcohol consumption declined in countries of southern Europe. *Addiction*, 92(Supplement 1), S21–S31.

Gupta, P.B. and Gould, S.J. 1997. Consumers' perceptions of the ethics and acceptability of product placement in movies: Product category and individual differences. *Journal of Current Issues and Research in Advertising*, 19(1), 37–50.

Hickey-Moody, A., Savage, G.C. and Windle, J. 2010. Pedagogy writ large: Public, popular and cultural pedagogies in motion. *Critical Studies in Education*, 51(3), 227–36.

Hill, L. and Casswell, S. 2004. Alcohol Advertising and Sponsorship: Commercial Freedom or Control in the Public Interest?, in *The Essential Handbook of Treatment and Prevention of Alcohol Problems*, edited by N. Heather and T. Stockwell. Chichester: Wiley, 339–62.

Hodgson, G. 2006. *More Equal than Others: America from Nixon to the New Century*. Princeton: Princeton University Press.

Loi Evin/Censure: La presse du vin s'inquiète. 2008. *L'Union*, 26 August 2008.

Gordon's Gin advertisement. 2002. Paris: Leo Burnett.

Mankekar, P. 1999. *Screening Culture, Viewing Politics: An Ethnography of Television, Womanhood, and Nation in Postcolonial India*. Raleigh: Duke University Press Books.

Martin, S.E., Snyder, L.B., Hamilton, M., Fleming-Milici, F., Slater, M.D., Stacy, A., Chen, M.-J. and Grube, J.W. 2002. Alcohol advertising and youth. *Alcoholism: Clinical and Experimental Research*, 26(6), 900–906.

Mosher, J.F. and Wallack, L.M. 1981. Government regulation of alcohol advertising: Protecting industry profits versus promoting the public health. *Journal of Public Health Policy*, 2(4), 333–53.

Nathanson-Moog, C. 1984. Brand personalities undergo psychoanalysis. *Advertising Age*, 18, 18.

OECD. 2012. Health Expenditure and Financing. *OECD. StatExtracts*. Paris: OECD.

Petersen, A. and Lupton, D. 1996. *The New Public Health: Health and Self in the Age of Risk*. London: Sage.

Rich, E. 2011. 'I see her being obesed!': Public pedagogy, reality media and the obesity crisis. *Health*, 15(1), 3–21.

Rigaud, A. and Craplet, M. 2004. The 'Loi Evin': A French exception. *The Globe*, 1(2), 33–6.

Robinson, T.N., Chen, H.L. and Killen, J.D. 1998. Television and music video exposure and risk of adolescent alcohol use. *Pediatrics*, 102(5), e54–e54.

Sandlin, J.A. and Milam, J.L. 2008. 'Mixing pop (culture) and politics': Cultural resistance, culture jamming, and anti-consumption activism as critical public pedagogy. *Curriculum Inquiry*, 38(3), 323–50.

Stewart, L. and Casswell, S. 1990. Creating a supportive environment for drinking: The alcohol industry as a drug educator. *Drug Education Journal of Australia*, 4(3), 225–31.

Sulkunen, P. and Ugland, T. 2005. The public health cycle. The Evin Law and the total consumption framework in French alcohol policy. Annual Meeting of the American Sociological Association, Philadelphia. Available at: http://research.allacademic.com/meta/p_mla_apa_research_citation/0/2/1/2/9/p21291_index.html.

Tones, K. 1996. Models of mass media: Hypodermic, aerosol or agent provocateur? *Drugs: Education, Prevention and Policy*, 3(1), 29–37.

Touillier-Feyrabend, H. 2006. Le dit sous interdits: l'expression publicitaire et la loi. *Ethnologie française*, 36(1), 55–63.

Tulloch, J. and Lupton, D. 1997. *Television, AIDS and Risk*. Sydney: Allen & Unwin.

Wilson, T.M. 2005. *Drinking Cultures: Alcohol and Identity*. Oxford: Berg.

Chapter 7

If I Am What I Eat, Who Am I? How Critical Shopping Teaches Adults about Food, Identity and Social Change

Kaela Jubas

This chapter is written from the perspective of somebody based in the field of adult education/learning. Rather than focusing on how food functions pedagogically, this piece focuses on how shopping for food can function pedagogically, particularly in relation to identity and social change. In other words, I am concerned with how shopping for food can help teach adults important things about themselves and their world. Although some adult education scholars call for greater attention to shopping and consumption (Jubas 2010; Sandlin 2000, 2004; Sandlin and McLaren 2010; Tisdell and Thompson 2007), very little research has explored shopping as a pedagogical process for adults. Moreover, much of the relevant adult education work remains conceptually, rather than empirically, oriented, and has not tended to involve participants (see Flowers and Swan's 2011 textual analysis of a documentary film, Sandlin's 2000 textual analysis of literacy education materials, Todd's 2010 study of American beef and milk marketing, or Walter's 2013 discussion of community gardens as pedagogical sites). I concur with Dawn Currie's (1999) assertion that participants help researchers deepen understandings of what culture means, and how it is enacted and embodied. As she writes about her inquiry into teenage girls' reception of magazines aimed at them, 'girls' lived experiences of adolescent femininity exceed the categories of its textual representation' (302).

In this chapter, I revisit data related to shopping and shoppers collected between 2005 and 2007 in the Canadian West Coast city of Vancouver, to draw out participants' thoughts and practices related to food, especially the varied movements related to food shopping and consumption (e.g., organic, fair trade, locavore). As I discuss below, participants in my study knew something about these movements, and attached themselves through their shopping understandings and practices to one or more of them. Participants responded to my research call for 'radical' shoppers who were concerned about consumerist pressures and their own consumption practices; participant recruitment and characteristics are discussed further below. In essence, I used shopping to spur conversations with individuals who had begun to see their own complicity in and potential to resist processes and structures of globalization which they saw as problematic. Although they raised different concerns and responses, they were all learning to see their own shopping as both part of 'the problem' and part of 'the solution'.

Because participants' food shopping was more frequent than their shopping for other items, food emerged as a primary concern in the study. This is consistent with Harriet Friedmann's (1999) statement that 'The most intimate daily practices of people around the world who are unknown to one another are connected – and disconnected – through growing, processing, transporting, selling, buying, cooking and eating food' (36). Confronted with lengthening chains from production to consumption, even the most critical shoppers find it difficult, if not impossible, to discern many items' composition, provenance or source and conditions of production. Food, especially when it remains unrefined, is relatively easy to 'know' and an obvious starting point for people interested in understanding what they buy and consume. Before I delve into these issues, I outline the theoretical framework and concepts which anchored my inquiry.

Understanding Shopping-as-Learning

My study was rooted in a constructivist notion of everyday life as a source of informal and 'incidental' or unanticipated adult learning. For constructivists, 'human beings do not "find" knowledge, but rather construct it' (Tisdell and Thompson 2007: 656); learning is understood as a process of building up knowledge through culturally and socially contextualized experiences, rather than as a process of information transfer from informed teachers to ignorant, individualized learners. While formal education refers to classroom-based, credentialed, assessed, deliberate and facilitated activities and processes, informal learning – which includes incidental learning – 'is usually intentional but not highly structured' (Marsick and Watkins 2001: 25). I am especially interested in critical or politically charged incidental learning which 'has to be uncovered … [because it is] embedded in other activities' (Foley 2001: 77) and contributes to people's understanding of, responses to and (re)constructions of social equities and practices.

I also see learning as multidimensional or holistic, involving emotions, senses and spirituality along with intellect (Dirkx 2001; Jubas 2010). In other words, learning and knowledge are based as much in what people feel, do, sense and experience spiritually as they are in what people think. In this case, I was most interested in how ordinary shopping practices – investigating, seeking, acquiring and, sometimes, refraining from buying goods, services or experiences – can help people learn about who they are, and how they encounter, understand and respond to contemporary problems.

As I establish elsewhere (Jubas 2010), shopping lends itself to a Gramscian perspective. In that view, democratic societies are constituted by a dialectic or a dynamic, irresolvable tension between cultural institutions and ideologies, and social structures (e.g., class, race, gender). Social conditions and ideas are always based in particular times and places, even as they retain traces of what has preceded them.

Another word used is consumption, from the verb which originally meant 'to take up completely, devour, waste, spend' (Williams 1983: 78). As capitalism developed, 'consumer' came to replace 'customer' or shopper. Over time, the original meaning of the word consumption has expanded. It retains its negative connotation of wastefulness and unsustainability, and has assumed a more positive meaning associated with consumer rights, information and activism. In this chapter, I alternate between the words consumption and shopping, although I concede that shopping does not extend to the use of items after they are acquired.

The Ideology of Consumerism

In its current mainstream or, to use Gramscian terminology, hegemonic iteration, consumerism is an ideology which plays off so-called free market capitalism to promote the ideas that people build identity and status through their shopping, and that consumer choice marks democratic freedom. As Gramsci recognizes, ideology both promotes and masks social and material relations that underpin everyday practice. Where and how individuals can and should shop, who is seen as responsible for shopping, and what to buy are lessons influenced jointly by cultural values, social norms, personal convictions and financial constraints (Bowlby 2001; Connelly and Prothero 2008; Jubas 2010; Sandlin, 2000).

In explaining how shopping-related teaching and learning occur informally, as well as formally, Jenifer Sandlin (2004) presents three options: 'embracing consumption', 'individually questioning consumption', and 'collectively politicizing and fighting consumption'. To complicate matters, individuals do not always shop in a singular, consistent way.

As people, products and money cross national and regional borders, new food-related opportunities and pressures are encountered. Materially, food producers, especially 'peasant farmers' reliant on subsistence farming to ensure a personal and community food supply, encounter directives to shift toward 'industrial export agriculture' (Friedmann 1999: 47). In the name of increasing international trade and the so-called free market, national governments worldwide are advised or choosing to dissolve subsidy programmes and marketing agencies which have supported small scale farms and local or national farming sectors. Culturally, shoppers (with material means) can buy and try new ingredients and test out cuisines from far-away places, and new culinary fusions are developed. Technological developments lead to changes in farming practices and genetic modifications, and create foods presented as new and improved! At the same time, movements such as locavore, Slow Food, organics and fair trade compete with a seemingly unending variety of products and experiences for shoppers' attention, and illustrate how shopping is a site of informal and incidental, multidimensional adult learning.

Meeting Some Critical Shoppers

The 32 participants in my qualitative case study self-identified as 'radical' or 'critical' shoppers. Expressions of interest in the study were invited through flyers in shops and cafes which featured local, organic, fair trade and/or natural products, emails sent to members of listservs of relevant organizations (e.g., a not-for-profit organization concerned with food security, a post-secondary education programme focused on the not-for-profit sector), and word of mouth. Participants chose between doing an individual interview or going on a shopping trip to a natural products grocery or clothing store. Five people attended a follow-up focus group session to explore ideas that surfaced in earlier conversations.

In terms of gender, all but three of the participants were female. Although I had hoped to attract more men, I was not entirely surprised by the way that gender representation was so skewed. From the early days of industrialization, shopping in Western societies has been connected to femininity, and the stereotype of women naturally suited to managing the tasks associated with shopping and consumption remains in place (Bowlby 2001; Jubas 2010).

Consistent with findings and assertions in other work about 'green' and other expressions of critical shopping (Connelly and Prothero 2008; Littler 2009), participants in my study largely described themselves, on a short demographics form that I asked them to complete, as middle class; however, several struggled to attach themselves to any class group, having come from working class families and moved into the middle class through education and employment. One participant described herself as having 'dropped out' of the middle class; for her, the material costs of taking lower paying work were outweighed by benefits of being part of a subculture that she admired, and her feeling of spiritual and personal satisfaction. For participants who were studying full-time and living fairly frugally, the disjuncture between what seemed affordable in their families of origin and during the study was considered temporary.

With regard to formal education, most participants had completed a post-secondary programme, in a range of disciplines. Over a third had completed graduate level education or were doing so, echoing participant profiles in other relevant research, including Connelly and Prothero's (2008) admittedly small study. Participants' employment involved them in a similar variety of jobs, in the corporate, not-for-profit and public sectors. Many of the participants who were studying did not have jobs or held part-time jobs that they saw as temporary; two people were retired, and one person was hoping to set up a business but was unemployed at the time. Three people were self-employed contractors or consultants.

Racially, most participants were white, four identified as Chinese or Japanese, and four as mixed race (e.g., white-Indian, white-Filipino, Metis-white). Ethnically, people reported various European backgrounds. As I explore in the following sections, these demographic characteristics help explain some of the comments that participants made in their conversations with me. Still other things – from age to family background and circumstance to social networks and communities to personal temperaments – suggest why their shared commitment to shopping in a critical way was understood and enacted in different ways.

Lessons Taught and Learned

The pedagogical function of participants' food shopping was apparent in several ways. First, participants pointed out that, even though they might enjoy food shopping, the process can become confusing and doubt-ridden. Contrary to common, idealized understandings of adult learning, this finding suggests that learning does not always lead to clear answers. In a complicated world, learning involves recognizing the complexities and uncertainties that confront people in even mundane activities of daily living. Second, shopping for food helps participants come to understand themselves in community, national and global contexts. Third, food shopping was understood as a process through which complex global issues were encountered on a daily, intimate level. In the remainder of this section, I outline these themes and what participants had to say about them.

Shopping for Food is Fun(!)(?)

There are some things – homes, cars, vacations – for which people shop rarely. Shopping for other things, such as clothing or home repair services or gardening supplies, might be seasonal. When it comes to food, shopping is a regular, perhaps even daily, process.

Not only did they shop for food more often than for any other items, participants often found food shopping the most enjoyable form of shopping. During her interview, Karen noted:

> If I'm doing grocery shopping, I tend to enjoy that more because I like food and I like choosing nice things to make for dinner. I like cooking. Other kinds of shopping, like shopping for clothes, you know, that's something I absolutely hate.

Another participant, Jody, agreed with my description of her as a 'foodie' during her shopping trip in a natural grocery store, after she commented that she tries to look at everything in the store and reads labels carefully. At a similar store, Theresa said that she likes 'to have the time to look at stuff' when she goes there. For participants such as these, who enjoy cooking and value wholesome, tasty, interesting foods, shopping can be the beginning of culinary discoveries and achievements for themselves and their families.

Participants especially enjoyed shopping at farmers' markets, where they could talk to producers, find out how products were grown and harvested, and ask for tips on how to store and prepare items. Kerri spoke about feeling 'really safe' at these markets, inferring the importance of trustworthiness of what vendors sell and say. Having to pay higher prices at the farmers' market was a consideration but, as long as prices were perceived as affordable, it was not seen as objectionable. As Sean explained, 'when I give … [the vendors] that 50 dollars … they get all of it. Whereas if I bought 50 dollars of stuff at the store, you know, they're getting, whatever, five dollars'. Participants typically saw prices at farmers' markets as reflective of the cost of production and a decent living standard.

Aside from farmers' markets, several participants described the enjoyment that they got from shopping at small, locally owned stores. Jocelyn was a dedicated patron of a coffee shop named Yoka's (since closed in Vancouver) near her neighbourhood. Not only did she trust the owners' skill in choosing and roasting coffee beans, she also appreciated their featuring of fair trade or organic beans. Just as importantly, she came to look at her visits there as a social time, shared with fellow community members, including the owners. According to her:

> We always talk about movies. I've wanted them to put a bulletin board so people could review movies …'cause if you look at the back of the schedule for the Hollywood [the neighbouring movie theatre, now also closed], it advertises Yoka's. Well there is a … local business that I go to. If it's closed and I didn't have any coffee I'd do without. I'm very religious about it.

On a similar note, Sharon offered these comments:

> I like to go to the local shops in my area, and if I've got time to do that I quite enjoy it. I take my little cart, you know, and I have my favourite little veggie store, and I have my, you know, bakery, and I have my other kind of places that I go to. And it's a bit of a, sort of, outing.

For participants who lived close to owner-operated shops where they could find specialized, fresh, affordable food, shopping became more than a chore; it became one of many experiences that helped ground them in community life, and illustrates how shopping and learning involve emotions and senses as much as intellect.

Intellectually, participants recognized a range of reasons for buying more expensive foods. Participants did not always feel able to make their preferred choices, but were clear that the price tag was never the only matter that informed their purchasing decisions. From personal health to food security to the environmental costs of long distance transport to producers' welfare, a range of concerns and convictions went into participants' shopping decisions. Claire was notably straightforward about her preference to buy locally produced food because she thought that it was better for her, the people growing the food, and the environment.

Shopping for food is neither fun and games, nor a matter of having and processing information in a matter-of-fact manner. Faced with varied options and messages, as well as their own financial limitations, participants developed hierarchies of values and considerations to guide them in their shopping. For example, Nicole explained methodically how, for her:

> I question where it's come from. That's one of my most important [considerations], where it's come from. Uh, I feel organic on specific things such as GMOs [genetically modified organisms] … Wheat, I know is not GMO, as of now in Canada, so I'm not as wary about that. Uh, and if it's fruit and vegetables I'll take local over organic because in some sense, like … anything that's grown in Vancouver, I feel it's lower in price but I know it's also coming from the local [farms].

Carla traced a similar process in her food shopping:

> There's no easy choices … If you can't afford these organic foods look closely at the label anyway, maybe you shouldn't be supporting that form of organic. If it's local and it's organic … and if you can afford it, you know, power to you. But there's definitely a hierarchy for me when it comes to buying things. Like, for food, if it's organic and local it's first, if it's local but not organic it's next, and so on down the line. I do try to follow some rules that way.

Vanessa remembered hearing an expert promote buying locally grown food whenever possible; however, her own experience with cancer motivated her to choose certain organic foods. Having had cancer helped her understand and consume food on an emotional and embodied, as well as an intellectual, level. For Vanessa, feelings, emotions, and psychological states such fear, anxiety or determination, as well as sensory memories of cancer treatments informed shopping and consumption decisions as much as any cognitive processing of information. All in all, these hierarchies illustrate how critical shoppers learn to engage in 'a kind of juggling, conceding on one aspect and holding fast on other issues' (Connelly and Prothero 2008: 126), and how their knowledge is constructed emotionally and sensually, as well as intellectually.

When participants expressed dislike for food shopping, many of their disparaging remarks were directed at large, multinational retail chains. Often seen as convenient and, sometimes, more affordable, shopping in these stores was not regarded as a pleasant experience. James was particularly articulate about this issue during his interview:

> James: I enjoy going to the grocery store. Um, some of them. I don't like Safeway.
>
> Kaela: Why don't you like Safeway?
>
> James: They lie about where their food comes from. Or maybe it's not lying, it's just, uh, laziness or carelessness. But you know, they'll say local and it's from California. Can you call California local to BC? Not really. And I'm a real trouble maker about calling that to their attention.

In short, larger stores associated with multinational chains lacked opportunities for participants to learn what they wanted to know about the food that they bought, and presented information that was seen as suspect.

Even in stores featuring natural, organic, locally produced or fair trade foods, participants experienced uncertainty and confusion. During her shopping trip at one such store, Kerri was puzzled by packaging which described the rice inside as 'nutra-farmed', and grapes labelled 'certified transitional'. On another shopping trip, Vanessa looked at bread, and cautioned that shoppers cannot assume that loaves labelled 'multi-grain' are completely whole grain. 'People get sucked in by that', she added.

For participants in my study, then, shopping for food presented an array of learning occasions. Sometimes, this learning helped them discover new products or find favourite ones, build a sense of connection and belonging in their communities, and feel that they were contributing to the welfare of themselves, their family members, and unknown producers in nearby or faraway places. Other times, the learning illuminated that shopping, like other social, cultural and material practices, is an arena of complexity and complication. Shopping for food could be fun and interesting, or irritating and frustrating.

I Shop; Therefore, I Am ...

Especially in a consumerist age, marketing ties 'social values with consumption of food products' (Todd 2010: 169). Learning how to shop for food in particular ways and places, assess options, and make certain choices helps people understand who they are and want to be, how to enact preferred identities, and how to recognize other people. Gender is one facet of identity which is constructed and expressed in the arena of shopping.

During the industrial revolution, shopping typically was attached to women who were excluded from much of the labour market and consigned to managing consumption in the home (Bowlby 2001). The stereotype of women as naturally amenable or culturally conditioned to oversee shopping was apparent in my study, and participants' experiences suggested that women are connected to shopping in particular ways in real-life as well as social imagination. In particular, participants agreed that their mothers were the earliest teachers related to shopping and food. Jocelyn, the oldest participant, shared this comment about her mother's long-lasting impact:

> So what I learned from her, for instance, she'd give me a list and some money ... And she would tell me how to pick out ... the best of the fresh vegetables ... I mean maybe some of the things I learned from her were good after all.

Amitah, a much younger participant, shared similar recollections:

> Okay, well where I did I learn about shopping? From my parents ... Usually from my mom ... When it came to food, um, she would always choose sort of

> fresh fruits and veggies. And she would cook a lot of things from scratch. We didn't buy packaged dinners. Um, so that impacted the way I looked at food.

Although a few participants came from families where eating organically or locally produced foods was the norm, several female participants noted that, as they approached and entered adulthood, their views of shopping and food diverged from their mothers' mainstream middle-class practices. Amitah traced her interest in eating organic food to a 'whole rebellion phase' of youth. Alice's general disdain for shopping was seen as 'ironic', given her mother's love of shopping and the family's habit of taking out-of-town guests to Canada's largest shopping mall.

Although Alice was a few years older than Amitah and they came from different places, they both grew up in middle-class families, and were exposed in their youth to an emerging critique of (over-)consumption and consumerism. Becoming an adult usually meant revising existing and adopting new values and practices, even though some of the early lessons about food shopping remained useful and valued. Regardless of their ages, participants opened themselves up to information and arguments from social movements, marketers, media reports, documentaries and non-fiction publications, trusted friends and, for some, religious doctrines. In so doing, they encountered and generated a combination of shopping-related concerns, claims and responses, which helped them develop a sense of themselves as unique, free-thinking adults. A couple of decades older than Amitah and Alice, Mary summarized these points:

> My mother taught me first, for sure … I mean the thing about frugality and not wasting, that's certainly from family of origin. So that remains. But the rest of my ideas about shopping are very much embedded in political analysis that's supported by the rest of my lifestyle … and the rest of my life experience.

The variety of influences, understandings and responses noted by participants was wide-ranging. Mary mentioned the importance of reading Hindu and Buddhist texts, and becoming involved in community-based sustainability networks. For Linda, having children – one of whom had a food allergy – brought her responsibility to protect other people and the planet to the surface in her food shopping.

Despite the range of shopping approaches that participants developed, many of their opinions and practices remained highly classed. In that regard, they suggest the 'social trajectories' (Bourdieu 1984) available to individuals on the basis of their initial class positions and identities, in ways that can appear both to fragment and reinforce class structure. Similarly, there have been drastic changes in gender roles and identities in Western societies over recent decades, even as social life remains gendered so that maleness and masculinity are accompanied by privilege that continues to elude femaleness and femininity. Women, specifically mothers, are still imagined as, and expected to be, the primary shoppers in Western societies. Because food choice and preparation are associated so closely with well-being and caring, shopping for food reinforces the image of women as caregivers and homemakers. Shopping, then, can become a process of new, critical possibilities and identities, at the same time as it can reinforce old hegemonic images and beliefs; I return to this paradox or dialectic between change and status quo in the final section.

Race and racial stereotypes, too, were inferred in participants' comments. Reesa, a white woman married to a Chinese-Canadian man, explained that, despite her commitment to a largely raw, organic diet, she sometimes bought packaged noodle dishes for her husband because he got 'tired of Caucasian food'. Linda, another white woman married to a Chinese-Canadian man, stated that her husband 'doesn't think of himself as Asian. He was raised very Western. His mom didn't even raise him in Chinese. He grew up speaking English'. Still, he made special trips to a supermarket known for its selection of Asian specialty foods.

Claire, who immigrated to Canada from Hong Kong as a toddler, talked about coming from 'a traditional Chinese family – we ate everything, right?' The insinuation here is that, in learning to approach food shopping like an imagined, idealized Canadian, Claire developed a more discriminating palate. Her comment recalls Aihwa Ong's (2004) notion that members of racialized minority groups are envisioned on a 'white-black continuum' (159), which ties race to class, and suggests how shopping involves identity construction and expression. Claire's middle-class status enabled her to shop in high status neighbourhoods and stores, in a more refined manner; in Ong's terminology, she was 'whitened' as a consumer and as a Chinese-Canadian.

A central part of Canada's social fabric, at least in rhetoric, is the platform of multiculturalism. Although Ellen, a participant of Indian descent, believed that multiculturalism allows culturally identifiable areas and practices to develop in response to the wants and needs of immigrant populations, contemporary hegemonic rhetoric of difference is troubling:

> Well … the biggest criticism of Canadian multiculturalism is that cultures get reduced to their most popular identifiable obvious … salient component, right? So Indian food gets reduced to samosas, Japanese food gets reduced to, um, sushi, Mexican food gets reduced to enchiladas.

Consumerism helps reduce racial and ethnic identities to commercializable differences which are marketed for the pleasure of members of other groups. Commenting on the connection between consumerism and race, bell hooks (2001) makes the following point about how social and cultural practices are tied to material conditions:

> When race and ethnicity become commodified as resources for pleasure, the culture of specific groups, as well as the bodies of individuals, can be seen as constituting an alternative playground where members of dominating races, genders, sexual practices affirm their power-over in intimate relations with the Other. (425)

Other scholars have extended and, sometimes, challenged hooks' understanding. For example, Flowers and Swan (2012) outline how an Australian cultural festival featuring 'ethnic' foods can be understood as an enlistment of white Australians into an official discourse of multiculturalism. More particularly, such a festival can recruit white working class male Australians into a more cosmopolitan, genteel version of masculinity. Moreover, it might advance the potential for members of racialized minority groups to influence the shaping of white consumers' culinary tastes and expectations.

For participants in my study who had lived or travelled abroad, notably in the Global South, food shopping reinforced feelings of national identity. Nicole, whose father's work took the family to Indonesia while she was a child, shared the following anecdote during her interview:

> I mean, the one thing I remember was the fruits and vegetables. Here in Indonesia, a tropical country, they grow amazing fruits and vegetables, and here I want … a McIntosh apple and an orange orange from Florida, you know, where, Indonesian oranges are small and green … Which is real but because they're not orange, you want an orange and I, like, I wouldn't be able to eat those things.

As an adult who has continued to travel abroad, Nicole grew out of her distaste for 'un-Canadian' foods, and came to appreciate the advantages of wholesome, unprocessed food produced on a local, small scale. Karen related her experience of travelling with her husband in another way:

> Karen: My husband and I were in Taiwan for a while and we were wandering around an open air street market and picking up, uh, we saw some apples that were grown in [British Columbia] …
>
> Kaela: So you can sort of have a taste of home?
>
> Karen: Yeah, yeah.

Participants also understood that food shopping has a material and a class-based reality, and that the financial costs of some options seem out of reach. In short, many participants echoed an understanding of identity as a dialectical construction. Approaches to and practices of shopping for food exemplify how gender, race, class and other aspects of identity are bought and sold, as well as inherited and assigned. Culture, materiality and personal preferences, and emotionally and intellectually sourced information coexist and, together, influence how adults understand themselves and others. Through their approaches to and practices of food shopping, adults learn not only how to shop, but also who they (can) become in that process. Foods themselves develop 'persona' (Todd 2010: 169), to which shoppers align or distance themselves, so that their choices become associated not only with immediate wellness and pleasure, but also with larger self-understandings and ambitions.

Learning to Change Shopping/Shopping to Make Change

As I explained earlier, my research focus was on adults who saw themselves as radical or critical shoppers. Participants had begun to link their shopping to new trends and long-standing conditions that they found troubling. For them, food shopping was more than a process of self-identification and self-expression; it was also a process of resistance to perceived problems.

Several contemporary movements use food as a focal point. Fair trade intervenes in the production-consumption chain, ensuring decent work standards for producers, promoting environmentally sustainable production practices, paying for wholesale purchases promptly and at fair prices, banning child labour, and investing in producers' workplaces and surrounding communities, primarily in the Global South. Generally accepted principles in fair trade point to a pedagogical purpose of building 'understanding by all participants of their role in world trade' (Fair Trade Resource Network no date: 3). Certified organic farmers do not use synthetic fertilizers, pesticides or herbicides, genetically modified organisms or synthetic additives and preservatives, and avoid keeping animals continually caged indoors (Certified Organic Associations of British Columbia no date). For locavores, 'knowing who made your food and where it hails from … is a political imperative' (Flowers and Swan 2011: 236). Slow Food is both an organization with branches around the world, and a more loosely structured network. It has developed 'ecogastronomy', 'an attitude that combines a respect and interest in … [food] culture with support for those battling to defend food and agricultural biodiversity around the world' (Slow Food Canada 2012, para. 2).

Participants were familiar with such movements, and aligned themselves in various ways with them. Active in the animal rights movement, Bonnie maintained a vegan diet, even avoiding leather clothes. When I asked whether her concern for animal welfare extended to people, she answered, 'Oh yeah, that's why I won't buy non-organic bananas or chocolate or coffee'. Sean favoured local production or fair trade, so that he was 'not visiting horrid crap on all these people living overseas'. Linda was willing to pay higher prices for organic food 'not [only] because I think it's good for my family, but because I think it's important in terms of farming and the land that we have access to and not putting so many pollutants into the soil'. Karen and Vanessa bought shares in community supported agricultural projects, and volunteered on affiliated farms. Clearly, the environmental concerns and social convictions that participants brought to their shopping went well beyond personal wellness.

Like some participants, Karen was explicit in naming corporations whose practices contravened her sense of justice and fairness. She remembered a conversation with her father, and his upset at Nestle's infamous promotion of infant formula to mothers living in poverty. 'Just the fact that they were … getting women hooked on this product but they didn't have clean water for it and … any kind of healthcare. So I haven't bought Nestle products since I was seven', she explained. Although her father was not the primary shopper in her family, her memories of his being 'incensed by it' stuck with her and taught her an important and lasting lesson about relating food shopping to social justice and change.

These anecdotes also illustrate the multidimensionality of adult learning (and shopping). Emotions – including upset and anger as well as satisfaction and pleasure – are especially apparent in food-related pedagogy and learning. Developing understandings of and commitments to food shopping in the service of social change are felt as much as reasoned.

Challenges for Radical Shopping Pedagogies

For the field of adult education, this chapter offers some interesting conceptual contributions. Just as adult learning can be described as informal or incidental, so too can pedagogy or teaching. Shopping does not have agency in the way that an instructor or any other person has; however, like learning, teaching can also be unanticipated, unrecognized and very much part of the everyday education of consumers.

As Sandlin (2004) establishes, the idea that well educated consumers can and will make the best decisions is problematic for several reasons. Personal wealth extends options to shoppers, irrespective of their knowledge. The reverse is also true: Building knowledge and understanding does not necessarily expand shoppers' options. Moreover, as I have noted, learning and shopping are holistic processes, motivated as much by emotional and sensual pressures and priorities as they are by reason. Marketers understand this reality, and develop advertising campaigns which associate 'emotional appeals and social values with the consumption of the product' (Todd 2010: 173). Products, brands, stores and neighbourhoods carry sociocultural messages, as well as what might be considered to be more pragmatic health, ecological and financial 'facts', which combine to teach adults about how and where to shop in a way that corresponds with who they are or want to be.

As various possibilities, expectations and preferences compete against one another, critical shoppers learn to assess their options. This self-education can be seen as simultaneously defiant of and consistent with hegemonic neoliberal rhetoric. On the one hand, participants articulated the personal, local and global importance of the production, purchase and consumption of food, and were troubled by the globalization of the agribusiness and its impacts on farmers, consumers, local economies, and the physical world. On the other hand, the idea that personal shopping can make large scale, structural differences reinforces elements of the consumerist discourse which represent the shopper as sovereign. As Max Haiven (2007) argues in his critique of the anti-consumerist non-profit publication AdBusters and associated campaigns, 'privatized' resistance encouraged by such contemporary shopping-related movements and organizations is 'not only inadequate for confronting the contemporary global political and cultural hegemony of neoliberalism, but in many ways [becomes a form of] rehearsing key tenets of neoliberalism' (86).

Moreover, as Jo Littler (2009) asserts, even though treating shopping as an arena of critical learning produces meaningful changes for and in individuals, it promotes the continual self-reflection expected within a neoliberal, hyper-individualized framework. As Littler continues to explain, reflexivity can become an opportunity to understand oneself in relation to other people and as participants in far-reaching social and material systems, or can be limited to self-indulgent, self-centred focus on oneself as the central actor in and author of a social narrative. The latter focus, emphasized in rhetoric and practice based on personal shopping decisions, overlooks the extent to which fair trade, organic, green and other desirable products increasingly are made, offered and promoted by the multinational bodies whose systems are seen as objectionable by critical shoppers in the first place. Because these products typically cost more than conventional products and shopping-related movements are often led by members of the middle class, critical shopping's primary appeal has been to the upper and middle (or aspiring-to-middle) classes; 'for those who are low in social or cultural [or material] capital, it can be hard enough to even get a foot in the pitch, let alone attempt to reconfigure the rules of the game' (Littler 2009: 79). Ironically then, critical shopping can consolidate rather than disrupt class-based and other inequities, and direct people's attention away from rather than toward problematic systems. These sorts of ironies point to the limitations of critical shopping as a form of social transformation.

This is not to conclude that trying to understand and practice shopping for food and other things in a critical manner is meaningless or undesirable, only that it is insufficient to achieve substantive, qualitative change. Some participants moved beyond a commitment to critical shopping and enacted forms of Sandlin's (2000) collective politicization of consumption and fighting back against consumerism. For example, Bonnie was active in the animal rights movement, and Vanessa was active in the cooperative and food security movements. Their version of critical practice extended beyond shopping to collective action and explicit sociomaterial purpose. The thoughts, feelings and sensations emerging in and resulting from shopping and consumption worked together with other influences – from varied sources of information to participants' identities and self-identifications as gendered, classed and raced individuals – to help participants learn about shopping, and what their shopping practices say about both them and the wider world. Ultimately, I contend, consumer power becomes truly meaningful when it is put to work as one part of a larger analysis and practice, including engagement with social and political movements and organizations that might use critical shopping as a tactic but not as a final aim. That, it seems to me, is the meatiest and most fruitful lesson to be learnt in the arena of shopping-as-pedagogy.

References

Bourdieu, P. 1984. *Distinction: A Social Critique of the Judgement of Taste*. Translated by R. Nice. Cambridge, MA: Harvard University Press.

Bowlby, R. 2001. *Carried Away: The Invention of Modern Shopping*. New York: Columbia University Press.

Certified Organic Associations of British Columbia. n.d. About Organic: What is Organic Farming? Retrieved 12 November 2012, from http://www.certifiedorganic.bc.ca/aboutorganic/whatis.php.

Connelly, J. and Prothero, A. 2008. Green consumption: Life-politics, risks and contradictions. *Journal of Consumer Culture*, 8(1), 117–45.

Currie, D.H. 1999. *Girl Talk: Adolescent Magazines and their Readers*. Toronto, Buffalo and London: University of Toronto Press.

Dirkx, J.M. 2001. The power of feelings: Emotion, imagination, and the construction of meaning in adult learning. *New Directions for Adult and Continuing Education*, 2001(89), 63–72.

Fair Trade Resource Network. n.d. 'What is fair trade?' Retrieved from http://www.fairtraderesource.org/wp/wp-content/uploads/2007/09/What-is-Fair-Trade.pdf.

Flowers, R. and Swan, E. 2011. 'Eating at us': Representations of knowledge in the activist film *Food, Inc. Studies in the Education of Adults*, 43(2), 234–50.

———. 2012. Eating the Asian Other? Pedagogies of food multiculturalism in Australia. *PORTAL Journal of International Multidisciplinary Study*, 9(2). Retrieved from http://epress.lib.uts.edu.au/journals/index.php/portal/article/view/2370/3288.

Foley, G. 2001. Radical adult education and learning. *International Journal of Lifelong Education*, 20(1/2), 71–8.

Friedmann, H. 1999. Remaking 'traditions': How we eat, what we eat and the changing political economy of food. In D. Barndt (ed.), *Women Working the NAFTA Food Chain: Women, Food and Globalization* (pp. 36–60). Toronto: Sumach Press.

Haiven, M. 2007. Privatized resistance: *AdBusters* and the culture of neoliberalism. *Review of Education, Pedagogy, and Cultural Studies*, 29(1), 85–110.

hooks, b. 2001. Eating the other: Desire and resistance. In M.G. Durham and D. Kellner (eds), *Media and Cultural Studies: Key Works* (pp. 424–38). Malden, MA and Oxford: Blackwell Publishers (first edn 1992).

Jubas, K. 2010. *The Politics of Shopping: What Consumers Learn about Identity, Globalization, and Social Change*. Walnut Creek, CA: Left Coast Press.

Littler, J. 2009. *Radical Consumption: Shopping for Change in Contemporary Culture*. Maidenhead: Open University Press.

Marsick, V.J. and Watkins, K.E. 2001. Informal and incidental learning. *New Directions for Adult and Continuing Education*, 2001(89), 25–34.

Ong, A. 2004. Cultural citizenship as subject-making: Immigrants negotiate racial and cultural boundaries in the United States. In L.D. Baker (ed.), *Life in America: Identity and Everyday Experience* (pp. 156–78). Malden, MA: Blackwell Publishers.

Sandlin, J.A. 2000. The politics of consumer education materials used in adult literacy classrooms. *Adult Education Quarterly*, 50(4), 289–307.

———. 2004. Consumerism, consumption, and a critical consumer education for adults. *New Directions for Adult and Continuing Education*, 2004(104), 25–34.

——— and McLaren, P. 2010. Introduction: Exploring consumption's pedagogy and envisioning a critical pedagogy of consumption – Living and learning in the shadow of the 'Shopocalypse'. In J.A. Sandlin and P. McLaren (eds), *Critical Pedagogies of Consumption: Living and Learning in the Shadow of the 'Shopocalypse'* (pp. 1–20). New York and London: Routledge.

Slow Food Canada. 2012. 'About'. Retrieved from http://www.slowfood.ca/about/.

Tisdell, E.J., and Thompson, P.M. 2007. 'Seeing from a different angle': The role of pop culture in teaching for diversity and critical media literacy in adult education. *International Journal of Lifelong Education*, 26(6), 651–73.

Todd, A.M. 2010. Happy cows and passionate beefscapes: Nature as landscape and lifestyle in food advertisements. In J.A. Sandlin and P. McLaren (eds), *Critical Pedagogies of Consumption: Living and Learning in the Shadow of the 'Shopocalypse'* (pp. 169–79). New York and London: Routledge.

Walter, P. 2013. Theorising community gardens as pedagogical sites in the food movement. *Environmental Education Research*, 19(4), 521–39.

Williams, R. 1983. *Keywords: A Vocabulary of Culture and Society*. Revised edition. New York: Oxford University Press.

PART III
Governance and Authority

Chapter 8
'Making it Local': The Rural Consumer, the Supermarket and Competing Pedagogical Authority

Bronwyn Isaacs and Jane Dixon

Introduction

Food historian, Michael Symons (2007), claims that since colonisation, Australia had been a nation of 'industrial feeders'. Lacking a peasant tradition, Australians relied for more than 150 years after European settlement on processed foods from venerable UK companies and purchases from small grocers to augment their backyard food provisioning activities (chickens for eggs, fruit trees, vegetable patches) along with weekly purchases of meat from the mobile vendor. Settling on the coastal fringe, these Australians viewed the rural heartland as inhospitable and harsh (Banwell et al. 2012); and although supplying national wealth from 'the sheep's back', the 'rural' was not deemed by households to be significant to food provisioning. In short, Anglo-Saxon Australians learned about food – its origins, uses, symbolic significance, tastes – from custom, an odd amalgam of company advertising and product labels and shopkeepers who could provide additional cooking tips and introduce novelties. These shopkeepers were well-known local identities, who provided hubs of social interaction, a foundational aspect of local community life.

While sources of food knowledge have exploded, over the last half century, in number and variety, and their teaching mechanisms have proliferated in range, arguably the two bedrocks of Australia's food literacy and engagement with food – company brands and shop keepers – endure as the most solid of food authority have been the most enduring. What has changed in this time is the nature of the food retailer, which has become the behemoth supermarket. Jane Dixon (2003; 2008) has described how supermarkets exert power to influence shopping practices, through enacting a particular form of market authority. They do this through controlling not only circuits of capital flow and accumulation (supply chain oversight, land and technology asset ownership) but also through orchestrating cultural circuits (loyalty programmes, shopping routines and advice about which foods are 'best' (cheap, easy, healthy, family friendly).

In Shepparton, Australia, supermarkets draw authority by merit of being the largest and most powerful retailers in town, implementing professional 'crackerjack' logistics, applying national business models, providing employment training and providing opportunities for consumers to make or aspire to a certain quality of life. In addition, supermarkets exert their authority by interrupting or redefining the pedagogies of 'local' and of 'community'. With the gradual decline of a food-based economy, and concern about the ability of Shepparton to make it with prosperity in the future, questions about job creation, commercial infrastructure, access to modern consumer items and the satisfaction of culturally diverse desires have been moving up the public's agenda. These are questions to which supermarkets provide ready and professional answers, exerting considerable influence over local space, politics and economy. Supermarkets promote themselves as local heroes: prioritising the family budget, providing convenience meals, and minimising shopping chores so time can be spent fulfilling other family obligations.

As a result, supermarket shopping becomes a daily life instruction in what behaviours are good, successful and important. Market authority is not immutable, however, as this study shows. The transformation of the town of Shepparton to a commercial regional centre has introduced new questions and new roles for old pedagogical authorities. Challenging supermarket authority are old actors with emotionally evocative pedagogical influence, such as small grocers and shops, the surrounding natural environment and enduring local histories. There are also meanwhile, two new types of food reflexive actor: the shopper empowered through having new sources of food provisioning knowledge and the citizen-consumer who understands that shopping can be a patriotic act of a newly conceptualised 'local' duty.

In this chapter, we explore the struggle for pedagogic authority between supermarkets, reflexive citizen-consumers and household food provisioners regarding food and the role it should play in social life. One discursive site of struggle is 'local food': who is best able to provide it, and its significance to 'quality of life' relative to the many other qualities promised by food and food practices. Our arguments are based on qualitative research in a community distinguished by being home to large numbers of food reflexive consumer citizens – a community that has grown up over 150 years around being a major food growing and processing centre. As a result, it is a community of food-learners: people who are keenly aware of the provenance of food, its economic value and its functional attributes in family harmony and collective well-being. In distinguishing between the reflexive consumer and the empowered 'local food' shopper, Josée Johnston and Michelle Szabo (2011: 316) suggest reflexivity has three attributes: a relative prioritisation of citizenship ideals over consumer desires; critical attitudes toward corporate knowledge claims; and, awareness of inequality in relation to food shopping and food system hierarchies. In the present Shepparton study, all three attributes are found to be present as rural consumers accept supermarkets as convenient public spaces supporting family desires but question their pedagogical values and authority, as well as the inequalities they foster and perpetuate in the food system. Consumers engage in daily practices that fit within the logics of the supermarket, but this does not preclude their ability to reflexively critique their presence or feel themselves conflicted.

As a useful point of departure for understanding the role of supermarkets as pedagogical authorities in a rural Australian community, we look to Nikolas Rose and Peter Miller's (1997) insights about the role of everyday products, advertising and experiences with instructive power. Rose and Miller suggest that corporate advertising works within a larger political economy of subjectification that draws upon diverse understandings of the consumer in order to create an 'apparently virtuous liaison of happiness and profit.' Elsewhere, Rose (1996: 151) explains this technique of subjectification by drawing on Michel Foucault's (1991) description of an enterprise culture of self-regulation. Power is asserted over a population via the necessity of teaching and improving the self, argues Rose:

> guidance of selves is no longer dependent on the authority of religion or traditional morality; it has been allocated to 'experts of subjectivity' who transfigure existential questions about the purpose of life and meaning of suffering into technical questions of the most effective ways of managing malfunction and improving 'quality of life'.

Supermarkets as 'experts of subjectivity' in rural Australia thus make shopping an emotionally loaded 'act of love' (D. Miller 1998), while operating with neoliberal assumptions about the guidance of an enterprising self. At the supermarket, 'the family becomes an important sphere in which moral and political principles are worked out' (Rose 1996: 162). In our chapter however, we suggest the rural context provides a particular rural influence over the moral and economic projects of 'making it' that conflicts with the authority of the supermarket. In Shepparton, reflexive citizen-consumers frequently reject the supermarket as 'experts of subjectivity' due to their own particular moral obligations rooted in the practice and value of local community.

The rural context therefore captures a perspective that is lost in vast majority of existing literature on consumption – a scholarship overwhelmingly enamoured by the city. In popular and academic literature, consumers are of interest when they appear as urban, post-modern citizens, a perspective frequently supported by a scale of analysis that focuses upon the family unit and networks of individuals (eg. D. Miller 1995; D. Miller 1998; Appadurai 1996). Meanwhile those who are problematising consumer identity with reference to the 'alternative' (organic, animal welfare, local or community box scheme) consumer, typically maintain their attention on the middle class and urban consumer (DuPuis and Goodman 2005; Kneafsey et al. 2008; Johnston and Szabo 2011). It is possible, that these scholars have been making some heroic assumptions about the supermarket-consumer relationship, while underappreciating the practices shared at the level of local community.

In order to understand the rural experience, we deploy the term 'local' as a spatial and social action referent – made meaningful through perception and practice of productive and consumptive activity in regards to a particular physical and geographical location taking place in a radius of approximately 100 km circumference around the regional centre of Shepparton. While the concept of local is rightly criticised as a place that does not exist outside international flows, trajectories, and change (Crang et al. 2003), we argue that relying upon Foucauldian analysis of governing family units and national political culture misses a vital perspective of scale, especially in regards to rural communities.

Community encompasses powerful social relationships between individuals, households and families which are based on shared values, practices, aspirations. Community is often expressed in terms of a 'we-feeling', and as an 'us-and-them' distinction, although this sense of community is based on assumptions about shared and distinctive interests, often masking conflicts and contradictions (Dixon 2011). For some households and individuals the 'we-feeling' encapsulates relationships based in identifying with a locality, or physically shaped social space, but this is not necessarily so with 'community' having a de-territorialised meaning for others. We believe that supermarkets enrol both 'the local' and 'community to perform pedagogic authority.

Supermarkets act as 'local pedagogues' when they (Dixon and Isaacs 2013):

- employ local people and training them to believe in the company ethos;
- sell produce from the local area, and publicising or extolling the value of this produce;
- sell products otherwise not available from the local area, increasing choices or quality available;
- make submissions to local government regarding planning ordinances, arguing a case for why rezoning land uses are in the interest of local people and the local economy.

Supermarkets act as 'community pedagogues' when they:

- publicise the community facilities and services to whom they donate money, thereby signalling the worth of particular community groups and goods and standing as a substitute for community ethical action;
- provide 'free' car parking facilities in contrast to local council parking spaces which require payment, thereby signalling they are on-side with motoring shoppers while council is not;
- appeal in advertising to shoppers who share the value of household budgeting, family time and generally who want to do the right thing by their families;
- structure store space and sell products that minimise effort and prioritise convenience on the part of the individual consumer.

As lifestyle pedagogues and powerful community actors, supermarkets thus influence household food provisioning and moral understandings of the rural community. These influences may in turn undermine existing, and often long-standing, popular perception of what 'the local' and a community lifestyle consist of. They also spur a reaction by reflexive consumers to seek and support alternative pedagogical authorities such as local farms, food businesses and farmers' markets.

The Study

The aim of this study, located in Shepparton, Australia was to understand how differently positioned consumers in a rural, food-producing region make sense of the supermarket in their food provisioning practices and in community life, and what this tells us about the authority of the supermarket. The participant observation for this study took place in and around Shepparton, with a population of around 29,000 residents. 'Shepp', as it is known by the locals, is the 'capital' or 'commercial centre' of the Goulburn Valley district, being the largest town and having a robust influx of 6,000 people in the 16 years prior to 2006: many of whom came from smaller surrounding towns. It provides major government services to the district population of 134,000 who reside over an area of 14,000 square kilometres, extending to the banks of the Murray River to the north and containing peri-urban settlements to the west, some 120 kilometres away from Melbourne. It is irrigation country, with agriculture being the top industry followed by retail and manufacturing. Until recently, food processing was the second most important employment activity based around the two long-standing canneries, SPC and Ardmona. When the canneries went through difficult times, local residents encouraged others to play their part by filling their shopping trolleys with cans. Numbers employed in agriculture have been declining steadily through dairy restructure, loss of orchards and greater capital intensity in all sectors; and it may be more correct to now think of Shepp as a major commercial and service centre (Dixon and Isaacs 2013).

Given that so many of our respondents had associations with orchards and local canneries, generally working on or in them at some point in their lives, they were understandably a food-engaged community. Locals were highly attuned to the area's history of food production, processing and retailing and they continued to identify as an agri-food community.

What we report on here is the outcome of a short ethnographic study, based on participant observation conducted over eight weeks in 2011. The data are the outputs from key informant interviews and five consumer focus groups and document analysis. Individual interviews were done with half a dozen 'community leaders' including peak horticulture bodies, a Member of Parliament, members of the local 'Ethnic Council' representing multicultural interests, two small business people and a fruit packing house manager. In addition, we interviewed: five former or present farmer/growers; organisers of three community-produce markets; managers of three of the major supermarket chains, plus two locally owned supermarket stores; a cafe proprietor; and five lots of young parents. Other data are drawn from living and shopping in the area over this time. The research was designed to canvas the broadest range of perspectives in the time available, and there were cleavages among our respondents in terms of life stage, age and whether old or new to the area.

The two researchers – one trained in anthropology and the other in sociology – drew out themes through repeated readings of transcripts. The theme list began with key terms adopted in the research protocol – healthy food, sustainable food and supermarkets. One of the major themes to emerge was that buying local produce and supporting local small store formats, such as butcheries, was more desirable than patronising supermarkets but that these practices were difficult for provisioners to maintain.

Findings

1. Positioning Food as Local: Competing Instruction from Corporate Processors, Supermarkets and Rural Citizens

Many people who were involved in local community food markets, or had at some time been involved in the processing food sector which relied on produce grown in the local area, shared a sense of loss of the 'good old days' associated with the once thriving and cooperatively owned food processing and dairy industries. In one of the focus groups, where several of the participants had worked for the Shepparton Processing Cooperative (SPC), the debate turned to why people would not buy local (and in this case, SPC products).

> I think it comes back to price. Prime example is steel goods, we make it, send it across China, get it manufactured and its shipped back here and its still cheaper than what we could make it. Similarly with fruit and vegies, a lot of the different imports are a lot cheaper. And a lot of cans come from China … and Thailand
>
> … Some of our ingredients at SPC, and goods, come from China
>
> … I remember back at my stint at SPC my job was to take the wrapper that was round the tin. Take the label off that said Thailand … That's what I did, take the labels off pineapples.
>
> … Which tin was that? the 18 pound?
>
> … Yes, so that would have been for our fruit cocktail, they weren't using the cans because they were reprocessing the fruit as a different product. It's all common practice
>
> … I worked at the cannery there too for 4 years, late life. We used to do it for the cherries. If they weren't in a big barrel they were in the drums

> … That's because cherries are the micro ingredients in fruit cocktail
>
> … He's right, but we still had to take the labels off.

The issue of supporting local producers through brand loyalty is today highly vexed, because once locally owned brands now belong to transnational corporations. One young couple, Maggie and Bob, who had grown up in the area put it thus: 'we are very much brand shoppers. We buy the stuff we used to eat when we were kids. For example we are more inclined to buy SPC rather than a supermarket brand or some product that's been imported from another country.'

Yet as Hattersley (2013) describes, SPC is not considered by everyone to be a local brand any longer. There is hair-splitting here though, for as Greg who worked for SPC points out: 'Of the large fruit companies, SPC Ardmona is the only one left owned by Australians'; to which Ed in the group exploded: 'I didn't know Coca Cola was Australian!', prompting Greg to respond, 'Coca Cola Amatil (CCA) is Australian owned. Only 30% of it is owned by Coca Cola in Atlanta …'. He proceeded to argue that CCA's ownership of SPC is positive: its 'the only company which is big enough to take [the supermarket duopoly] on.'

Not only was company origin and domicile contestable among local people, but how to source and whether to choose local food were points of debate. As Brett said: 'everyone wants to buy local, but it's confusing to know how to do so.'

Brett continued by explaining his statement. In the face of uncertainty around what is badged as local food, 'In the end it comes down to price. That's why there needs to be regulation. You might look at a packet of nuts that says 'mixed and imported ingredients' and its only 1 per cent imported'. Brett believed that because price could be easily quantified and compared, it was taking precedence for consumers over the issue of food origin. Trustworthy information regarding food origin had become difficult to access. There was no debating however, the technical question of the price of a tin of soup or packet of nuts.

In addition to 'local food' being destabilised by who 'owns' the food, where it comes from and whether you can trust the badging as 'local', numerous respondents also discussed how with migration and modernisation, what they understood food to be, the food that local people ate, had changed. One older woman from the women's focus group described how,

> … in my lifetime, I've had new foods I've been broadened by – different ethnic foods I mean … when I was growing up Italian food was very strong. And to a lesser extent Greek migrants when they first come to Australia. And each wave of migration to Australia has brought its own style of food and enriched the whole lot. I mean a few years ago, most people wouldn't have known what a nice Thai green curry was. Now they love it! I'd say it changes with each group of people as they come to Australia and bring their food, Depending on where you live, there is Lebanese and Turkish food getting around.

Indeed, new immigrants not only brought new foods that had been incorporated into local diets, they also brought diverse family pedagogies, broadening the community repertoires in which food values were pursued. Changes in preference which followed links to the global world such as a 'nice green curry' were not necessarily viewed as negative, but could be folded into existing perceptions of an enduring local community. So while we did not hear consumers describe supermarkets as supporters of local produce – although supermarket managers (from the big and small supermarkets) proffered their stocking of locally grown produce as evidence of supporting the local community – we heard from consumers that supermarkets made preferred family meals possible because they were a convenient way to source necessary and interesting ingredients.

Supermarket managers were quick to claim that their stores were valued local institutions because of their employment of large numbers of local people, the small business opportunities they generated, as well as their financial support of community enterprises (Dixon and Isaacs 2013). Local residents rarely spoke of employment or commercial enterprise but valued their provision of free car parking in contrast to the local council introduction of pay parking. Older residents were almost unanimous in reasoning that they shop at large supermarkets because 'it's quick and easy'. … 'Car parks are a very important now. It's all about where can you find a free car park, having to pay for a car park is a very important issue.' They told stories about getting parking tickets and how unfair that is … 'I wrote a rude letter to the council, I've never been so cross in all my life.'

By providing free and easy parking, supermarkets appear to uphold cherished local values regarding entitlement and enjoyment within town space. In contrast to this perception however, supermarkets were also described as having a predatory or destructive effect on local space in terms of their consequential effect upon the environment. Residents commonly observed supermarkets to be making life harder for local farmers who may have once supplied ingredients to local processed products. Tragic tales of fields of tomatoes 'rotting on the ground' and desperate dairy farmers were well known and repeated as accusations against supermarket sourcing strategies.

The widespread concern in regards to this issue was reflected in a written submission from the then local Member of Parliament in response to the Australian Government National Food Plan Issues Paper. Sharman Stone, Member for Murrain, presented a jaundiced view of the economic power of the supermarket in supply chains and their lack of support for local producers, (referring both to Australian and her area's food producers), because of their home brand policy.

> Coles and Woolworths are both pursuing a policy of increasing their home brands, which typically consist of the cheaper imported or local and imported ingredients. The labelling laws in Australia do not allow consumers to easily identify what part or proportion of their purchase consists of imported ingredients …

She continued to argue that the Australian government was failing in its responsibility to protect the preferences of Australia's consumers for home grown product through administering 'slow, expensive and inadequate anti-dumping laws' (Stone 2011).

Alongside, and intertwined with, supermarket supply chain trends MP Stone criticised the Australian government (at the time of interview, she belonged to the opposition Liberal-National Party coalition) for not doing more to protect her constituents who work for the Australian based Heinz factory which closed its tomato sauce factory in 2011. The US owned Heinz is relocating to the relatively cheaper labour site of New Zealand where it will import tomato paste from China, thus denying Shepp district tomato growers an income when they 'had no problem, historically, growing enough tomatoes ... even during the drought'. In this point she, like so many of our respondents, weaves a story about multiple and intersecting pedagogical influences, the logics and affective power of environment, industry and governmental regulation, all impacting on the possibilities in rural Australia for agri-food enterprises.

Almost no one we spoke to was opposed to buying 'local food', but what was considered to be 'local food' varied considerably. However, even when people could agree on what constituted 'the local', an inability to support the local – due to factors including time, food cost, and the convenience of the supermarket format which did not appear to support local products – fostered resentment among consumers, denting the authority of the supermarket to shape the complex relationships around food, food provisioning and 'quality of life'.

2. Shopping Spaces of Pedagogical Formation: The Moral Instruction of Behaviour, Social Relationships and Quality of Life

In Shepparton both old and young consumers lamented that a process was in place in which social interactions in public and commercial spaces was being displaced by the increasing demands of financial savings, personal time-saving and desires of the immediate family. Many respondents spent a lot of time talking about paying for parking. While this seems trivial, it is perhaps indicative of a concern about the shifting temporal pace at which social and commercial actions are conducted in the town and the fear of being dislocated from public and commercial space. Among those residents who had grown up in the area, there were shared stories and values which conflicted with those offered by supermarket logics. These shared histories and values exerted considerable pedagogical authority, telling a story about locality and their identity which at times harmonised, and at time conflicted, with the logics of the supermarket.

While supermarkets were recognised to donate funds to the community, they were also seen as robbing it of more intangible qualities of community spirit. Some Shepp consumers were acutely aware that supermarkets gradually displaced small shopkeepers when the latter could not compete with their wages and as shopping hours were extended. In part because the retirees had more time for shopping and community engagement than the young parents, they often supported farmer market formation and shopped there. At one of the farmer's markets, Ted told us:

> It used to be that the supermarkets were able to sell meat until 5.30pm – but when there was a change it was a big destroyer for butchers: people could get their meat at any time … It'll be 24 hours a day soon – it's all going that way … Grocers too – the same thing: they all lost out.

A sense of the local being intertwined with familiar people and strong social bonds was palpable. Phillip, who had worked for SPC, reminisced:

> When I was younger, the local baker was one uncle, the local butcher was another uncle, the local general store was owned by two cousins. So we had a very personal experience doing the shopping … Certainly [with supermarkets] the variety available became much greater and distribution systems were put in place … But, I think that's starting to cycle around now and I think that people are prepared to pay a little more for personal service.

Familiarity with the people serving and the quality of service from small, independent supermarkets were intertwined. Reanne, a young mother, explained:

> Well, service isn't number one at the supermarket – you're constantly waiting and that's probably the difference between a local and a big conglomerate. Help is just non-existent at Safeway whereas if you go to IGA [a popular independent called 'Fairleys'] and go up at the counter and say 'I can't find something' they will say 'oh no worries, we'll go and get someone to help you' … But you weigh it up, having to go somewhere else to get everything you want? Nup, I'll go and get the job done.

Time and again we heard glowing reports about Fairley's supermarket, established in the 1920s. Cheese producers, Tom and Betty, identified Fairley's as a local institution because it stocked local produce, employed friendly staff over a long period and provided a site for social interaction:

> You see a lot of local people meeting there, and they stock a lot of local products. And the other thing that's really noticeable about that supermarket is that the staff have been there for a long time … and the aisles are wide, you can get around … and the staff are lovely, they are actually genuine people. Now that sounds awful doesn't it?

An owner-manager of a small supermarket, established by local people 30 years earlier, also believed that there is an important role for small supermarkets in providing a community service. He explained that he had 'never done anything else like this before. I'm a farmer, here in the Goulburn Valley; we had a dry land farm. And I did truck driving, delivering around Shepp.' Things were hard on the farm and he sold up. He enjoys what he's doing now: 'It's a lot different – I've always worked by myself out on the farm, by myself, just talk to the sheep. Very quiet ....' In contrast, he sees his new role as a small grocer playing

> a bit of a social role, plenty of people tell you stuff. They get it off their chest. I don't know if they mean to or not but they come in and certainly spill their guts and tell you what's going on. And what's going on in the neighbourhood. If there's a drug bust or a murder – you certainly do hear what's going on. I don't know why, but they do.

Many participants from the Goulburn Valley Environmental Group believed that existing supermarkets did not reflect the desires and values of local community. There was criticism of a lack of 'social conscience', illustrated by supermarket logistic practices such as making farmers pay additional costs for the pallets on which their products were transported. The supermarkets themselves were described as out of line with the desires among locals to see their historically iconic food producing region flourish. Cassie, a landscape gardener, explained that a good proportion of her job was intended to help families and schools start backyard gardens, a practice at odds with supermarket sourcing strategies. As she explained, 'We don't have a strictly organic supermarket in Shepparton. We don't have that alternative. We get three new supermarkets a year but none of them are organic.' Shane went on: 'At the baker at Benalla I hang out. A lot. They know my name, they know the kids and you kind of keep track of your life by going there everyday.' The group imagined a Shepparton farmers market with 'real local produce' and lamented so much produce was wasted when tomato growers and orchardists had no buyer for their produce. For this group whose ages ranged from young adults to grandparents, the community social bonds which formed through an imagined farmers market would allow local people to express the food values that were important to them.

The area's older residents were especially vocal about supermarkets imperilling a range of valued local features: small family owned and operated businesses, social relationships and civility. Thus it is not surprising that older residents appear to be the main organisers of the community-produce markets. They recounted memories of home deliveries: an exchange where the food was grown or processed mattered less than the face-to-face contact with a familiar retailer. Sandra recalled a time before supermarkets and the need for car parks.

> I can remember how Mum used to ring up the store and they used to have the groceries ready for her, and lots of groceries were delivered ... You know what we used to have? I'm going back over 60 years now, but the old Indian hawker used to come around, with the veggies! And I think he delivered the ice, because we had an ice chest, And he would have this great big knife that he used to cut

> off the veggies – I was terrified of him. And the bread would be delivered and you'd break it in half … He came in the horse and cart.

While the energy for running community markets principally came from older residents, all young parents we interviewed said that they would prefer to go to the green grocer and the independent butcher. In part this decision was about the fresh quality of the fruit and vegetables, but in part it was about supporting local businesses because they knew the owners and they would prefer to shop differently and to support different values. As a result, there was a muted resentment towards the 'Big Two' supermarkets in particular. Reanne contrasted the atmosphere of the large and 'local' supermarket:

> That's not the way with the local IGA – a family friend of ours owns it and I know people who work there, and they hire local people, the families are local – so that's a whole different deal to the whole Coles/Safeway aspect.

The value assigned to supermarkets, small grocers and markets as sites of local social interaction was contested, even within the family group. For instance, Reanne talked about how she practised different kinds of 'shops'. While a 'casual shop' meant being able to go to a friendly local IGA supermarket, 'in your trackie [sportswear]', and buy whatever was available, by contrast, a 'proper shop' involved making a list, wearing nicer clothes and taking her son on a 'trip' to Coles or Woolworths, where a greater variety of food products were available. Going to a Woolworths complex with its bright lights and energy was not about talking with the people who worked there, but rather about sourcing all the necessary ingredients with which to provide the family with healthy meals that week. The larger supermarkets, by providing 'everything in one place,' allowed Reanne to confidently achieve certain goals she had set for herself such as using supemarkets to source diet products or the ingredients featured on TV shows such as *Master Chef*.

Consumers like Reanne, were conflicted by the supermarket retail format. While the format makes being a modern shopper and parent possible, it makes being a 'good local' difficult. On the one hand, the one-stop shop format is valued by all for its convenience, which often is equated with having to get in and out of the car only once and being able to do large volume purchases occasionally rather than frequently. On the other hand, it is an unsociable retail format, resulting in lost civic virtues of service and conversation. For this reason, many of the senior citizens with more available time to shop, augmented supermarket shopping with fresh food small shops and visits to community markets and farm-gate sales.

3. Making 'the Local' through Community: Negotiating the Authority of Neoliberal Institutions

Some citizens were responding to the current crises by attempting to build spaces and support for new food pedagogues: community food markets where strong social ties might be sought but which played a role in further complicating what local food is constituted by, or home environments where backyard gardening and or traditional family meal events could take place. Like much of urban and regional Australia, the Shepparton district is home to numerous what many would call 'farmers markets.' However as we learned these are not tightly defined 'farmers markets' because the grower/producers do not have to be present to sell the produce and the principle of locally produced food has been sidelined. The conundrum facing these community-auspiced events was explained by the organisers of the Girgarre food market, set up in 2005 after years of drought.

> So we sat around at our little development group and what we wanted to have was an event. Nobody in the country is going to drive half an hour [for produce] and that's where our biggest draw card is from: Shepparton, Echuca … Our market is different to a farmers market … ours is a community event.

> When we started, 5 people said they'd help … [Now] We have 50 people helping us. If anyone of us gets sick we have people walking in the door saying 'Can we help?' … The Country Fire Authority probably has 15 volunteers each market … they organise the BBQ, tea and coffee … The cottage manages the craft market and the craft market funds the community car. The school is also involved.

They stressed that if they sold only 'local' produce there would not be enough variety to attract return attendances,

> So we lifted our ban that to sell at the market you had to be from Victoria. You can bring in regional produce; and as far as I'm concerned regional produce starts at Hobart and ends at Cooktown. We promote Australian made produce... about 90% of it is Goulburn Valley.

The organisers were proud to distinguish themselves from markets, where the farmer gets the profit minus the stall fee: 'We make a profit but it comes back to the community.'

At another small local market located within the Shepp town centre, older residents selling home-made jams, pies and local produce reflected on the new dominance of the supermarket. In their conversation, both Aussie brands and local grocers had disappeared:

> The supermarkets are open till midnight now aren't they?

> It'll be 24 hours a day soon – its all going that way.

> Grocers too – the same thing – they all lost out …

> Now they've deleted all the Aussie brands in the supermarket. They must do it deliberately. You can't get good food any more, you can't get Aussie brands.

Conversation then moved to the simultaneous loss of certain expressions of domestic and community relationships:

> People also don't eat together any more: that's another tradition that's gone.
>
> It used to be that everyone worked 8–5 and once weekends were free and all the shops were closed. No one had to work.
>
> When that changed it ruined the markets – they lost about half their income: here in Shepparton that was about the late 70s, early 80s.
>
> It used to be that the football was only on Saturday afternoon. Now it's every Thursday, Friday, Saturday, Sunday, Monday night.

In contrast, Richard who had worked for a horticulture peak body for many years was highly critical of these food markets and was more positive about the role of the supermarkets in supporting local producers. He alerted us to the fact that despite popular perceptions, many of the area's local markets were sourcing produce from as far afield as Queensland, some 3,000 kilometres north. He wondered if the reputation of the whole horticulture sector was being jeopardised:

> Part of the popularity of farmers markets comes from a sometimes misguided assumption that they carry a small carbon footprint. The idea is that the food is also fresher and safer, but sometimes it isn't … Some supermarkets have great efficiency in their logistics. Their logistics are crackerjack.

He was particularly concerned with quality supply issues.

> Originally most farmers markets were set up to avoid legality and because they were not able to sell elsewhere – a way to offload dodgy produce and there is no integrity in that. For example the [popular] market out at Violent Town … requires no certification.

In a certain twist of irony given the relaxed attitude of the community market towards local produce, a manager for one of the Big Two supermarkets expressed a personal goal to 'get local produce in the store. For example, kiwi fruit and salad from Echuca.' He saw this goal as important symbolically and economically.

> We've had articles published in the local paper for our concern for local farmers … Last year we tried to get local tomatoes, but we couldn't get the local hydro tomatoes because they had a contract with [the opposition supermarket].

However, in the remarks which followed there was a sting in the tail with the suggestion that local food would receive support only if it could be provided by large firms: 'Customers want local produce but everything local is supported by agribusiness. If you're not in agribusiness, you're just not there.'

While positioned through their affective attachments to local community and the natural environment, there was little falling into the trap of 'unreflexive localism' (DuPuis and Goodman 2005) on behalf of the Shepparton market organisers, although this may be present among some shoppers. Unexpectedly, the older Shepp respondents who are active in the non-local produce community markets shared the attributes of reflexive consumers as described by Johnston et al. (2011). Unlike the participants in the Johnston study, this older Shepp generation were not affluent, and perhaps for this reason were genuinely concerned with people's capacity to pay for fresh produce and with suppliers' capacity to earn a decent income in the face of brutally unfair supermarket prices. By being familiar with the practical realities of engagement with industrial supply chains and having experienced the closer social bonds they associated with rural society in the past, they were also mindful of local citizenship ideals: that they had a responsibility to create and recreate participative democracy at the local level.

In contrast to a sense of loss related to the displacement of small and familiar shops by large anonymous supermarkets among the older and long-term Shepp residents, several of the 'New Australian' migrants, who met as part of the Ethnic Council focus group, expressed sadness regarding not being able to source their ethnic foods at all; or when they could (generally from supermarkets and one specialist Lebanese grocer), that these foods still tasted different from back 'home'. The conversation went thus:

> When I go to Iraq I feel and taste like the taste is different. The meat is different, the fish and the chicken is different. The food here does not taste the same.
>
> For us it is bananas! When we eat the bananas here it is not the same, sometimes I find good bananas here but it is not everyday.
>
> When I buy potatoes you often find that many of them are not good, they are a bad colour and they have started to grow, and it is a fruit shop, it's not fresh!

For this group, the specific retail format was not a key concern, except when for Muslim consumers meat had to be halal; and for that they were grateful to the opening of two halal butchers in town. Prior to their opening they would travel to Melbourne to get meat.

Within the discussion, some migrants explained their issues were not related to a lack of time for food preparation, but being able to afford to have enough home-cooked food each day in case visitors dropped by. The migrants made much fewer references to the importance of a productive natural environment, or the devastation of wasted produce and difficulty of the drought. The migrants also did not typically expect social contact taking place around shopping trips, because social interaction centred on their homes and shared meals. Thus the desires and histories shaping pedagogical influences for migrants, as opposed to those who had grown up in Shepparton, were very different. However, in common with the older residents from the community market who had bemoaned the trend towards convenience eating patterns, the migrants discussed how eating together continued to be of great importance. David, from the Democratic Republic of Congo explained how his family thought about food:

> It is important to us to cook for ourselves, to check_what is going into the meal. For example, the level of oil and the level of salt. In our culture it is not common to eat food that you have not prepared. People who eat in the restaurant are people who are living in the town, where you don't have time to cook but when you are living with your family and with your culture, you don't need to eat out … African solidarity is different to English [Anglo Australian] solidarity.

Conclusion

Although a long-standing institution (Humphery 1998), the supermarket's pedagogical authority is contested in rural Australia by both existing and emerging actors. One the one hand, the supermarket is perceived as a powerful institution that makes everyday habits and practices possible. With fresh produce transported via crackerjack logistics, a broad variety of products on sale and assurance of easy parking, supermarkets provide a way of making 'humans thinkable', a space in which life choices become technical questions of consumption (Rose 1996: 151). It is at the supermarket that consumers obtain ingredients to prepare, or purchase a pre-prepared, 'nice green curry,' with the minimal effort that meets the moral-economic strategy of 'getting everything done.' However while supermarkets are promoted as pedagogues of convenience, able to align corporate profit with the consumer's self-actualisation of happiness, in Shepparton, the harmony of such an alignment was frequently contested. Citizen-consumers scrutinised and challenged supermarket authority, questioning their business operations and their commitment to Australian farmers. In conscious rejection of supermarket logics, Shepparton household food provisioners sought to continue their support for local food-producing businesses and associated social ties.

In our research, we find citizen-consumers who experience community obligations intrinsically rendered by the specifically rural context. Consumers do not merely live upon the environment and its history, but 'dwell' within it (Ingold 2000). Daily life habits and practices are folded within various obligations to and experiences of local environment, historical identity and community. The surrounding rural environment was one emotionally evocative pedagogical influence, a once (believed) productive natural environment stressed by the contemporary reality of drought and tough economic decisions often exacerbated by supermarket sourcing strategies. The history of the Goulburn Valley as a food-producing region was another old and powerful authority. With the exception of new migrant arrivals, who were beginning to form local histories of their own, for most Shepparton consumers, identification with local food production issues, natural conditions and common hardship, was key to being a local resident. Such community concerns were clearly evident in MP Stone's parliamentary submission as they were in the commonly stated preference to shop at the small, independent supermarket praised as most 'local' and 'genuine'.

The pedagogical authority and specificity of the rural was made pertinent within flexible flows and connections to spaces further afield. While identifying 'locally', was employed as a rural identifier, a way to assert an identity over that of the national or global, the 'local' itself was a fluid term involving geographically distant connections and could be moulded to fit competing groves of moral expectations. The increasing ambiguity of the local was evident in the conceptualisation of globalisation and confusion about who owns iconic Australian brands, the cynicism regarding 'local food' credentials, and in the lack of independent retail outlets for local produce. Thus farmers markets, the very institutions considered to support local food systems did not find it inconsistent to re-define 'regional' to the extent that, 'starts at Hobart and ends at Cooktown'. The priority of the Girgarre market organisers was the vitality of their local community, and for that reason, they transformed the farmers market into a produce market which supported various and competing community economic and social goals. They, along with older, family owned and operated food retailers, were enlisting their definitions of 'local food' retailing to serve the community through fostering social bonds between people from the local area.

Our research uncovers a state of pedagogical transition underway in rural Australia, repositioning the links between 'local food' and rural community well-being. The community ideal of supporting 'locally' owned businesses, farming, produce and civic conventions was however elusive, and consumers resented the supermarkets for not making it easier to support 'local' people and products. It is in these powerful local conventions that we locate a distinctively rural influence over consumption and pedagogical authority. The valuing of social community ties is, of course, not precluded in the supermarket and many of the goals of Shepparton consumers – saving money, reducing environmental footprint, accessing or creating foods that are appropriate for the family – are not unique to rural life. Yet a critical knowledge and daily experience of supermarket-exacerbated food crises, the affective power of the local environment, and the instructive importance of a historical identity built around food production, demonstrates the leverage of rural pedagogical influences to make a difference at the scale of the local and of community. As a community of food-learners Shepparton consumers were highly aware of fluctuations in the natural environment, in the ownership and volumes of local food production, and the power of the supermarket over all aspects of the supply chain. Their daily unceasing education, received from the conflicting pedagogical authorities of everyday life, speaks of the particular reflexivity and potentially empowered position of rural consumers who are distinctively placed to recognise, contest and re-fashion pedagogical food authorities.

References

Appadurai, A. 1996. *Modernity at Large: Cultural Dimensions of Globalization*. Minneapolis: University of Minnesota Press.

Banwell, C., Dixon, J., Bambrick, H., Edwards, F. and Kjellstrom, T. 2012. Socio-cultural reflections on heat in Australia with implications for health and climate change adaptation. *Global Health Action*, 5(19277). Available at: http://dx.doi.org/10.3402/gha.v5i0.19277 [accessed 16 January 2014].

Crang, P., Dwyer, C. and Jackson, P. 2003. Transnationalism and the spaces of commodity culture. *Progress in Human Geography*, 27(4), 438–56.

Dixon, J. 2003. Authority, power and value in contemporary industrial food systems. *International Journal of the Sociology of Agriculture and Food*, 11(1), 31–9.

———. 2008. Operating upstream and downstream: How supermarkets exercise power in the food system. In J. Germov and L. Williams (eds), *A Sociology of Food and Nutrition: The Social Appetite*, 3rd edn. Oxford: Oxford University Press, 100–24.

———. 2011. Diverse food economies, multivariant capitalism, and the community dynamic shaping contemporary food systems. *Community Development Journal*, 46(suppl 1), i20–i35.

——— and Isaacs, B. 2013. There's certainly a lot of hurting out there: Navigating the trolley of progress down the supermarket aisle. *Agriculture and Human Values*, 30(2), 283–97.

DuPuis, E.M. and Goodman, D. 2005. Should we go 'home' to eat?: Toward a reflexive politics of localism. *Journal of Rural Studies*, 21(3), 359–71.

Foucault, M. 1991. Governmentality. In G. Burchell et al. (eds), *The Foucault Effect: Studies in Governmentality*. Chicago: University of Chicago Press.

Hattersley, L. 2013 Agri-food system transformations and diet-related chronic disease in Australia: A nutrition-oriented value chain approach. *Agriculture & Human Values*, 30(2), 299–309.

Humphery, K. 1998. *Shelf Life: Supermarkets and the Changing Cultures of Consumption*. Cambridge and New York: Cambridge University Press.

Ingold, T. 2000. *Perception of the Environment: Livelihood, Dwelling, and Skill*. London: New York: Routledge.

Johnston, J. and Szabo, M. 2011. Reflexivity and the whole foods market consumer: The lived experience of shopping for change. *Agriculture and Human Values*, 28(3), 303–19.

Kneafsey, M. 2008. *Reconnecting Consumers, Producers and Food: Exploring 'Alternatives'*. Oxford and New York: Berg.

Miller, D. 1995. *Acknowledging Consumption*. London and New York: Routledge.

———. 1998. *Theory of Shopping*. Ithaca: Cornell University Press.
Rose, N.S. 1996. *Inventing Our Selves: Psychology, Power, and Personhood.* Cambridge and New York: Cambridge University Press.
——— and Miller, P. 1997. Mobilizing the consumer: Assembling the subject of consumption. *Theory, Culture & Society*, 14(1), 1–36.
Stone, S. 2011. *Editorial Opinion: National Food Plan.* Published 5 September 2011 on the website of the Hon Dr. Sharman Stone, available at http://www.sharmanstone.com/MediaandSpeeches/OpinionPieces/tabid/93/articleType/ArticleView/articleId/438/National-Food-Plan.aspx.
Symons, M. 2007. *One Continuous Picnic*. Carlton: Melbourne University Press.

Chapter 9
'Just Say No to Pies': Food Pedagogies, Health Education and Governmentality

Deana Leahy and Jo Pike

Introduction

The past decade has witnessed a proliferation and intensification of food pedagogies across a range of sites (Flowers and Swan 2012). As such the contemporary food classroom now stretches beyond what might be considered to be traditional school sites and can include cookbooks (Gray and Leahy 2013), TV shows (Rich 2011a), movies (Flowers and Swan 2011), kitchen gardens (Leahy 2010) dining halls (Pike 2008) and even school lunch boxes (Pike and Leahy 2012). Each new site serves as a place whereby children, parents, cooks, the overweight, the underweight, the activist, the gourmet (and the aspiring gourmet) amongst others can be taught 'something' about food. Within traditional educational sites too, the food curriculum and its associated pedagogies have been transformed. Although the transformations are motivated by divergent interests, many contemporary anxieties related to food and specifically school food are driven by the perceived threat associated with rising levels of overweight and obesity within the OECD countries. According to the Australian National Health Medical Research Council (NHMRC) there has been a steady increase in the prevalence of obesity and overweight among Australians for the last 30 years. 'In 2011–12, around 60% of Australian adults were classified as overweight or obese, and more than 25% of these fell into the obese category' (ABS 2012). While the overall rates of adult obesity and overweight have reportedly increased, it appears to be the rising prevalence of childhood obesity and overweight that has caused the most consternation among public health professionals and academics. Childhood obesity and overweight is thought to contribute to a greater likelihood of adult obesity and the earlier onset of diseases such as diabetes and coronary heart disease while the direct and indirect economic costs of obesity are frequently cited to legitimise a range of different interventions (NHMRC). Whilst several scholars have critiqued the basis on which such claims are made about the prevalence and effects of the so-called 'obesity epidemic' (see Campos 2004: Gard and Wright 2005), the idea that we are in the midst of a pandemic persists and such 'truth claims' have significant effects.

The renewed focus on food in schools appears to be predicated on the belief that schools are perfectly placed to act as a key site for obesity prevention and intervention to improve the health knowledge and behaviours of young people in relation to what they eat (Gard and Wright 2005; Rich 2010; Vander Schee and Gard 2011). Consequently, the obesity epidemic has had a profound effect on schools and the ways they deal with the 'problem' of food which is evident not only in Australia, but also in New Zealand (see Burrows and Wright 2007), the United Kingdom (see Evans, Evans and Rich 2003; Pike 2010; Rich 2010), the US (see Vander Schee 2009) and Canada (see Rail 2009).

The flurry of food-related activity in schools has significant implications not only for the schools themselves, but also for the children, young people, parents and families currently targeted by such initiatives. Directly related to efforts to regulate food in school is the recent proliferation of programmes and other activities that seek to directly 'intervene' in students', and their families', lives. Both school and state-level policies in Australia for example, offer guidance in some cases, and explicitly dictate in others, what kinds of food can be bought at school, as well as brought into school from home. In some cases, parents risk being sent home with their children's lunches in hand if they contravene the accepted wisdom that cake is no longer an appropriate food item to bring to school (O' Flynn, forthcoming). As we have argued elsewhere, parents are frequently subjected to campaigns about appropriate food items for inclusion in their child's lunchbox. Lunchboxes, ergo parents/carers, may be subjected to scrutiny by teachers and other school staff mandated to inspect the nutritional value of the contents of lunchboxes as children sit poised ready to eat their lunch (see Pike and Leahy 2012).

In addition to the 'policing' of the school lunchbox, other initiatives require students to participate in an increasing number of lessons about food, health and eating across a range of different curriculum areas along with further optional extra curricula activities. Most notably, the subject area of health education has been recruited in the fight against obesity in an attempt to explicitly shape young people's food-related desires and practices so that they align with healthy governmental eating imperatives (Leahy 2012; Pike and Leahy 2012; Rich 2011b; Vander Schee and Gard 2011). However, what is less clear is how these particular imperatives manifest themselves within the classroom and how such attempts are received by young people themselves.

Throughout this chapter we interrogate the ways in which food pedagogies, are developed and implemented within school health education spaces. Drawing on governmentality studies, we consider the conditions that 'make possible' a range of different food pedagogies within the context of the school. Additionally, we consider the possibilities that these food pedagogies offer to students in terms of how they might view themselves in relation to food and health and further, the range of practices these pedagogies offer up as ways for students to improve their diets and consequently, their health. The chapter draws on empirical data from two studies undertaken in secondary schools in Victoria, Australia to illustrate some of the food pedagogies that are assembled within health education classrooms. Both studies were conducted using a range of ethnographic methods including, observations of health education lessons and interviews with teachers, together with a critical analysis of health education curriculum documents and teaching resources.

In order to engage with the layers of complexity involved in understanding food pedagogies in school health education we divide the chapter into three sections. The first section provides an overview of the theoretical terrain of governmentality studies that informs our analyses. In this section we work on the premise that school-based health education is a key governmental site for the enactment of broader health imperatives (Leahy 2009, 2012: Lupton 1999). Given this, we consider the implications this has for health education, and the food pedagogies that ensue. In the second section we examine three different food pedagogies that seek to shape young people's food choices. We discuss a number of common classroom scenes and the pedagogical strategies that make up the scenes, including the use of food diaries, dietary analysis and role play. We conclude by suggesting that the lessons learned in health education about food, its consumption and practices have implications for perpetuating some potentially problematic understandings about the self and others.

Governmentality and School Food Pedagogies

Michel Foucault understands government as 'the conduct of conduct' and the 'way in which the conduct of individuals or groups might be directed: the government of children, of souls, of communities, of families, of the sick' (Foucault 1982: 220–21). Government, for Foucault, refers not only to disciplinary power that shapes the range of possibilities open to individuals within a field of action, but also to the ways in which individuals are encouraged to act upon themselves, to regulate their own conduct with particular ends in mind. Contemporary approaches to shape the conduct of individuals involve various programmatic attempts 'to foster and shape such capacities so that they are enacted in ways that are broadly consistent with particular objectives such as order, civility, health or enterprise' (Rose 2000: 323). We suggest that school-based health education seeks to govern the health-related conduct of the population and to cultivate young people's capacities so that they align with [healthy] governmental imperatives (Leahy 2012). Given that in the contemporary moment 'we' are waging war on an obesity epidemic (Gard and Wright 2005) it is little surprise that school-based health education has been called upon to do 'governmental' work that seeks to explicitly shape conduct in the form of cultivating 'appropriate' food-related understandings, desires and practices of children and young people.

Health education classrooms operate as essential 'contact points' for government (Burchell 1996). They effectively provide a space that permits connections to be forged between questions of government and the space of bodies, lives, selves and persons (Dean 1999) via the deployment of various food pedagogies. Given its positioning within broader governmental assemblages, health education and the attached governmental food-related expectations, we want to suggest by drawing on Peter Miller and Nikolas Rose (1990) that 'technologies' of government – in this case food pedagogies – do not simply come into being, they are developed with a specific purpose in mind. These purposes might be termed 'the pedagogical force' (Ellsworth 2005) – a force that is both behind, and woven through, pedagogy. The forces shaping food pedagogies in contemporary health education classrooms are fuelled by the 'urgent' need to curb the obesity epidemic. As a result the ensuing pedagogies are shaped in particular ways for this specific purpose. In conceptualising food pedagogies though we need to extend our analysis beyond simply contemplating the forces that sit behind the pedagogy, in other words the governmental imperatives. To do this we draw on the concept of governmental pedagogical assemblages (Leahy 2009, 2012) to grapple with the multiple and complex discourses and techniques that are at play within contemporary classrooms. The analytic concept of pedagogical assemblages evolves out of the field of governmentality studies, in particular the work of Rose (2000) and Mitchell Dean (1999). Dean suggests that practices of government and for our purposes here, pedagogy cannot be conceived of as a coherent whole, and instead 'should be approached as composed of heterogeneous elements having diverse historical trajectories, as polymorphous in their internal and external relations, and as bearing upon a multiple and wide range of problems and issues' (1999: 29). In adding to understandings of current practices of government, and thus pedagogy, Rose suggests that:

> current control [pedagogical] practices manifest, at most, a hesitant, incomplete, fragmentary, contradictory and contested metamorphosis, the abandonment of some old themes, the maintenance of others, the introduction of some new elements, a shift in the role and functioning of others because of their changed places and connections with the 'assemblage' of control. (2000: 322)

Given the messiness of government, we suggest that the conceptualising, and enacting, of food pedagogies is not as straightforward as curriculum writers, text books and resources might have us believe. Furthermore, much goes on in what Elspeth Probyn (2004) refers to as the 'hurly burly' of classrooms where different actors, rationalities and technologies converge to create a complex assemblage. In drawing attention to these levels of complexity we suggest that we can better understand how food is both thought and taught about in classrooms. In what follows we present three classroom scenes which offer a snapshot of the contemporary health education classroom and illustrate how this assemblage of control functions through different pedagogical strategies.

Scene One/Strategy One: Risky Beginnings

A Year 10 Health and Physical Education class is covering the topic of nutrition which is introduced via the screening of a condensed version of Morgan Spurlock's

(2004) movie 'Supersize Me' available on YouTube. In this well-known movie, Spurlock eats nothing but McDonald's for one month in order to prove that doing so causes health problems – he gains weight and sustains liver damage during the course of the movie. In the seven-minute clip students watch Spurlock binge, vomit, and go from fit to fat in quick time. At the end of the clip, the teacher switches the media off and turns to the class and says, 'Look what happens when you eat McDonald's every day. So who's going to still eat McDonald's? It's silly to, don't you think?' Several members of the class raised their hands and others called out, attempting to respond to both questions simultaneously. One student said, 'I work at McDonald's, another said, 'Yeah but we don't eat it every day for every meal' and another said, 'You turn into a fat cunt.' The teacher responded to the latter comment by expelling the student from the room, the rest of the class were directed to the textbook to read about nutrition, whilst the teacher went out to 'deal' with the student.

Scene Two/Strategy Two: Food Diaries and Dietary Analysis

A year 10 Health and Physical Education class was focusing on nutrition. The first move made by the teacher was to get students to record what they ate yesterday and today already. Essentially they were being asked to make a food diary that they could then analyse. The class begins:

> Ms Murray: Okay today we are going to be looking at nutrition, and I want you to write everything down that you ate yesterday and today already.
>
> Class: (General groan)
>
> Ms Murray: Now once you've done that I want you to go through and make a note of the following things. I'll put them on the board and go over them in a minute. Start writing down what you ate, and be honest with yourself. Be sure to note quantity.
>
> Class: (Another groan)
>
> Ms Murray: (turns to the board and writes down the following list: Fibre. Calcium. Cholesterol. Salt. Sugar)
>
> Can I have your attention for a moment please? Now this is for when you have finished noting down what you have eaten. I want you to go to your text and look up each of these on the board [points to board] and find out what they do for you or to you and make some notes. Um, I want you to focus on the following [writes on the board as she is talking]. What is the RDI [Recommended Daily Intake]? Are you eating the RDI? And what will happen if you don't eat the RDI? [stops

> writing]. So girls, basically the consequences of not eating properly, eating the things that you should be eating. So what are the risks to your health? So whether it be related to cancer, CVD [Cardio Vascular Disease] [asks question] Who knows what CVD is? [no one answers] Mmm, well it is in the book. So you might want to organise it under some goals for yourselves like this in your books, like this. (compiles the following list on the board)
>
> *Goals*
>
> - Reduce fat intake
>   - Problems which may occur if this goal is ignored:
> - My personal goal:
>   - I will lower my fat intake by …
>
> [turning back to the class] So if you can do that for the others here [pointing to the list]. You can see why you might need to change your eating habits, if you can see what the risks are to you, yeah? [Field notes, year 10 HPE class]

Scene Three/Strategy Three: Life Skills

A Year 8 health education class is covering nutrition and the focus of the lesson is the humble pie. In selecting the pie as a key focus for this particular lesson, the teacher drew on a class discussion the previous week. Previously students had researched what constitutes good food and why and how they might make good food choices. They also learnt about what constitutes bad food and bad food choices. The pie had been discussed at length and at the end of the discussion the teacher passed judgement on the pie and proclaimed that it fell into the category of a 'bad food' choice (though in passing sentence some in the student jury were not convinced; students last week had queried the status of a pumpkin and leek pie and mentioned it again as the teacher began the discussion). The pie lesson aims to build on students' understandings of good and bad food, and help students develop the necessary life skills to make good food choices. The lesson for today is to learn and practice, pie refusal skills. Students are put into pairs and asked to work out who was number one and who was number two. Student number one is then asked to pick something up, and both students are asked to imagine that the object selected was a pie. Number one is then asked to convince number two to take the pie. Number two must practice saying 'no'. The activity begins. After a short period of time the teacher calls stop and asks which students took the pie. Most hands go up. Her face is distorted with apparent shock and she asks with horror 'What, you all took the pie? Really? Why?' Without waiting for a response she announces that the activity must be repeated. Once again, student number two must practice refusal skills but this time they must communicate their response assertively. The teacher demonstrates by lifting her hand into a stop sign and saying 'No thank you I do not want the pie'. She asks all the students to copy her as a test run before putting it into action. She then asks the students to practise that in their pairs. Which they do; some earnestly, some quizzically, some giggly and some with looks of disinterest and possibly disdain.

School Food Pedagogies

The pedagogical strategies deployed within each vignette are put to work in the health education classroom for the explicit purpose of shaping young people's food choices and practices. These attempts generally unfold in a series of stages that often follow a similar plot line. The first stage attempts to alert students to risks of bad food choices and the health and social consequences of these as the 'Supersize Me' exercise illustrated. In the second stage, students are led to understand that they are themselves at risk of becoming obese and developing diet related diseases as the second vignette demonstrates. Finally, students are encouraged to develop sufficient skills to counter the risks to their health, i.e. the ability to just say no to pies. We are interested here in unpacking the three stages and the plot lines to understand the pedagogical ambitions and the various techniques that are assembled in order to realise these ambitions. Our discussion focuses on the presence of risk and how it powerfully shapes both the selection and enactment of food pedagogies. A second, and related theme, is that of governmental self-formation. Both are interwoven through the vignettes and serve to simultaneously render young people as perpetually 'at risk' of overweight and obesity and responsible for ensuring that they prudently manage the threat.

Health education and the food pedagogies that are brought to life in its classrooms, are saturated with discourses of risk (Leahy 2012). This is not surprising given that risk is considered to be a central rationality and technology of contemporary government (Dean 2010; O'Malley 2004) and thus it permeates the fields of youth studies (Kelly 2003), health promotion and public health (Fox 1999; Lupton 1995) education and public pedagogies (Hickey-Moody 2012; Rich 2011a). The dominance of risk, and the expert knowledges that work alongside risk, are crucial in the pedagogical assemblages in a number of ways. In the first scene medical knowledges are drawn on throughout the YouTube clip to tell a cautionary tale warning people of the disastrous health effects that will be experienced if they were to follow a similar path and eat McDonald's every day. In the second vignette scientific nutritional knowledge provides the foundations for the lesson of the day in the form of knowledge about various nutrients, their Recommended Daily Intake and their effects. Expert knowledges are also integral to the 'Just say no to pies' activity in that life skills are considered to be crucial if people are going to be healthy.

However, as we have suggested earlier on in the chapter, attempts to govern, and thus pedagogies, are not as straightforward as teachers simply drawing from, or adding expertise and stirring the pedagogical pot. There is always more in the pedagogical mix than just expertise. Here we heed Moore and Valverde's (2000) counsel that calls for governmentality scholars to look beyond the deployment of expert rational and objective risk knowledges to consider the non-rational aspects at work. For example, in the YouTube clip medical knowledges are accompanied by images of Spurlock surrounded by super-sized fries and sodas, followed by him vomiting out of his car window. The sheer visual size of the meal accompanied by the noise of the vomiting works on a different register to for example the health risk of adult onset diabetes. The YouTube clip incorporates techniques that are meant to disgust us, to make us feel revulsion and repel us. To teach us that eating fast food is disgusting. This lesson is not lost on the teacher who states 'So who's going to still eat McDonald's? It's silly to, don't you think?' Without giving students a chance to respond, she answers her own question by stating it is silly to eat McDonald's. This pedagogical move is not about reinforcing expert knowledges, but rather is about making an explicit and seemingly unquestionable judgement about the rational capacities of people who consume junk food. Admittedly the judgement was called into question by the students, and the one student who managed to catch the intended message was ejected from the class for bad language.

The 'Just say no to pies' scene too is based on expert knowledges that tell us that 'peer group pressure' is one of the reasons why young people might make bad health-related decisions (in this case being persuaded to accept a pie against their better judgement). However the actual strategy of cultivating pie refusal skills to resist peer pressure is a hybridised pedagogical strategy that replaces drug pushers with pie pushers. Thus pies are afforded the same status as other toxic and addictive substances and those that consume, sell or give them away are analogous to addicts and dealers. What is interesting too in this assemblage is that when students failed to refuse the pie, the teachers' shocked reaction and visible disbelief added to the pedagogic force. Like the disgust and repulsion at Supersize me, the teacher's affective response again endeavours to galvanise a different register, one that does not rely on rational thinking alone. In both examples governmental pedagogies are made up of more than expert risk knowledges. They are assembled together from a range of diverse knowledges, and affects that enables the pedagogy to 'get right in there in your brain, your body, your heart, your sense of self, of the world, of others, and of the possibilities and impossibilities of all of those realms' (Ellsworth 1997: 6). We want to turn now to consider another technique that was put to use in the vignettes: food diaries and analysis. In many ways as a strategy, it enables the pedagogy to get in, in that it calls on a level of self-surveillance and self-formation.

In the second classroom scene the teacher encourages young people to reflect upon their food intake for the previous day, to consider the effects of their diet upon their future health and to formulate goals in order to ameliorate the worst of these effects. While this strategy may follow a format familiar to many readers, particularly those with experience of slimming groups or diet related self-improvement programmes in the media, there is nothing natural or given about this strategy. Rather, it might be understood as a part of a process of 'governmental self formation' that is specifically constructed to develop a sense of self-care in students. This self-care is dependent upon a student's self-knowledge which is elicited above through the teacher's invocations to 'Start writing down what you ate, and be honest with yourself.' If taking care of yourself involves first knowing yourself, then knowing yourself is dependent on your ability to tell the truth about yourself, to confess to oneself and others (Besley 2005) about your food intake. Once the students have written down as honestly as possible what their food intake is, this is subjected to scrutiny by individual students and measured against the normative framework of RDI. For those students who perceive themselves to fall outside this normative distribution, self-regulation is required to achieve a set of self-formulated diet related goals. The monitoring and regulation of food intake and the practice of dieting is one of a number of 'disciplinary practices played out on the body through forms of *assujetissement* – the process of at once becoming a subject and becoming subjected' (Heyes 2006: 127). The use of food diaries as a pedagogical tool can be understood as a practice which renders the body docile in terms of being subjected to a range of disciplinary practices, but in other senses is seen to construct the subject in a more active or productive sense. For Cressida Heyes, this ambivalence is one that is frequently overlooked by feminists seeking to critique the current preoccupation with diet.

> On the one hand, deliberately losing weight by controlling diet involves the self-construction of a docile body through attention to the minutest detail. On the other hand, becoming aware of exactly how and what one eats and drinks, realizing that changing old patterns can have embodied effects, or setting a goal and moving toward it, are all enabling acts of self-transformation. (2006: 128)

The pedagogical use of food diaries cannot simply be understood then as a technology of domination since they 'emphasize the importance of making one's own choices, initiating transformation, and approaching food (and other things) with wisdom and flexibility' (Heyes 2006: 144). Thus, they offer students a way of transforming themselves into particular types of self-regulating subjects, albeit within a set of tightly bound parameters. And the particular types of enticements to take up these kinds of subject positions are associated with a higher moral status gained through techniques of self-mastery and ascetic practice. Foucault defines an ascetic practice in the following way.

> what one would call an ascetic practice, taking asceticism in a very general sense – in other words, not in the sense of a morality of renunciation but as an exercise of the self on the self by which one attempts to develop and transform oneself, and to attain a certain mode of being. (2000: 282)

Mastery of the self or *askesis* involves the subject governing her own conduct through a variety of different techniques of the self. The regulation of appetite, avoiding excess, selecting appropriate food items, refusing to accept pies, can all be regarded as practices of the self that support the attainment of certain modes of being aligned with governmental imperatives of health. While the YouTube clip alerts students to the potential risks of unhealthy eating, use of food diaries as a pedagogical tool encourages students to consider themselves as perpetually at risk. Such practices then entice young people to operate in a constant state of vigilance, continuously monitoring themselves to ensure they implement their knowledge of healthy eating practices and make the correct choices related to what they eat. Consequently, despite Foucault's suggestion that practices of self-government do not reflect ascetics in the sense of 'a morality of renunciation', in relation to school food pedagogies there *are* tangible rewards for those young people demonstrating their moral character through their ability to resist the temptation of pies, everyday McDonald's and other bad food choices. The renunciation of pies it seems is central to the formation of the healthy self and the achievement of a higher moral mode of being. There are a number of ways in which 'the art of self-government is explicitly connected with morality' (Foucault 2002: 206) and the ways in which practices of consumption, particularly food choices are framed is an example of this. Students that make 'bad' food choices are regarded as irrational, ill-disciplined and susceptible to temptation whereas those making 'good' food choices are regarded as virtuous, disciplined and capable of resisting the lure of the pie pusher. Dean suggests 'morality is understood as the attempt to make oneself accountable for one's own actions' and when food selection and consumption is understood as a choice, individuals are held accountable for the repercussions of those choices. Thus, the health status of young people, their nutritional status and body fat percentage can be understood as the inevitable consequence of the food choices they have made. The possibility of being overweight, obese, healthy or ill then represents only one potential option in a field of different possibilities for young people's physical development (Rose 2007). However, such choices are never value neutral. Since good food choices are the only rational choice to make, bad food choices attract moral judgement and the accusation of irrationality.

Conclusion

Throughout this chapter we have attempted to illustrate the ways in which school food pedagogies seek to shape the aspirations and food practices of young people. And while we do not claim to know what students were thinking during their lessons about food, or what they took away from each of the classes they attended, it is possible to consider how, drawing upon dominant discourses of risk, food pedagogies shape students' possible fields of action and encourage them to act upon themselves in a project of self-formation. The classroom scenes reveal how school food pedagogies are shaped by broader social, political and economic forces (see Lupton 1995; Coveney 2000). Thus at the present moment, these forces are generated and sustained by an overriding concern with obesity. But there are other forces at play that work to shape each of the pedagogical moments that ultimately mean that pedagogy, and the art of governing, is much messier than policy, curriculum or the range of expert knowledges might have us believe. Throughout this chapter we have argued that risk powerfully circulates within pedagogical assemblages, both expert risk knowledges and hybrid knowledges. Additionally though notions of the unhealthy, abject and morally corrupt other permeate the pedagogical assemblage. As students learn about food, they also learn about what is deemed acceptable (desirable) consumption patterns, acceptable (desirable) bodies and acceptable (desirable) practices. The learning extends beyond lessons in what is acceptable and desirable though. As Beausoliel suggests:

> Purposely, or inadvertently, campaigns to promote healthy eating and active living have the effect of reinforcing dominant discourses of the ideal body as lean and thin. Not surprisingly, fat hatred and discrimination against people deemed fat flourish. (2009: 104)

What is concerning, is that research is revealing that the lessons are being heard loud and clear. Burrows and Wright (2007) in their analysis of national assessment data of the Health and Physical Education curriculum area in New Zealand show that children at Year 4 and Year 8 are making connections between health, morality and character in their assessments. More recent research, again from New Zealand, has reported that children as young as five are developing distorted body images, with some measuring their waists, watching their weight and believing that they won't get married if they are fat (Cosgriff et al. 2013). Other scholars from the UK have also queried school food pedagogies that encourage the surveillance of diet and that cultivate/celebrate lean bodies (whilst demonising non-lean bodies). They argue that such pedagogies may be implicated in the production of disordered eating and ill-health (Evans, Rich and Holyroyd 2004). Health education is not entirely to blame here as we recognise that there are a multitude of other public food pedagogies at work, reinforcing similar messages. We want to suggest though, that health education should be providing a space whereby such messages are interrogated rather than reproduced unproblematically.

References

ABS. 2012. *Australian Health Survey: First Results, 2011–12*. ABS cat. no. 4364.0.55.001. Canberra: Australian Bureau of Statistics.

Besley, T. 2005. Foucault, truth telling and technologies of the self in schools. *Journal of Educational Enquiry*, 6(1), 76–89.

Beausoleil, N. 2009. An impossible task? Preventing disordered eating in the context of the current obesity epidemic, in *Biopolitics and the Obesity Epidemic: Governing Bodies*, edited by J. Wright and V. Harwood. New York: Routledge, 93–107.

Burchell, G. 1996. Liberal government and techniques of the self, in *Foucault and Political Reason*, edited by A. Barry et al. Chicago: University of Chicago Press, 19–37.

Burrows, L. 2009. Pedagogizing families through obesity discourse, in *Biopolitics and the Obesity Epidemic: Governing Bodies*, edited by J. Wright and V. Harwood. New York: Routledge, 127–40.

———. 2010. Kiwi kids are weetbix kids: Body matters in childhood. *Sport, Education and Society*, 15, 235–51.

——— and Wright, J. 2007. Prescribing practices: Shaping healthy children in schools. *International Journal of Children's Rights*, 15, 1–16.

Campos, P. 2004. *The Obesity Myth: Why America's Obsession with Weight is Hazardous to Your Health*. New York: Penguin.

Coveney, J. 2000. *Food, Morals and Meaning*. London: Routledge.

Dean, M. 1999. *Governmentality: Power and Rule in Modern Society*. London: Sage.

Ellsworth, E. 1997. *Teaching Positions: Difference, Pedagogy and the Power of Address*. New York: Teachers College Press.

———. 2005. *Places of Learning: Media, Architecture, Pedagogy*. New York: Routledge.

Evans, J., Evans, B. and Rich, E. 2003. 'The only problem is, children will like their chips': Education and the discursive production of ill health. *Pedagogy, Culture & Society*, 11(2), 215–40.

———, Rich, E. and Holroyd, R. 2004. Disordered eating and disordered schooling: What schools do to middle class girls. *British Journal of Sociology of Education*, 25(2), 123–42.

Flowers, R. and Swan, E. 2011, 'Eating at us': Representations of knowledge in the activist documentary film *Food, Inc. Studies in the Education of Adults*, 43, 234–50.

———. 2012. Pedagogies of doing good: Problematisations, authorities, technologies and teleologies in food activism. *Australian Journal of Adult Learning*, 52(3), 532–72.

Foucault, M. 1982. The subject and power, in *Michel Foucault: Beyond Structualism and Hermeneutics*, edited by H. Dreyfus and P. Rabinow. Chicago: University of Chicago Press, 208–26.

———. 2000. The ethics of the concern for self as a practice of freedom, in *Michel Foucault: Essential Works of Foucault 1954–1984*, Volume 1: *Ethics*, edited by Paul Rabinow. London: Penguin, 281–302.

———. 2002. Governmentality, in *Michel Foucault: Essential Works of Foucault 1954–1984*, Volume 3: *Power*, edited by James. D. Faubion. London: Penguin, 201–23.

Fox, N. 1999. Postmodern reflections on risk, hazards and life choices, in *Risk and Sociocultural Theory: New Directions and Perspectives*, edited by D. Lupton London. London: Routledge, 12–34.

Gard, M. and Wright, J. 2005. *The Obesity Epidemic: Science, Morality and Ideology*. New York: Routledge.

Gray, E. and Leahy, D. 2013. Cooking up healthy citizens: The pedagogy of cookbooks. M-*C Journal*, 16, 1–8.

Heyes, C. 2006. Foucault goes to weight watchers. *Hypatia*, 21(2), 126–49.

Hibsta, 2009. Supersize me in 7 minutes: How too much of McDonalds will make you feel [video file] Retrieved from http://www.youtube.com/watch?v=N2diPZOtty0.

Hickey Moody, A. 2012. *Youth Arts and Education: Reassembling Subjectivity through Affect*. New York: Routledge.

Kelly, P. 2003. Growing up as risky business? Risks, surveillance and the institutionalized mistrust of youth. *Journal of Youth Studies*, 6, 165–80.

Leahy, D. 2009. Disgusting pedagogies, in *Biopolitics and the Obesity Epidemic: Governing Bodies*, edited by J. Wright and V. Harwood. New York: Routledge, 172–82.

———. 2010. What's on (or off) the menu in school? *Text: Rewriting the Menu: Dynamics of Contemporary Food Choices*, 9, 1–12.

———. 2012. Assembling a health[y] subject. Unpublished PhD thesis, Deakin University, Victoria, Australia.

Lupton, D. 1995. *The Imperative of Health: Public Health and the Regulated Body*. London: Sage.

———. 1999. Developing the whole me: Citizenship, neo-liberalism and the contemporary health and physical education curriculum. *Critical Public Health*, 9, 287–300.

Miller, P. and Rose, N. 1990. Governing economic life. *Economy and Society*, 19, 1–31.

Moore, D., and Valverde, M. 2000. Maidens at risk: 'Date rape drugs' and the formation of hybrid risk knowledges. *Economy and Society*, 29, 514–31.

O'Flynn, G. 2015. Food, obesity discourse and the subjugation of environmental knowledge. *Australian Journal of Environmental Education*. Available at: http://dx.doi.org.ezproxy.lib.monash.edu.au/10.1017/aee.2015.13.

O' Malley, P. 2004. *Risk, Uncertainty and Government*. London: Glasshouse Press.

Cosgriff, M., Burrows, L., Petrie, K., Keown, S., Devcich, J., Naera, J. and Duggan, D. 2013. 'You'll feel fat and no one will want to marry you': Responding to children's ideas about health. *Set: Research Information for Teachers*, 1, 21–8.

Pike, J. 2008. Foucault, space and primary school dining rooms. *Children's Geographies*, 6, 413–22.

———. 2010. 'I don't have to listen to you! You're just a dinner lady!': Power and resistance at lunchtimes in primary schools. *Children's Geographies*, 8, 275–89. Accessed 7 August 2013. DOI: 10.1080/14733285.2010.494867.

——— and Leahy, D. 2012. School food and the pedagogies of parenting. *Australian Journal of Adult Education*, 52(3), 434–60.

Probyn, E. 2004. Teaching bodies: Affects in the classroom. *Body and Society*, 10, 21–43.

Rail, G. 2009. Canadian youth's discursive constructions of health in the context of obesity discourse, in *Biopolitics and the 'Obesity Epidemic*, edited by J. Wright and V. Harwood. New York and London: Routledge.
Rich, E. 2010. Obesity assemblages and surveillance in schools. *International Journal of Qualitative Studies in Education*, 23(7), 803–21.
———. 2011a. 'I see her being obesed': Public pedagogy, reality media and the obesity crisis. *Health*, 15, 3–21.
———. 2011b. Exploring the relationship between pedagogy and physical cultural studies: The case of new health imperatives in schools. *Sociology of Sport Journal*, 28, 64–84.
Rose, N. 1999. *Powers of Freedom: Reframing Political Thought*. Cambridge: Cambridge University Press.
———. 2000. Government and control. *British Journal of Criminology*, 40(2), 321–39.
———. 2007. *The Politics of Life Itself*. Oxford: Princeton University Press.
Vander Schee, C. 2009. Fruit, vegetables, fatness, and Foucault: Governing students and their families through school health policy. *Journal of Education Policy*, 24(5), 557–74.
——— and Gard, M. 2011. Editorial: Politics, pedagogy and practice in school health policy. *Policy Futures in Education*, 9, 307–14.

PART IV
Ethics and Critique

Chapter 10

What Do Food Labels Teach People about Food Ethics?

Heather J. Bray and Rachel A. Ankeny

> If I looked at the label I would have no idea what it meant. I could read it until the cows come home, it doesn't mean anything to me … I'd like to be able to, but I actually don't know what I'm looking for … I'm not educated in label-reading I suppose. (Fiona, Adelaide, 2011)

Introduction

We are increasingly aware that our food choices are more complex than simple responses to our empty stomachs (at least in the developed world). We are encouraged in various ways to buy and eat 'responsibly'. Although texts that examine food ethics in general (e.g., Mepham 1996, Coveney 2006; Singer and Mason 2006; Pollan 2006; Nestle 2006) provide useful theoretical frameworks, they do not explore in any detail how most consumers deal with the often conflicting knowledge claims with which they are presented when making everyday food choices. Shifting cultural attitudes, belief systems, and habits together with increasing concerns about the ethics of food production pose a challenge for the food industry as there is limited understanding in the business world (even among those who promote 'ethical products') of who the ethical consumer is and what he or she wants (Chant 2008). Hence this chapter draws on ongoing qualitative research focused on explicating Australians' understandings of what we term 'ethical' food choices such as organic, 'green' or sustainable, fair-trade, low food miles, carbon-neutral, free-range, regional and local, and genetically modified (GM) foods.

Although our research explores these issues in the Australian context, we contend that there are many similarities to other developed countries which have experienced greatly increased uptake of ethical foods in recent years and which have some form of legislated labelling. Some differences in food habits have been documented: Australians are not as strongly opposed to GM foodstuffs (Biotechnology Australia 2005) as those in the EU, but are not as broadly accepting as those in the US. Australia tends to have lower rates of vegetarianism (and most define this category differently than, for instance, the British, cf. Beardsworth and Keil 1992), and though declining in comparison to historic norms, have higher average rates of intake of meat, as well as a deep cultural identification with being meat eaters (Ankeny 2008). Australians have growing interests in environmentally sustainable food products, given the country's biodiversity and frequency of severe weather events such as drought, and about the implications of their relative geographic isolation for the safety and security of the food supply. As a highly multicultural nation, Australian policy-makers are concerned with promoting culturally appropriate public health policies relating to nutrition and food.

Most Australian food labels are currently adequate to allow basic discrimination between products, particularly regarding core ingredients, nutritional content, and food safety (via proxy measures such as use-by-dates). Many manufacturers also include information that allows consumers to identify products that claim to be produced 'ethically', which has contributed to the recent and considerable growth in this market segment. Some have argued that these categories often are not reflective of consumer values but instead represent attempts by producers, retailers, and others in the supply chain to construct definitions according to commercial realities (e.g., Parker et al. 2013). We define food labels as all of the information provided on packaging or for unpackaged food at the point of sale. We consider this definition to cover not only ingredient and nutritional panels but also place-of-origin designators and details of processing or production methods (e.g., official accreditation or more informal markers). When considering food labels, we include all of the product descriptions provided, including 'stories' told about the product or manufacturer and images on the label. Our focus is on the average consumer's contact with information within the context of choosing products at a standard retail outlet. Of course other devices not explored here – such as the Internet, consumer guides, or food policy debates – may provide more detailed and higher-quality information than labels as well as the needed time and space for discourse and deeper understanding of key issues. Nevertheless, it is clear that many busy consumers rely primarily on labels when making food choices.

Some scholars have argued that choice of ethical food products should be viewed as a political act of 'resistance' to globalisation and capitalism (e.g., Guthman 2004; Holzer 2006; Hartleib and Jones 2009). According to them, ethical consumers choose to buy (or not to buy) products based on their political, religious, spiritual, environmental, and/or convictions in concert with their knowledge (Sandlin and Walther 2009). The growth of this market sector is viewed as representing increased community support as a result of growth in knowledge about various product categories. The validity of this 'cause and effect' relationship relies on the assumption that these transactions are in fact based on knowledge, and that such knowledge is readily available and interpreted in similar ways by consumers, producers, and retailers.

In contrast, our ongoing research has revealed that many people who report they wish to eat 'ethically' are frustrated when they try to make 'good' choices about what to buy, and feel that they have inadequate information and knowledge about the available products. They want more specific information on the origins of products (beyond legislated country-of-origin labelling), processing or production methods and their moral implications, and impacts on the producers or the environment in the production or distribution processes, to name a few examples. Hence we contend that the observed increase in purchasing in these 'ethical' food categories cannot be taken at face value as an indicator of increased knowledge (and in turn as evidence of choice of ethical foods as an act of resistance even in the weakest sense). Instead, as we will argue via two case studies, people often choose 'ethical' foods for reasons not directly related to typical ethical rationales and despite labels not providing the information that they view as essential to their purchasing choices.

Our interdisciplinary research is located at the intersection of several fields including food studies, bioethics, and public understanding of science. In this chapter, we utilise these perspectives to focus the lens of pedagogy on the types of product knowledge that are assumed and transferred via 'ethical' food labels, particularly scientifically based knowledge claims. Understanding how labels associated with ethical food categories are interpreted and what meanings are constructed by consumers is critical to developing a richer understanding of what consumers are seeking in 'ethical foods' and how labels could be improved to enable informed decision-making.

Food Labels as Pedagogical Devices

> most meat you'd assume would be local but you never really know what the cow ate or what the chicken ate and so you tend to think … they could have eaten something that was GM modified [*sic*] especially if it's a chicken … if you want to take that the next level back you look at the cow, where was the cow located, where was it eating? Was the farmer using you know pesticides or whatever, and you just don't know and it gets to the point where it's just too hard, you just buy it, and you turn into a creature of habit … I just can't find myself analysing all this stuff. I just want a couple of steaks and you give up, it's just too much information. (Darren, Adelaide, 2009)

Rick Flowers and Elaine Swan (2012b) define pedagogies as 'the sites, processes and technologies of learning and teaching that happen outside of formal educational systems' (after Sandlin et al. 2010; Luke 1996; see also Sandlin and McLaren 2010). We focus on one key type of informal pedagogy, the information presented on food labels at point of sale, to explore how food and the market serve as teachers via labels. It is undeniable that public, informal food pedagogy including labelling has influences on identity formation and also serves as a mechanism of cultural transfer, both of which are key themes in the literature (Burdick and Sandlin 2013).

Our focus on labels allows us to narrow our analysis to the knowledge at the core of the transactions within ethical food choices. Flowers and Swan (2011, 2012a) have emphasised the importance of not only the content-knowledge claims in food pedagogy but also who produces them and who is 'in the know'. Several ethical issues in food production have scientific issues at their core, and hence consumers' responses to scientific knowledge as compared to other types of knowledge claims are of particular interest. We take 'knowledge' to go beyond mere information, and do not assume that scientific knowledge should be privileged over other forms or types of knowledge, such as knowing through personal experiences or values. While there has been a move away from the deficit model of public engagement with science which holds that the public needs to be 'better educated' (or to have 'better knowledge') to make 'better decisions', we are yet to develop deeper understandings of how the scientific information that people receive is constructed and reinterpreted, especially in the case of food.

One study within public understanding of science that has specifically explored food labels (Eden 2011) examines them through the lens of *boundary objects* (Star and Griesemer 1989) which are objects that form an interface between one group and another. They are interpreted differently across communities and hence are plastic, but have enough immutable content to maintain integrity, remain recognisable, and serve as interpreters between communities. It is the messenger, and not just the message, that matters because boundary objects are given meaning according to their contexts, origins, and associations, rather than being free-floating bundles of information. It is the sense that users make of boundary objects that affects whether and how these objects communicate across multiple social worlds.

Sally Eden (2011) suggests that viewing food labels as boundary objects allows us to see that labels are sometimes given different meanings by producers and consumers which fail to facilitate the 'collective work' of reconnecting consumers with producers and promoting purchase. Thus the failure of food labels is less about the public's failure to receive and act on information provided by 'experts', but instead is a relational product of heterogeneous actors. Specifically with reference to organic versus fortified food labelling, Eden finds that most consumers reduce labelling information to a simple binary division between whether the product is viewed as science/technology/processed food or natural/raw/unprocessed food, especially where they feel they do not have enough knowledge to understand the information provided. Her research participants believe that food that is modified in some way (in this case, processed) *requires* labelling to explain the (negative) modifications involved, while raw food does not. They believe labels are only needed where they cannot make 'sense' of the raw food without such labelling. These ideas about labelling are at the core of contemporary labelling debates.

To further explore the notions of multiple knowledge/s that are in contest in the case of food labels, we present two 'ethical food' case studies from our own research together with relevant literature from a range of disciplines, including public understanding of science and behavioural economics. We explore the nature of knowledge on these labels viewed as 'boundary objects' and the meanings of these knowledges which are constructed socially and culturally by consumers, producers/manufacturers, retailers, and policy-makers.

Humanely Produced Animal Products: 'Happy Animals', Happy Consumers

> If I'm a consumer and I'm standing in the aisle of my supermarket and I look down at a box of eggs and there's a picture of a happy chicken outside with long grass, trees and lakes, than that is my expectation of what a free range egg is. (ACCC chair Sarah Court, 2012)

Rising demands for food and increasing urbanisation over the last 50 years have led to increased intensification of livestock production. Pig and poultry production in particular are predominantly intensive, vertically integrated industries in western societies such as Australia, where the biological efficiency of the animal has been maximised through manipulation of genetics, nutrition, and housing conditions. In response, increasing attention has been paid to the welfare of animals raised for food, both by producers hoping to maximise returns by maintaining healthy herds/ flocks (Hemsworth et al. 2009), and by the wider community who are concerned about animals (Fraser et al. 1997; Taylor and Signal 2009) and increasingly interested in 'ethical' food production and consumption. Recent Australian media reports and activist campaigns by groups such as Animals Australia have focused on practices that some consumers believe are unethical, such as sow stalls, caged hens, bobby calves, and live export of beef cattle and sheep. Industries and retailers are using labelling (some in association with prominent animal welfare groups such as the RSPCA) to identify products produced with higher standards of animal welfare. However there is little research on what meanings consumers construct from this additional information provided or whether these strategies alleviate or exacerbate concerns about animal welfare.

Currently, there is no legislated requirement in Australia to label products according to the type of animal production system utilised. However there are a number of non-regulated labels that make direct (or indirect) claims that a labelled product has been produced under a higher standard of animal welfare. Although 'certified organic' includes minimum standards for animal welfare, it is the term 'free-range' which has been most recently contested in Australia (Parker et al. 2013). While there is no legally enforceable definition of 'free-range', the current egg industry code limits free-range egg producers to 1,500 hens per hectare. The Australian Competition and Consumers Commission (ACCC) recently rejected a certification trademark application from the Australian Egg Corporation on the basis that they planned to use 'free-range' to describe birds kept at stocking densities of up to 20,000 birds per hectare and routinely practice beak trimming which was not viewed as congruent with the definition of 'free-range', noting that 'these practices and standards do not accord with consumer expectations about the free range production of eggs' (ACCC 2012).

The growth of the Australian 'humane' animal product market in recent years (e.g., 'free range' egg lines have nearly doubled between 2005 and 2011, according to Australian Egg Corporation reports) indicates that producers and retailers believe that there is increasing interest in these products and that consumers are seeking to influence production practices through their purchasing decisions (Dixon 2003; Kehlbacher et al. 2012). So as the conventional wisdom runs, people are buying more animal-friendly products because they 'care' about animals. We *do* know that consumers 'care' about animal welfare in theory: a number of studies reveal that a significant percentage of consumers believe that society has a moral obligation to maintain high standards of animal welfare for production animals (Frewer et al. 2005; Brom 2000; Vanhonacker et al. 2008; Taylor and Signal 2009). To date there has been little research on whether consumers are in fact seeking to influence animal production methods when they choose humanely produced products, although some claim that consumer purchases generally constitute a form of collective political action (e.g., Holzer 2006, Hartleib and Jones 2009, Parker et al. 2013). In most markets, humanely produced products attract a premium price because it is argued that these products cost more to produce, and therefore most studies of consumer choice in this domain examine 'willingness to pay' relative to other factors such as price and taste (e.g., Elbakidze and Nayga 2012).

Our research suggests that motivations to buy humane products are complex and interrelated with other food attributes, which is supported by other findings; for instance in a study by the consumer advocacy organisation Choice, its members (who presumably are a particularly concerned group of consumers) reported buying free-range eggs primarily for animal welfare reasons but also ranked taste, health/nutrition, and environmental reasons as secondary considerations (Clemons 2012). Participants in our focus groups who were motivated to avoid animal-based foods because of concerns about how livestock animals are treated were much more likely to be vegetarian or vegan. Few participants chose welfare-friendly products solely because these animals are kept in 'better' conditions; some who had removed animal products from their diet had done so not for reasons of animal welfare but because of the perceived impacts of meat production on the environment. For these latter participants, kangaroo meat (seen as more 'suited' to the Australian environment) was viewed as preferable to pasture-raised beef, as well as healthier and lower in fat.

One of the clearest observations from our research is that people who are willing to eat animal products (including meat) believe, quite strongly, that free-range meat is of better quality and is more nutritious and tastes better than non-free-range meat; because of these attributes, they are prepared to pay more for the products. As with other ethical characteristics, humane production is a credence attribute of food which cannot be directly discerned from the product itself at purchase or after consumption (although some consumers claim to be able to taste the difference with various ethical products). This connection drawn by many consumers between high animal welfare standards and higher quality also is correlated with positive assumptions about other attributes such as food safety and healthiness. Parallel conclusions have been drawn in a study of Italian participants tasting yoghurt products with and without animal welfare labelling who indicated that high welfare products failed to meet their quality expectations (Carlucci et al. 2009).

Further evidence that favouring a product labelled as humane often is the result of reading the label as a proxy for quality (rather than with consumer participation in a dialogue about the most ethical or appropriate animal production methods) comes from the limited knowledge base of most consumers about animal production methods. Australians report being concerned about animal welfare (Taylor and Signal 2009) but self-report wide variability of knowledge about farming practices. Interestingly, higher levels of self-rated knowledge do not increase 'willingness to pay' among rural participants, but do result in greater 'willingness to pay' among those from metropolitan areas. This finding suggests these groups of consumers are working with different types of knowledge, or that the knowledge which they have has led to different perspectives and hence diverse conclusions. Additionally, Australian consumers often do not perform better than chance when asked factual (but not highly scientific) questions about farming practices (Coleman 2010), suggesting that they know little of the detail of animal welfare-related practices and hence that they are likely to construct their own meanings from labels. In turn then it should be unsurprising to us that these meanings differ widely, and may go well beyond or outside the animal-friendly standards that are explicitly being labelled. A similar conclusion has been drawn in a US study where many consumers interpreted the term 'all-natural' on meat products as equivalent to 'free-range' when USDA standards in fact permit the former term only to indicate a lack of artificial ingredients, colours, and preservatives, and minimal processing (Abrams et al. 2010).

In the case of animal products, it may be more than background understandings and the words on the label that provide consumers with the basis for alternate constructed meanings. Anne Marie Todd (2010) explores how anthropomorphism, in particular the talking cows in the (USA-based) Happy Cows campaign, educate consumers that 'happy cows' make 'healthy' cheese. Cathy Glenn (2004) goes further in critiquing the same campaign as an example of factory farm discourse that uses 'Nature as Virtual Reality', removing the consumer from the realities of animal production by objectifying animals and appearing to enable them to give consent to being used for human purposes. Christine Parker and her colleagues (2013) deconstruct 'happy hen' pictures on Australian labels, noting that while some are clearly idyllic and not likely to be taken as actual representations of hens' living conditions, some labels of this type are presented as a form of 'evidence', replete with weblinks to 'chook cams', while still others provide textual defences of their portrayals (see also Miele 2011). While it may be doubtful that a consumer would choose one product over another because the animals featured on the label look 'happier' (despite the quote provided above), images of animals in idyllic locales are often used to market products to consumers and may collectively contribute to diverse views about how the majority of animal products are produced.

GM Foods: Blinded with Science?

> It's kind of a perception that … you get food from the lab or food from the garden and genetically modified to me is kind of food from the lab whereas food from the garden is the fresh, natural kind of stuff. (Sophie, Adelaide, 2011)

Although food containing GM ingredients has been available on Australian shelves for many years, the labelling of GM foods in Australia is hotly contested. Industry groups maintain that current standards are adequate; however, many advocacy and consumer groups claim that labelling laws are insufficient to allow consumers to make a 'choice' when purchasing food. 'Choice' in this usage implies that consumers are not provided with enough information to avoid GM foods, should they wish to do so. It is assumed in this discourse that consumers who choose to consume 'ethically' are avoiding GM products to some extent for political purposes such as to influence policy on growing GM crops (cf. Roff 2007), as well as for reasons relating to perceived health risks associated with GM ingredients. Our research (supported by existing scholarship on related topics) suggests that current GM labelling does not allow consumers to make purchasing choices that align with their ethical beliefs nor does it permit them to participate in a dialogue about the role of GM in food production through their purchasing decisions.

In Australia, food containing GM ingredients must be labelled as such as legislated by law [Australia New Zealand Food Standards Code – Standard 1.5.2 – Food Produced Using Gene Technology – F2012C00771]. However, there are notable exceptions including:

- highly refined food (other than that with altered characteristics) where the modified DNA or proteins resulting from it are removed during processing (e.g., canola oil from GM plants);
- a processing aid or food additive, where no modified DNA or protein resulting from it remains in the final food;
- flavours where the concentration in the final food is less than 0.1 per cent;
- unintentional presence, where the ingredient is less than 1 per cent of the food; and;
- any foods consumed at the point of sale (e.g., in restaurants or cafes).

These requirements reflect a position that (legislated) food labelling is about what a food contains, not how it is produced. Approval of GM products for sale by the regulating authority Food Standards Australia New Zealand (FSANZ) is based on the principle of 'substantial equivalence'; products deemed to have similar physical and chemical properties as their conventional counterparts are treated in the same manner with regard to health and safety and subjected to little, if any, additional testing (Lockie et al. 2005). Critics claim that this labelling regime shifts the responsibility for demonstrating safety away from industry and the need to establish riskiness onto its opponents; this in turn facilitates rapid approval of GM foods (Levidow and Carr 2000) and suits the needs of industry more than those of consumers, resulting in regulation *for* industry rather than regulation *of* industry (Lockie et al. 2005).

While there is strict regulation about labelling to indicate the *presence* of GM ingredients, there is currently no legislation regarding labelling to indicate the *absence* of GM ingredients. Consequently many products available for sale in Australia carry a 'GM-free' or similar label, even where there are no GM ingredients equivalent to those contained in the product available in Australia or globally. Food producers and manufacturers may be using this label in some cases for export compliance purposes. However, in Australia this type of labelling communicates values to local consumers, particularly by serving as a point of differentiation in the marketplace by implying that by choosing the non-GM product, you are *not* choosing or even are explicitly rejecting another (hypothetical but non-existent) GM product.

Our research has revealed several trends: first, many consumers tend to consider all non-GM foods as 'ethical', without disentangling the other values that might or might not be present in such products (such as local, sustainable, organic, and so on). Those who are not particularly concerned about eating GM ingredients often view their decisions as a function of a hierarchy of values where other ethical issues, such as buying local or environmentally sustainable products, are more important to them. Most research on attitudes to GM foods asks participants whether they purchase GM foods, and there is little further exploration of how consumers actually think they are identifying GM foods at the point of sale. Australian studies do indicate generally high levels of consumer support for GM labelling (Dietrich and Schibeci 2003; Lea 2005), although it is not clear whether participants in these studies were aware of the current labelling requirements (and their limitations). These studies indicate that the current labelling regime does not mitigate consumers' fears that they might be eating GM foods (Lea 2005), and they report anger over inadequate labelling. Our qualitative research supports these findings: the absence of a GM label is not considered by many consumers to be a sufficient indicator that a product is in fact not GM, at least according to their own definitions. For example, although there are no fresh GM fruit or vegetables for sale in Australia, seedless watermelons and 'overly large' strawberries are often viewed with suspicion as potentially GM by many of our research participants.

Activist groups claim that this labelling regime is insufficient to allow consumers to choose food that does not contain GM ingredients or has not been produced using GM ingredients, particularly because of the exemptions outlined above. In 2002 Greenpeace Australia launched the True Food Guide in large part to help shoppers avoid GM foods. The guide is based on whether companies 'have a clear policy on excluding GE [genetically engineered]-derived ingredients, including oils derived from GE crops, and animal products from animals fed on GE crops (but not processing aids and yeasts that are processed in a laboratory setting rather than in the open environment)' (True Food Network 2011). The contested definition of what a GM food is (e.g., something that contains modified DNA at a concentration of greater that 1 per cent versus something that has been produced with the use of GM technology at some point from paddock to plate) remains one of the main issues for labelling and a point of difference between supporters and opponents of GM foods.

The involvement of the retailers in this space has become increasingly important as they play critical roles in how food products come to be valued (Dixon 2003).

Many retailers are introducing their own labelling schemes; some of the largest retailing chains have removed GM foods from their own-brand products and have begun to increase lines of organic and other certified GM-free foods. Thus they create opportunities to represent themselves as champions of consumer interest and demands (Lockie 2002) through voluntary labelling which is promoted as more transparent.

Despite repeated calls for better labelling to allow consumers to make choices about whether to consume GM foods, questions remain about the most appropriate form of labelling and what information should be included. Meanwhile, consumers are making decisions to purchase (or not to purchase) GM foods based on *their own* understandings of what these labels mean. Given that the technological interventions associated with labelling are difficult to understand (Eden 2011), consumers must construct their own meanings and adapt the new information on the label to fit within decision frameworks which are more familiar to them. In the case of GM, our research has found that one way in which many consumers do this is by reconceptualising GM ingredients as a form of 'additive', and avoiding anything with additives as a way to avoid GM; this trend is particularly apparent among mothers with young children who may have behavioural or medical problems thought to result from or be exacerbated by 'additives'. Understanding how and by whom meanings associated with labels will be created, and whether they will actually allow consumers to make the decisions that they wish to make, is vital if consumers are to actively participate in food policy debates.

Learning to Choose Food Ethically: The Role of Food Labels

> I'm interested in promoting more sustainable agriculture and really the only sort of certified produce system that we have in place in Australia is the organic one … but I also buy the sustainable apple juice even though I'm not sure what thing it's certified under, in the hopes that at least they're making an effort to do something that's a more sustainable way of producing food. (Sally, Adelaide, 2011)

Food labels have evolved via legislation and practice to be more than descriptions of products hidden by packaging. They include a range of mandated information such as nutritional claims, ingredients, food safety information, and standardised terminology for health claims (in Australia, a recent set of reforms occurred; see the report 'Labelling Logic' by Blewett et al. 2011). But labels typically also contain a range of unregulated statements ('green' is a particularly important category currently undefined in Australian law) which are only disputable when they constitute false advertising (as with free-range). In addition, there are various voluntary or membership certifications in use, particularly for ethical categories such as organic, fair-trade, and sustainable.

From a non-regulatory viewpoint, labelling is a market-based construct. Thus 'ethical' labelling is arguably an oxymoron, particularly given current food chain structures. Many ethical categories are aimed at reducing the impact of market forces on agricultural systems and the environment, while using market forces to encourage people to act 'ethically'. Although on the surface ethical food labelling enables consumers to identify products and make purchases aligned with a preference for ethical modes of production, increasingly these 'special circumstances' attract price premiums or competitive advantages for participating firms. For organisations using ethical labels, economic factors often are as important (or more important) as enviro-social ones in choosing to label (Hartleib and Jones 2009; Parker et al. 2013).

Hence if one of the key purposes of 'pedagogy' is to educate and disrupt existing assumptions, particularly binaries between good and bad, current labelling regimes for ethical foods have limited abilities to do this. Similar to the paradox noted in 'green consumerism' (Kahn 2010), labelling leads to consumers making assumptions about the motivations underlying such labels (e.g., that the producer or retailer is more socially responsible and concerned about the same issues as the consumer). Consumers thus are absolved of the responsibility of figuring out which products are truly 'ethical' or of taking political action to correct unethical practices: '... the take-home message of green consumerism is largely to stop worrying about the big problems and to instead do one's little part for sustainability through endless repetitions of spending on behalf of "the planetary good"' (Kahn 2010: 49). Hence as Richard Kahn argues, green consumerism is limited pedagogically as it encourages a false sense of control over larger processes of production via purchasing; a similar point is made in Julie Guthman's 2007 critique of voluntary food labelling as a form of 'neoliberal governance'. In reality, these products obscure the critical knowledge that might be necessary to truly behave in a 'green' manner, or in the case of ethical foods more generally, 'ethically'.

Public understanding of ethical food choices must be viewed as shaped by scientific and non-scientific knowledge claims and 'embodied experiences' (Lyons 2006: 156), as has been illustrated via our two case studies. To focus merely on the need for more education about the 'facts' about various types of food categories is to overlook the context within which food choices occur, and the diverse values that people bring to these choices. Our approach contends that people's eating habits and food choices do not occur in a cultural, social, or historical vacuum: for example, people do not buy 'junk food' simply because they lack of knowledge about nutrition (as might be claimed under a deficit model of public understanding) or due to economic or other limitations to the access of foodstuffs, but within broader sociocultural, moral, and historical contexts that oftentimes go unrecognised in conventional approaches to these questions. Consumers may wish to make 'ethical choices', but struggle to do so within the context of real shopping which is limited by time as well as economic and other resources. Many consumers cannot achieve the high levels of 'ethical competency' necessary to make the 'right' decisions as this requires large amounts of time and investment to seek out information and shop accordingly (Miele and Evans 2010; Vecchio and Annunziata 2012) or what some term 'reflexively' (Roff 2007; Hartleib and Jones 2009).

It is these complex contexts that interact with the information presented on food labels whenever consumers make purchasing choices and create new meanings through their interpretations of labels and the products they describe. Understanding attitudes and values associated with food choice and consumption requires a deeper examination of the diverse factors that have influenced people's perceptions of their obligations and ethical choices with regard to food without presupposing that there is one correct answer (and hence we do not believe it is appropriate to describe a single model of 'ethical' decision-making with regard to food) or even an agreed-upon language for discussing food choice.

This chapter proposes that food labels should be viewed as a form of informal pedagogy because they are explicitly designed to inform consumers and provide them with some form of useful knowledge. Using the pedagogical lens then provides us a novel frame for considering not only what knowledge is contained (or is absent) on food labels, but also what forms of knowledge are privileged, who is providing the knowledge, and how consumers interpret and understand labels based on their own experiences, values, and background knowledge. As our case studies illustrate, consumers construct their own meanings based on food labels and these meanings may be (strictly speaking) factually incorrect (e.g., an absence of indicators regarding GM content may be taken as evidence for no GM ingredients) or may not be related to the label's original intent (such as the ways in which 'free-range' is a proxy for quality). Rather than viewing these diverse meanings simply as incorrect or labels as misleading, we have argued instead that labels should be considered as boundary objects that cross several worlds inhabited by stakeholders with diverse perspectives, and therefore are a rich source of data for the complex values at issue in relation to food ethics. Labels can allow people to choose between products by identifying those which are seemingly aligned with their values, but often result in products being understood as simply 'good' or 'bad' without engagement with key underlying issues that relate to whether the product in fact is aligned with particular values. This gap is marked given that many consumers have limited understandings of various ethical food categories and even less awareness of the limits of current labelling regimes or of the range of products actually available in a particular market.

The most sceptical critic might note that what results from this situation is a kind of political consumerism 'lite': labels make it easy for a consumer to think that he or she is doing something 'good' in choosing one product over another when in reality labelling is often unregulated and increasingly driven by the mainstream commercial sector. Hence labelling on products appears to teach people (or perhaps dictate to them) what is 'good' without allowing them to engage in a deeper dialogue about the multiplicity of factors and the broader contexts that influence whether a product is in fact 'good' in terms of their values.

Therefore, labels are a critical avenue for informal pedagogy about food and its associated attributes and it is necessary to develop a framework and a language for debating issues associated with food ethics in contemporary

Australia in order to foster more productive public involvement in food policy. Evidence from consumer studies indicates that our current labelling regimes and practices are not in fact leading to these deeper forms of engagement. Rethinking current approaches to labelling by viewing it as a form of pedagogy allows us to reconsider how to foster more effective and just food-related policies, and also provides opportunities for better alignment of consumer values and needs with industry marketing strategies.

Acknowledgements

The authors would like to acknowledge the assistance of Susie Chant, Joanne Givens, and Kelly McKinley with the pilot work, which was partially funded by a small grant from the Adelaide Faculty of Humanities and Social Sciences. This research has been supported by an Australian Research Council grant DP110105062 and NETS/DFEEST.

References

Abrams, K.M., Meyers, C.A. and Irani, T.A. 2010. Naturally confused: Consumers' perceptions of all-natural and organic pork products. *Agriculture and Human Values*, 27, 365–74.

ACCC. 2012. *ACCC not satisfied with proposed free range egg standards. Media Release*. [Online] Available at http://www.accc.gov.au/media-release/accc-not-satisfied-with-proposed-free-range-egg-standards [accessed: 5 September 2013].

Ankeny, R.A. 2008. The moral economy of red meat in Australia, in *Food and Morality: Proceedings of the Oxford Symposium on Food and Cookery 2007*, edited by S. Friedland. Totnes: Prospect Books, 20–28.

Beardsworth, A. and Keil, T. 1992. The vegetarian option: Varieties, conversions, motives and careers. *The Sociological Review*, 40, 253–93.

Blewett, N., Goddard, H., Pettigrew, S., Reynolds, C. and Yeatman, H. 2011. *Labelling Logic: Review of Food Labelling Law and Policy*. Canberra: Commonwealth of Australia.

Biotechnology Australia 2005. *What You Really Need to Know about What the Public Really Thinks about GM Foods* [Online]. Available at: http://www.biotechnology.gov.au/assets/documents/bainternet/GMFood20052005111516025 4.pdf [accessed 12 February 2010].

Brom, F.W.A. 2000. Food, consumer concerns, and trust: Food ethics for a globalising market. *Journal of Agricultural and Environmental Ethics*, 12, 127–39.

Burdick, J. and Sandlin, J.A. 2013. Learning, becoming and the unknowable: Conceptualizations, mechanisms, and process in public pedagogy literature. *Curriculum Inquiry*, 43, 142–77.

Carlucci, A., Monteleone, E., Braghieri, A. and Napolitano, F. 2009. Mapping the effect of information about animal welfare on consumer liking and willingness to pay for yogurt. *Journal of Sensory Studies*, 24, 712–30.

Chant, S.M. 2008. Solefoods: An Opportunity Assessment. Adelaide University Incubator (unpublished research).

Clemons, R. 2012. *Free range eggs: What does 'free range' really mean, and are consumers being misled?* [Online: CHOICE] Available at: http://www.choice.com.au/reviews-and-tests/food-and-health/food-and-drink/organic-and-free-range/free-range-eggs-2012.aspx. [accessed 5 September 2013].

Coleman, G.J. 2010. Educating the public: information or persuasion? *Journal of Veterinary Medical Education*, 37, 74–82.

Coveney, J. 2006. *Food, Morals and Meaning*. London: Routledge.

Dietrich H. and Schibeci, R. 2003. Beyond public perceptions of gene technology: Community participation in public policy in Australia. *Public Understanding of Science*, 12, 381–401.

Dixon, J. 2003. Authority, power and value in contemporary industrial food systems. *International Journal of Sociology of Agriculture and Food*, 11, 31–9.

Eden, S. 2011. Food labels as boundary objects: how consumers make sense of organic and functional foods. *Public Understanding of Science*, 20, 179–94.

Elbakidze, L. and Nayga, R.M. 2012. The effects of information on willingness to pay for animal welfare in dairy production: Application of nonhypothetical valuation mechanisms. *Journal of Dairy Science*, 95, 1099–1107.

Flowers, R. and Swan, E. 2011. 'Eating at us': Representations of knowledge in the activist documentary film Food Inc. *Studies in the Education of Adults*, 43, 234–50.

———. 2012a. Pedagogies of doing good: Problematisations, authorities, technologies and teleologies in food activism. *Australian Journal of Adult Learning*, 52(3), 532–72.

———. 2012b. Why food? Why pedagogy? Why adult education? *Australian Journal of Adult Learning*, 52(3), pp. 419–33.

Food Standards Australia New Zealand. 2007. *Annual Report 2006–2007*. Canberra: FSANZ.

———. 2010. *Australia New Zealand Food Standards Code. Standard 1.5.2. Food Produced Using Gene Technology*. [Online]. Available at: http://www.comlaw.gov.au/Series/F2008B00628 [accessed 30 September 2013].

Fraser, D., Weary, D.M., Pajor, E.A. and Milligan, B.N. 1997. A scientific conception of animal welfare that reflects ethical concerns. *Animal Welfare*, 6, 187–205.

Frewer, L.J., Kole, A., Van De Kroon, S.M.A. and de Lauwere, C. 2005. Consumer attitudes towards the development of animal-friendly husbandry systems. *Journal of Agricultural and Environmental Ethics*, 18, 345–67.

Glenn, C.B. 2004. Constructing consumables and consent: a critical analysis of factory farm industry discourse. *Journal of Communication Inquiry*, 28, 63–81.

Guthman, J. 2004. *Agrarian Dreams: The Paradox of Organic Farming in California*. Berkeley: University of California Press.
———. 2007. The Polanyian way? Voluntary food labels as neoliberal governance. *Antipode*, 39, 456–78.
Hartleib, S. and Jones, B. 2009. Humanising business through ethical labelling: Progress and paradoxes in the UK. *Journal of Business Ethics*, 88, 583–600.
Hemsworth, P.H., Barnett, J.L. and Coleman, G.J. 2009. The integration of human-animal relations into animal welfare monitoring schemes. *Animal Welfare*, 18, 335–45.
Holzer, B. 2006. Political consumerism between individual choice and collective action: Social movements, role mobilization and signalling. *International Journal of Consumer Studies*, 30, 405–15.
Kahn, R. 2010. Producing crisis: Green consumerism as an ecopedagogical issue, in *Critical Pedagogies of Consumption*, edited by J.A. Sandlin and P. McLaren. New York: Routledge, 47–57.
Kehlbacher, A., Bennett, R. and Balcombe, K. 2012. Measuring the consumer benefits of improving farm animal welfare to inform welfare labelling. *Food Policy*, 37, 627–33.
Lea, E. 2005. Beliefs about genetically modified foods: A qualitative and quantitative exploration. *Ecology of Food and Nutrition*, 44, 437–54.
Levidow, L. and Carr, S. 2000. Unsound science? Transatlantic regulatory disputes over GM crops. *International Journal of Biotechnology*, 2, 257–73.
Lockie, S. 2002. 'The invisible mouth': Mobilizing 'the consumer' in food production-consumption networks. *Sociologia Ruralis*, 42, 278–94.
———, Lawrence, G., Lyons, K. and Grice, J. 2005. Factors underlying support or opposition to biotechnology among Australian food consumers and implications for retailer-led food regulation. *Food Policy*, 30, 399–418.
Luke, C. 1996. Introduction. In C. Luke (ed.), *Feminisms and Pedagogies of Everyday Life*. Albany: State University of New York Press, 2–31.
Lyons, K. 2006. Environmental values and food choices: views from Australian organic food consumers. *Journal of Australian Studies*, 87, 155–66.
Mepham, B. 1996. *Food Ethics*. London: Routledge.
Miele, M. 2011. The taste of happiness: Free-range chicken. *Environment and Planning A*, 43, 2076–90.
——— and Evans, A. 2010. When foods become animals: Ruminations on ethics and responsibility in care-full practices of consumption. *Ethics, Place and Environment*, 13, 171–90.
Nestle, M. 2006. *What to Eat*. New York: North Point Press.
Parker, C. Brunswick, C. and Kotev, J. 2013. The happy hen on your supermarket shelf: What choice does industrial strength free-range represent for consumers. *Journal of Bioethical Enquiry*, 10, 165–86.
Pollan, M. 2006. *The Omnivore's Dilemma*. New York: Penguin Press.
Roff, R.J. 2007. Shopping for change? Neoliberalizing activism and the limits to eating non-GMO. *Agriculture and Human Values*, 24, 511–22.

Sandlin, J.A. and McLaren, P. 2010. *Critical Pedagogies of Consumption: Living and Learning in the Shadow of the 'Shopocalyse'*. New York: Routledge.

Sandlin, J.A. and Walther, C.S. 2009. Complicated simplicity. Moral identity formation and social movement learning in the voluntary simplicity movement. *Adult Education Quarterly*, 59, 298–371.

Singer, P. and Mason, J. 2006. *The Ethics of What We Eat: Why Our Food Choices Matter*. New York: Rodale.

Star, S. and Griesemer, J. 1989. Institutional ecology, 'translations' and boundary objects: Amateurs and professionals in Berkeley's Museum of Vertebrate Zoology, 1907–39. *Social Studies of Science*, 19, 387–420.

Taylor, N. and Signal, T.D. 2009. Willingness to pay: Australian consumers and 'on the farm' animal welfare. *Journal of Applied Animal Welfare Science*, 12, 345–59.

Todd, A.M. 2010. Happy cows and passionate beefscapes: Nature as landscape and lifestyle in food advertisements, in *Critical Pedagogies of Consumption*, edited by J.A. Sandlin and P. McLaren. New York: Routledge, 169–79.

True Food Network. 2011. *True food guide. How we rated companies*. [Online]. Available at http://www.truefood.org.au/truefoodguide/HowWeRate/ [accessed 20 December 2012].

Vanhonacker, F., Verbeke, W., Van Poucke, E. and Tuyttens, F.A.M. 2008. Do citizens and farmers interpret the concept of farm animal welfare differently? *Livestock Science*, 116, 126–36.

Vecchio, R. and Annunziata, A. 2012. Italian consumer awareness of layer hens' welfare standards: A cluster analysis. *International Journal of Consumer Studies*, 36, 647–55.

Chapter 11
Learning to Eat with Attitude: Critical Food Pedagogies

Jennifer Sumner

Introduction

In the winter of 2011, I began teaching a master's-level course called The Pedagogy of Food at the Ontario Institute for Studies in Education of the University of Toronto. The decision to develop such a course in the Adult Education and Community Development (AECD) Program where I work was based on a number of parameters: the growing coverage of food in mass media such as newspapers and online blogs; the formation of the interdisciplinary Canadian Association for Food Studies; the burgeoning popular and academic literature on food issues; and my personal observation that, when searching for a topic for a final paper, many students chose a food-related one.

Teaching this course for the last three years has inevitably raised questions about food pedagogies in the classroom – what are they, why are they important, who should they be aimed at, what curricula should they have? In this chapter, I engage with these questions by first discussing the nature of pedagogy itself before moving on to explore food pedagogies, including critical food pedagogies and their place in an increasingly neoliberal context. I also reflect on the nature of the teaching and learning activities I have used over the last three years, and how they have affected students' relationships to food.

Pedagogy

The English term pedagogy has its roots in the ancient Greek words for child and leader, and was linked to the slave who escorted the children to school (*Websters* 1990) and the room in the school where the slaves waited for the children being taught (*OED* 2013). From this inauspicious beginning, the term evolved into 'the art, occupation or practice of teaching', including the theory or principles of education (*OED* 2013).

Despite attempts to replace pedagogy with the concept of andragogy to differentiate the teaching of adults from the teaching of children (e.g., Knowles 1989), pedagogy has remained the term of choice regarding the 'art, science or profession of teaching' (*Websters* 1990) people of all ages. Associated with the classroom for many years, the term has recently moved beyond these confines with what Rick Flowers and Elaine Swan (2012: 424) refer to as 'the pedagogical turn', which involves using pedagogy:

> in a broader sense beyond classroom teaching practices in schools and universities to examine the proliferation and intensification of teaching, learning, curricula, training and education outside of educational institutions.

The pedagogical turn has multiple influences, including the work of Paulo Freire (1996) with the poor in the streets of Brazil, the recognition of social movements as sites of learning (Miles 1996; Sumner 2008a), the valorization of lifelong learning (Longworth and Davies 1996) and the educational role of public institutions such as museums (see, for example, Chadwick and Stannett 1995). This turn was reinforced by the explicit use of new understandings of pedagogy, such as Carmen Luke's (1996) pedagogies of everyday life, Henry Giroux's (2004) use of public pedagogy, Greg Noble's (2013) ideas about cultural pedagogies and pedagogies of civil belonging, and Anna Hickey-Moody et al.'s (2010) pedagogy writ large. The pedagogical turn has inspired a number of theorists including Giroux (2002) and Jenny Sandlin et al. (2009) to, in the words of Flowers and Swan (2012: 424), 'conceptualise pedagogy on different terms than in traditional educational theory where typically pedagogy is defined in terms of formal curricula, classroom processes and educational institutions'. In contrast, they define pedagogy as 'the sites, processes and technologies of learning and teaching that happen outside of formal educational systems' (424). For Flowers and Swan, pedagogical sites

> are now seen to include mass media, popular culture, museums, art galleries, public policy projects, welfare institutions, health, community activities, reality TV, psychological practices, the internet, screen technologies and media, and social networking sites. (424)

This broad conceptualization has provided the opportunity for a particular focus of learning and teaching – food pedagogies.

Food Pedagogies

A new concept in the educational and food studies lexicon, food pedagogies represent the introduction of pedagogical issues to the realm of food. Food is a natural candidate for this synthesis because 'not only is food an *object* of learning, but it is also a *vehicle* for learning' (Flowers and Swan 2012: 423). This observation emphasizes the fact that food is not only a worthy object of study in itself, but also, as Mustafa Koç et al. (2012) observe, an entrée into larger issues that concern humankind: sustainability, development, globalization, governance and power.

To date, few people have directly examined the concept of food pedagogies, but Flowers and Swan (2012, 2013) have recently opened a whole field of study in the area. For these authors, the term 'food pedagogies' refers to:

> Congeries of education, teaching and learning about how to grow, shop for, prepare, cook, display, taste, eat and dispose of food by a range of agencies, actors and media; and aimed at a spectrum of 'learners' including middle class women, migrants, children, parents, shoppers, and racially minoritised and working class mothers. (2012: 425)

In this way, Flowers and Swan (2013) have created a conceptual space that is:

> capacious enough to denote a range of sites, processes, curricula, 'learners' and even types of human and non-human 'teachers' but tight enough to refer to some kind of intended or emergent change in behaviour, habit, emotion, cognition, and/or knowledge at an individual, family, group or collective level. (4)

The creation of such a conceptual space encourages a spectrum of applications – hence 'pedagogies' in the plural – that allows for breadth while also focusing on the kinds of change anticipated by Flowers and Swan. Many of these applications address questions of power and thus open up the possibility for critical food pedagogies.

Critical Food Pedagogies

In this chapter, I am using the term 'critical food pedagogies' as a subset of Matthias Finger's (2005: 167) understanding of critical pedagogy, which is based on a 'rational theory of emancipation, conceived as a cognitive consciousness-raising process among socially interacting individuals'. From this perspective, critical pedagogy regards education as a political, not a neutral, process and 'seeks to illuminate how education and learning (teachers as well as learners) are implicated in structures and practices that both reinforce and challenge injustices' (Butterwick 2005: 257). According to Finger (2005: 167):

> critical pedagogy has two meanings, namely (a) the fact of being or becoming aware of non-emancipatory institutions and worldviews, which is a form of ideology critique, and (b) the process of reasoning critically, which is a form of awareness raising.

The ideology critique and awareness raising associated with Finger's (2005) understanding of critical pedagogy bring certain issues of power to the forefront of pedagogical inquiry. Early iterations of this perspective on critical pedagogy focused on issues of class (e.g., Freire's critical approach to literacy), but feminists challenged the gender and race-blind elements of the term, along with other issues implicated in inequality, such as sexuality and able-bodiness (Butterwick 2005).

If this perspective on critical pedagogy raises some questions about power, and food pedagogies allow for breadth while also focusing on change, then we can understand that critical food pedagogies entail a range of approaches that are not just concerned with any type of change, but with change that addresses power and injustice – what might be termed progressive change, understood by Alan Bullock and Stephen Trombley (1999: 690) as change that is characterized by a search for four factors:

> for a new balance in the relationship between increasingly remote global corporations and the interests of the worker, consumer and environment; for improved means to secure greater equality for women and minorities; for a redistribution of political power from corporate capital and from a vast federal government; for a tolerance which embraces the nation's growing ethnic and cultural diversity.

Examples of critical food pedagogies based on Finger's (2005) perspective would include the educational work of the social movement Food Not Bombs (FNB), which is concerned with not only 'drawing attention to the immediate food security needs of individuals and communities', but also challenging 'notions of democracy and social justice through a critique of the corporate global food system as well as engaging issues of food access for individuals living in poverty' (Mair et al. 2008: 388). Activists in the Kitchener-Waterloo chapter of FNB worked to inform themselves and others about the environmental and social impacts of power-laden processes of food production, marketing and distribution, challenged notions of public space and fostered public awareness by making visible serious social problems including poverty, homelessness and poor nutrition (Mair 2005).

These types of critical food pedagogies are overtly political – that is, they follow Leslie Lipson's (1981) observation that politics is the process in which a community confronts a series of great issues and chooses between opposing values. In this way, they reflect Freire's (1976) timeless observation that education is never neutral but highly political, whether recognized or not. They are also consciously critical because they involve 'questioning the pretensions of organized power' (Innis in Neufeld and Whitworth 1997) – in particular the power associated with the state and the market. And these critical food pedagogies can be found at a range of scales, from the individual through the local to the national and the global. In addition, they aim to promote progressive change through more balanced relationships, greater equality, redistributed power and cultural tolerance.

Such critical food pedagogies also involve what has been termed 'dangerous knowledge' (Welton 1991), knowledge that challenges the status quo in terms of food. According to Chris Argyris et al. (1985: xi), the status quo involves a pattern created by the interdependence among norms, rules, skills, and values 'that becomes so omnipresent as to be taken for granted and to go unchallenged'.

With respect to food, the norms, rules, skills, and values of the status quo are created by powerful corporate players in the global market. These critical food pedagogies valorize the knowledge that challenges the industrial food system by disseminating it through workshops, blogs, email lists and courses. An example of the latter is the course called The Pedagogy of Food.

Critical Food Pedagogies in Action: Teaching The Pedagogy of Food

Courses focusing on food are sprouting on university campuses, exhibiting both a conscious and an unconscious understanding of food pedagogies. From Marion Nestle's (2010) inspired teaching in the early 1990s to Julie Guthman's current work at the University of California, Santa Cruz, courses about food are being gobbled up by students eager to engage with food issues. But few, if any, of these courses focus on the pedagogical aspects of food. This aporia begged to be filled as I developed a course focused on food in an institution dedicated to education.

The inspiration for the course came from a comment I had read by the American essayist Wendell Berry, who argued that eating is an agricultural act. As someone with an agricultural background, I immediately felt this comment exploding in my mind with possibilities. Not only did it link food from field to fork, but it also opened up a multiplicity of other considerations. His comment prompted me to write a conference paper, which was later published as a journal article (Sumner 2008b). In that article, I concluded that:

> Eating is not only an agricultural act. It is also a social act, a political act, a cultural act, an economic act and an environmental act. And it is, above all, a pedagogical act. By eating, we can learn to adapt to a dysfunctional industrial food system that benefits a privileged few and downloads never-ending, unsustainable costs onto people, communities, nation-states and the environment. But eating can also help us to learn to think, to resist and to build an alternative future. (36)

This article was on my mind while I developed the course during 2010. As I struggled to come up with a resonant title for the course, I realized that I already had all the necessary components, so I named it The Pedagogy of Food.

In the beginning, pedagogical components were woven into the course design but did not constitute an overt part of it, due to the dearth of writings on the subject. Over the years, this has changed, particularly because of the pioneering work of Flowers and Swan (2012, 2013). But the lack of literature did not preclude conscious engagement with the pedagogy of food. For example, during the second or third class, I bring in oranges to open up a discussion of commodity fetishism. Holding up an orange, I ask, 'if this orange could speak, what could it tell you?' Initial looks of incredulity are quickly followed by thoughtful comments: how it was grown, how those who picked it were treated, how far it had travelled, how much the people who unpacked it at the supermarket were paid. Such an exercise 'removes the veil' (Hudson and Hudson 2003) that obscures the social, economic and environmental relations behind the final product that we purchase. Students also seized the pedagogical moment, like the woman who brought in a loaf of Russian black bread to share with the class, so she could teach us about her childhood in the Soviet Union. In this way, to reiterate Flowers and Swan (2012), food is truly a vehicle for learning. Such integrated pedagogy is consistent with the spirit of adult education, where students often learn by doing. As I tell students in the Introduction to Adult Education course I also teach – you will not learn the 10 top tips for teaching adults in this course, but by the end of the semester, you will have been exposed to, and participated in, many ways of teaching adults.

Curriculum

The course combined two of my central interests – education and food. The pedagogical aspects were clearly present in the curriculum, but the main focus began as food. This was partly due to the dearth of readings on food pedagogies, and partly due to the wealth of books and articles on the subject of food.

From the beginning, the course was designed from a critical perspective, which mirrors the overall perspective of the Adult Education and Community Development Program where I teach. I told the students that I expected them to critically engage with the readings, classroom discussions and assignments – mere description was not enough. In essence, they needed to learn to develop an open, questioning attitude toward the subject matter, question the pretensions of organized power and take nothing for granted. The overall goal of the course was to help students gain a basic understanding of the critical pedagogy of food, while the objectives included cultivating an understanding of the interface between the field of adult education and food; appreciating the importance of this interface within the global and local context; gaining familiarity with issues associated with food; and raising awareness of the importance of food in any pedagogical endeavour. To guide student thinking, I chose three themes: eating is an agricultural act (Berry 1990); food is an edible dynamic (Belasco 2007); and eating is a pedagogical act (Sumner 2008b). In particular, eating can be understood as a pedagogical act because it involves:

> teaching, learning, inclusion, enculturation, etiquette, environmental awareness, sharing, alliances, celebration, and transcendence. Food catalyzes the potential for experiential learning, social learning, lifelong learning, transformative learning, informal learning, incidental learning, embodied learning and collective learning. (Sumner 2008b: 35)

The readings for the first year were a mix of academic and popular literature, with three of the authors coming to the classroom to discuss their work with the students. The readings dealt with a range of issues: the power of food, the political economy of food, food justice, the local food movement and global food. Student feedback at the end of the course encouraged me to be even more focused in my approach to readings the following year, with greater emphasis on the academic side. As a result, the second iteration of the course featured readings that focused on introducing food, the politics of food, the pedagogy of food, global food, local food, organic food and several food issues. In the third year, I presented yet another new set of readings, partly inspired by the advice of the students in the second year of the course and partly due to the publication of my co-edited book on critical food studies (Koç et al. 2012).

The assignments, however, have not varied over the three years. The first is always a personal reflection about the role of food in students' lives, their understanding of what we can learn from food and their vision of the role that food can play in the search for a more sustainable world. This assignment does not require any academic referencing, but simply kick-starts the thinking processes about food and food pedagogies, and creates a personal benchmark for student learning over the semester. In this assignment, students have reflected on such subjects as comfort food, memories of grandparents' vegetable gardens, mom's cooking and struggles with food and body image. The second assignment involves a group presentation – a critical analysis of a programme or organization that focuses on food. At the Masters' level, group assignments are of a high calibre and become not only learning journeys for the presenters, but also teaching opportunities for them – in essence, they spend an hour teaching the rest of the class what they learned about a local, regional, national or international food programme or organization. Over the years, there have been presentations on such programs/organizations as a local, mobile food distribution business, the provincial food certifier called Local Food Plus and a new food co-op. The third and fourth assignments are tied together, with the latter being a final paper and the former being a poster of the final paper. The third assignment sprang from my realization that I was the only one who read the students' final papers and it seemed a shame to waste the pedagogical opportunity they offered. Doing a poster presentation of their final paper allowed students to share their research and learning with peers, while also creating a teaching tool that others at OISE could study and enjoy – all posters are hung on the walls of the department for a number of months. The final papers use the readings as a basic resource and concentrate on a chosen focal area. Over the years, students have written about such topics as the Hawaiian pineapple industry, eco-villages, worm composting, coffee production in Jamaica, permaculture in Cuba and indigenous food sovereignty.

In addition to the presentations associated with assignments, a number of structured activities also take place during the semester. On the first day of class, after some discussion about the pedagogy of food, I involve the students in an exercise I call conceptualization. After forming them into groups of three or four and giving them flip-chart paper and markers, I ask them to draw the relationship between food and learning. The purpose of the exercise is to get them thinking about the subject matter of the course and to work together to create of vision of what it might entail. Each group negotiates the concepts to illustrate this relationship, then works on the drawing, hangs it up and explains it to the class, prompting comments and suggestions from fellow students. On the last day of class, I hang the pictures back up and ask each group if they would draw the picture differently, given what they have learned over the semester. Most suggest changes, some of a radical nature. All can see the learning journey they have made during the 12 weeks of the course.

As mentioned above, I always try to bring in guest speakers, preferably authors who are on the reading list. In addition, the myriad films on the subject of food provide excellent pedagogical fodder. Twice, a student has led a mindful eating exercise, which encourages people to slow down and become more aware of their food. Some activities are relatively unstructured, as when students pass around a newspaper or magazine article about food, which sparks an impromptu discussion or they bring in food that they share and talk about. In the first class, I usually pass around fair-trade chocolate, using it as a springboard for talking about the issues behind fair trade: the poverty of the farmers who grow our food, the chronic unfairness of the global food system and the dialectical interplay between bottom-up personal choice and top-down government policy. Using chocolate as a pedagogical tool produces instantaneous results – those who may have doubted the pedagogical impact of food feel it viscerally during this exercise.

Students

Canada is very multicultural, with one in five people born outside the country, and Toronto is even more so – 45 per cent of the city's population were born outside Canada (Chui et al. 2007). The OISE student body reflects this diversity, which makes for an enriched classroom experience. Amidst this diversity, however, the students who apply to the Adult Education and Community Development Program have a number of commonalities: they are middle class, they are predominantly women, they are somewhat older than the average graduate student, they have a wealth of work and volunteer experience that they bring to the classroom, and they have a social-justice perspective.

It is clear from the end-of-term student evaluations that most students enjoy the class and learn a great deal. It also seems to leave a lasting impression on a number of them. For example, one student approached me after the second class to explain that she was very uncomfortable with a critical perspective – it was not familiar and she had never encountered it before. But she was willing to learn, even though she realized it would bring her into conflict with her job. Over the semester she worked hard and not only received an 'A' in the course, but also decided to apply to transfer from the non-thesis M.Ed programme to the MA programme. She successfully transferred and went on to produce an acutely critical thesis on the effects of the private Global Food Safety Initiative on public food safety in Canada. In the acknowledgements of her thesis, she credited The Pedagogy of Food as having a profound impact on her understanding of the food system.

When taking the course, another student became aware of the good work of a non-profit organization in Toronto called The Stop, which offers an array of services and initiatives, including community gardens and kitchens, after-school cooking and gardening programmes, a farmers' market, and community advocacy training, as well as a nutrition and support programme for new and expectant mothers and a sustainable-food-systems education centre (Saul 2011). An aspiring pastry chef, she not only began volunteering to bake for The Stop, but also created a website to encourage others to do the same (Seiw 2011).

Teaching a course like The Pedagogy of Food raises questions about the ultimate aim of critical food pedagogies. Why is it important to teach this way? What is the point of the knowledge that is shared, created and diffused beyond the classroom? In the next section, I will describe some of the projects carried out by the students, which will help to illustrate what they learned about the politics of food in a neoliberal world.

Critical Food Pedagogies in a Global Context

Critical food pedagogies do not occur in a vacuum. They are carried out within a larger context that has been given a variety of names: turbo capitalism, globalization and neoliberalism. I will work with the last term because it has traction among critical pedagogues who work from Finger's (2005) perspective (see, for example, Youngman 2000; Collins 2006; Sumner 2008c) and conveys the theoretical framework behind the cumulative disasters we are facing around the world.

Critical geographer David Harvey (2006: 145) has defined neoliberalism as:

> a theory of political economic practices which proposes that human well-being can best be advanced by the maximization of entrepreneurial freedoms within an institutional framework characterized by private property rights, individual liberty, free markets, and free trade. The role of the state is to create and preserve an institutional framework appropriate to such practices.

Harvey (2006) goes on to point out that neoliberalism has entailed a great deal of destruction, not only of prior institutional frameworks and powers, but also of 'divisions of labour, social relations, welfare provisions, technological mixes, ways of life, attachments to the land, habits of the heart, ways of thought, and so on' (146). This destruction has resulted in the cascading social, environmental and economic crises we face today. I use Harvey's description of neoliberalism on the second day of class to establish the larger context for the pedagogy of food, and continue to refer to it over the course of the semester as questions arise about various food crises. In response, some students did their group presentation on the global beverage giant Coca-Cola, critiquing its role in the obesity epidemic and its marketing programmes in developing countries. Another group dissected Canada's food guide, finding its 'nutritionism' approach reduced food to its constituent parts, without consideration of such issues as culture, spirituality or community, which ultimately helps multinational food processors promote their largely unhealthy products. And a third group presented on food waste and linked it to neoliberal globalization and food crises in communities. In terms of posters of final papers, there were projects on cancer and the food system, meat eating and climate change, the commodification of water and the impacts of the industrial food system across international borders.

With reference to food, Guthman (2008) maintains that neoliberal policies have fostered the restructuring of the agriculture and food sectors through the privatization of land and water rights, the use of free trade agreements to dismantle national-level food safety regulations and the protracted dismantling of food-oriented entitlement programmes set up to combat hunger. Further, she argues, neoliberalism has become so pervasive that it has even had a lasting influence on attempts to oppose these policies in the food and agricultural sectors. In other words, neoliberalism has also shaped the 'politics of the possible' (1180) in that efforts to develop alternatives and/or to redress some of the negative implications of neoliberal policies are still framed within its worldview, thus continuing to condition our relationship to food and significantly narrowing how we imagine the future. In response to her work, one group of students gave a presentation on fair trade, and criticized the dominant free trade regime, which exploits farmers around the world. And a number of groups did their projects on NGOs that have stepped in to fill the gaps in dismantled food programmes, such as FoodShare and The Stop. In terms of posters of final papers, there were projects on such subjects as unsustainable fishing practices and the exploitation of migrant farm workers.

Critical pedagogies of food critique the narrowing of the politics of the possible and raise awareness of how neoliberalism contributes to what Harvey (2006: 153) describes as 'accumulation by dispossession', that is, modes of accumulation that dispossess the majority of their means of life, which can range from enclosing the commons to the privatization of public healthcare. The concept of accumulation by dispossession not only applies fruitfully to food issues. It also provides a framework for conceptualizing what can be understood as a *pedagogy of the dispossessed*, based on Freire's (1996) classic creation – pedagogy of the oppressed. According to Freire (1996: 30), the pedagogy of the oppressed:

> must be forged *with*, not *for*, the oppressed (whether individuals or peoples) in the incessant struggle to regain their humanity. This pedagogy makes oppression and its causes objects of reflection by the oppressed, and from that reflection will come their necessary engagement in the struggle for their liberation. And in the struggle this pedagogy will be made and remade.

Following Freire, the pedagogy of the dispossessed

> must be forged with, not for, *the dispossessed* (whether individuals or peoples) in the incessant struggle to regain their humanity. This pedagogy makes

> *dispossession* and its causes objects of reflection by *the dispossessed*, and from that reflection will come their necessary engagement in the struggle for their liberation. And in the struggle this pedagogy will be made and remade.

This transformational pedagogy mirrors Guthman's (in Stoneman 2010) concept of radical food pedagogy, understood as a pedagogy that 'must go beyond self-satisfying food choices and have students reflect on potential levers of transformation'. Such transformation would entail the broadening of the politics of the possible that is embedded in critical food pedagogies – a kind of pedagogy of the possible. Pedagogies of the possible were reflected in some of the group projects, such as the presentation on the NGO called Women's Health in Women's Hands, which uses feminist popular education to deal with women's health issues, and in some of the poster projects, including learning food citizenship, decolonizing indigenous diets, critical food literacy, the pedagogy of baby food, intuitive eating and radical homemaking.

Conclusion

The group presentations and poster projects provided learning opportunities for both the presenters and the whole class. Students not only learned the theoretical underpinnings of critical food pedagogies, but applied that learning through their assignments and then taught the rest of us, thus setting the stage for ongoing, iterative learning long after the course finished. Through critical food pedagogies, the students have had the opportunity to gain crucial knowledge about food: where it comes from; why over a billion people do not have enough to eat while an equal number are obese; who benefits – and who loses – when they purchase food sourced from all parts of the globe; what is genetically modified food and why is it being promoted; and whether it is better to buy local food or organic food. They have also come to know what dispossesses them of this knowledge so they can learn to work toward a permanent liberation from this ongoing dispossession. Such knowledge gives new meaning to Anthony Winson's (1993) contention that food is the 'intimate commodity' – it has allowed students to know more about themselves and the wider world. In this way, critical food pedagogies has helped them to understand that eating is indeed a pedagogical act – that it is more than the immediate consumption of food and involves 'a situated, multifaceted and complex process, involving multiple relationships with special and often conflicting purposes, power relations and interests' (Zukas 2005: 467). Unsustainable fish, fair-trade chocolate, bottled water, organic carrots, industrial meat, local food, genetically modified organisms, biodynamic cookies, the *Western* diet – the food on the table will never be the same for these students. By taking the course, they will have learned to eat with attitude, consciously asking questions, broadening their knowledge, engaging with the present neoliberal reality and practising the pedagogy of the possible.

References

Argyris, C., Putnam, R. and Smith, D.M. 1985. *Action Science*. San Francisco: Jossey-Bass.

Belasco, W. 2007. *Appetite for Change: How the Counterculture Took on the Food Industry*, 2nd Edition. Ithaca and London: Cornell University Press.

Berry, W. 1990. *What are People For?* San Francisco: North Point Press.

Bullock, A. and Trombley S. 1999. *The New Fontana Dictionary of Modern Thought*, 3rd Edition. London: HarperCollins.

Butterwick, S. 2005. Feminist pedagogy, in the *International Encyclopedia of Adult Education*, edited by L.M. English. New York: Palgrave Macmillan, 257–62.

Chadwick, A and Stannett, A. (eds). 1995. *Museums and the Education of Adults*. Leicester: National Institute of Adult Continuing Education.

Chui, T., Tran, K. and Maheux, H. 2007. *Immigration in Canada: A Portrait of the Foreign-born Population, 2006 Census* (Statistics Canada Catalogue No. 97-557-XIE). Retrieved 31 August 2008, from http://www12.statcan.ca/english/census06/analysis/immcit/pdf/97-557-XIE2006001.pdf.

Collins, M. 2006. The critical legacy: Adult education against the claims of capital, in *Contexts of Adult Education: Canadian Perspectives*, edited by T.J. Fenwick, T. Nesbit and B. Spencer. Toronto: Thompson Educational, 118–27.

Finger, M. 2005. Critical theory, in the *International Encyclopedia of Adult Education*, edited by L.M. English. New York: Palgrave Macmillan, 165–8.

Flowers, R. and Swan, E. 2012. Introduction: Why food? Why pedagogy? Why adult education? *Australian Journal of Adult Learning* 52(3): 419–33.

———. 2015. *Food Pedagogies*. Farnham: Ashgate.

Freire, P. 1976. Literacy and the possible dream. *Prospects* 6(1): 68–71.

———. 1996. *Pedagogy of the Oppressed*. New York: Continuum Press.

Giroux, H. 2002. Neoliberalism, corporate culture and the promise of higher education: The university as a democratic public sphere. *Harvard Educational Review* 72(4): 425–64.

———. 2004. Public pedagogy and the politics of neoliberalism: Making the political more pedagogical. *Policy Futures in Education* 2(3/4): 494–503.

Guthman, J. 2008. Neoliberalism and the making of food politics in California. *Geoforum* 39: 1171–83.

Harvey, D. 2006. Neo-liberalism as creative destruction. *Geografiska Annaler* 88B(2): 145–58.

Hickey-Moody, A., Savage, C.S. and Windle, J. 2010. Introduction: pedagogy writ large: public, popular and cultural pedagogies in motion. *Critical Studies in Education* 51(3): 227–36.

Hudson, I. and Hudson, M. 2003. Removing the veil?: Commodity fetishism, fair trade, and the environment. *Organization and Environment* 16(4): 413–30.

Knowles, M.S. 1989. *The Making of an Adult Educator*. San Francisco: Jossey-Bass.

Koç, M., Sumner, J. and Winson, A. (eds). 2012. *Critical Perspectives in Food Studies*. Toronto: Oxford University Press.

Lipson, L. 1981. *The Great Issues of Politics*. Englewood Cliffs: Prentice-Hall.
Longworth, N. and Davies, W.K. 1996. *Lifelong Learning: New Vision, New Implications, New Roles for People, Organizations, Nations and Communities in the 21st Century*. London: Kogan Page.
Luke, C. 1996. *Feminisms and Pedagogies of Everyday Life*. New York: SUNY Press.
Mair, H. 2005. A mouthful of change: Eating and acting for food democracy. Paper presented at *Two Solitudes: Isolation or Impact?* The Eleventh Canadian Congress on Leisure Research, Nanaimo, B.C. CD-ROM.
———, Sumner, J. and Rotteau, L. 2008. The politics of eating: Food practices as critically reflective leisure. *Leisure/Loisir* 32(2): 379–405.
Miles, A. 1996. Adult education for global social change: Feminism and women's movement, in *Toward a Transformative Political Economy of Adult Education: Theoretical and Practical Challenges*, edited by P. Wangoola and F. Youngman. DeKalb: LEPS Press, 277–92.
Nestle, M. 2010. Writing the food studies movement. *Food, Culture and Society* 13(2): 160–8.
Neufeld, M. and Whitworth, S. 1997. Imag(in)ing Canadian foreign policy. In *Understanding Canada: Building On the New Canadian Political Economy*, edited by W. Clement. Montreal and Kingston: McGill-Queen's University Press, 197–214.
Noble, G. 2013. Strange familiarities: A response to Ash Amin's Land of Strangers, *Identities: Global Studies in Culture and Power*, 20:1, 31–6, DOI: 10.1080/1070289X.2012.752373.
Oxford English Dictionary. 2013. *Pedagogy*. Available at www.oed.com.
Sandlin, J.A., Schultz, B.D. and Burdick, J. 2009. *Handbook of Public Pedagogy: Education and Learning beyond Schooling*. New York: Routledge.
Saul, N. 2011. No stopping The Stop. *Alternatives Journal* 37(2): 11.
Seiw, A. 2011. Bake for The Stop. Available at http://bakeforthestop.wordpress.com/2011/03/22/welcome-to-the-pedagogy-of-food-class-members/.
Stoneman, S. 2010. Julie Guthman: On globalization, neoliberalism, obesity, local food and education. *Politics and Culture* 2009 (2). Available at http://www.politicsandculture.org/2010/10/27/an-interview-with-julie-guthman.
Sumner, J. 2008a. Protecting and promoting indigenous knowledge: Environmental adult education and organic agriculture. *Studies in the Education of Adults* 40(2), 207–23.
———. 2008b. Eating as a pedagogical act: Food as a catalyst for adult education for sustainability. *Kursiv - Journal fuer politische Bildung* 4: 23–37.
———. 2008c. Governance, globalization and political economy: Perspectives from Canadian adult education. *Adult Education Quarterly* 59(1): 22–41.
Webster's Ninth New Collegiate Dictionary. 1990. *Pedagogy*. Springfield: Merriam-Webster.
Welton, M. 1991. Dangerous knowledge: Canadian workers' education in the decades of discord. *Studies in the Education of Adults* 23(1), 24–40.

Winson, A. 1993. *The Intimate Commodity: Food and the Development of the Agro-Industrial Complex in Canada*. Toronto: Garamond Press.
Youngman, F. 2000. *The Political Economy of Adult Education and Development*. London: Zed Books.
Zukas, M. 2005. Pedagogical identity, in the *International Encyclopedia of Adult Education*, edited by L.M. English. New York: Palgrave Macmillan, 476–69.

Chapter 12

Food Consciousness: Teaching Critical Theory through Food Narratives

Meredith E. Abarca

I still remember the anxiety I experienced when as a graduate student I struggled to simply decipher words in the texts of my critical theory, feminist theory and postcolonial theory courses. Comprehension of what Gayatri Spivak, Judith Butler, Homi Bhabha, Michel Foucault, Jacques Derrida, and Henri Lefebvre argued about subalternity, performativity, hybridity, omnipotent power, *différance*, and symbolic mediation of space escaped me leaving only a feeling of intellectual inadequacy. Yet, through the ethnographic research for my dissertation on food narratives of working-class Mexican women I not only understood these concepts, but these food stories helped me go beyond the limits of such theoretical implications. Food narratives made theory concrete. I understood *how* subalterns speak through food; *how* they perform their gender and sexuality as well as their class and ethnic positionalities through the language of their cooking, a language that communicates beyond the limits of words; *how* the ingredients and cooking methods of their recipes epitomize historical, intercultural, and diasporas realities of hybridity, and *how* they manoeuvre socio-economic and cultural power relations in order to empower themselves by transforming the kitchen into a creative space of their own. Gathering and analysing food narratives began my journey towards what I now understand as the transformative theory of food consciousness.

This memory captures why food narratives are my pedagogical approach to engage student with different aspects of critical theory. While critical theory aims at interpreting, challenging and reshaping our social and cultural realities, such comprehension is often hindered by intangible abstractions produced by and surrounding theory. Perhaps the argument that food can function as a medium for deciphering existing theories and creating new ones may sound paradoxical given the abstract nature of theory and the practicality of food related activities. Food, however, as philosopher Lisa Heldke aptly states, is a 'thoughtful practice': a cognitive process inseparable of action (Heldke 1992: 214).

Pedagogically I translate Heldke's theory into the critical analysis of food narratives that described activities such as cooking, eating, serving, producing, distributing, gathering or withholding food. I do this by asking questions such as: who speaks?; what genres are employed?; how are food moments communicated?; what emotions are evoked and invoked?; where are these texts produced?; who is the audience?; what do these narratives suggest about production, distribution, and consumption of food? The answers to these questions aim at three goals: examine the social, cultural, political, economic and epistemological implication embedded in food narratives; show how theories have concrete manifestations and relevance to people's everyday food practices; and, encourage students to engage in self-critical reflection of their knowledge about food (its history; its social and cultural value; its geopolitical and ecological implications) and their eating habits. Through critical analysis of food narratives and assignments of self-reflection, I guide students toward the development of their own food consciousness.

Food narratives are food-centred texts that frame the design of my undergraduate and graduate courses where food is the focal point of theoretical discussions. These courses have ranged from Introduction to Literary Studies, to Theory and Practice, to Multicultural Literature, and Special Topics in Women's Studies. In these classes, food narratives include: personal stories, those of students' and those found in culinary memoirs; food images and passages kneaded into the pages of literary works (novels, poems, short stories, autobiographies); food moments that move the plot or provide the setting in films; food representations in popular culture and advertisements. To further contextualize these food stories, depending on the theme of the course (memory, the body, de-colonization), I include substantial scholarly material form the interdisciplinary field of Food Studies.

The reading selection for my courses changes substantially from one semester to the next. Due to this tendency in this chapter I offer not a model to design a course with the goal of helping students develop a food consciousness. Instead I conceptualize the ways in which I use the study food narratives to practice what bell hooks calls 'engaged pedagogy' (1994) where the classroom becomes a 'contact zone of engagement' (Pratt 1991) that provides venues for students' development of a food consciousness. Through this form of consciousness, students begin to understand that their food choices are never neutral, but governed by social, political, economic, and cultural ideologies that continuously (re)shape their individual, familial, and cultural sense of self (Counihan and Van Esterik 2013; Julier and Lindenfeld 2005).

Food Narratives as Engaged Pedagogy

I first used food narratives as a pedagogical tool to engage students into the field of critical theory in 2003. My syllabus for an undergraduate Introduction to Literary Theory justified the inclusion of food related material by stating that food knowledge helps transform theoretical ideas into personal realities. For example, to study Marxism in terms of food production and distribution, to study Psychoanalysis in terms of food's emotive elements, to study Structuralism in terms of food rituals, etc. allow students to see that these theories argue for or against things that affect their daily lives. It is through making this personal connection where engaged pedagogy takes place.

For students to actively engage at a critical personal level with new knowledge, such knowledge must be presented from that which is familiar to that which is unfamiliar. Food is familiar to students: they eat it; share it; have memories of it; make judgements about it. But the analysis of food narratives through an interdisciplinary theoretical approach is usually not familiar to them. For example to stress this point I introduce students to the fact that the organ responsible for judging the taste of food is not our tongue but our brain, 'a culturally (and therefore historically) determined organ through which [judgments] are transmitted and learned' by a given set of 'criteria for evaluations' (Montanari 2006: 61). With this knowledge the critical questions to ask are what and who defines the evaluative criteria? Or as food historian Massimo Montanari puts it 'whose taste' influences our own judgement of food? (2006: 61). The more we learn about food's holistic impact in terms of its effects on issues ranging from health to environment, from culture to politics, from economics to ethics, etc. through the analysis of food narratives and reflections on our own eating habits, the harder it becomes to stay disengaged from thinking critically about food. Furthermore, due to food's materiality and our daily consumption of it, thinking critically about food goes beyond the level of discourse and enters into the realm of action.

Heldke, as mentioned above, explains this praxis through her conceptualization of cooking as a 'thoughtful practice' which requires the 'need of thoughtful, reflective attention from everyone who cooks and eats'. Heldke further argues that reflection affects personal attitudes, which are 'individual embodiments of cultural-wide ideologies,' which turns individual actions as carriers of 'potential moral weight' (2003: xxix). In other words, attitudes about food and food choices are not free of ideological and possibly moral implications. Students see the concreteness of Heldke's philosophical argument through the analysis of food narratives and the relevance it has to their lives by reflecting on culinary daily logs that they keep during part of the course.

As mentioned earlier, bell hooks' 'engaged pedagogy' and Louise Pratt's 'pedagogical arts of the contact zone' have greatly influenced my ideas of critical engagement through food. Underscoring some of their basic principles, therefore, is in order. For hooks engaged pedagogy is 'progressive [and] holistic education'; it emphasizes 'well-being [… as] a process of self-actualization' by connecting the 'will to know with the will to become' (1994: 15–19). Engaged pedagogy leads to a consciousness that intertwines mind, body and spirit; it challenges the compartmentalization created by the boundary between public (objective) discourses and private (subjective) emotions. Engaged pedagogy 'allows students to assume responsibility for their choices' (1994: 19). For her part, Pratt defines the classroom as a 'contact zone of engagement' when it includes:

> exercises in storytelling and in identifying with the ideas, interests, histories, and attitudes of others; experiments in transculturation and collaborative work in the arts of [critical analysis]; the redemption of the oral; ways for [students] to engage with suppressed aspects of history (including their own histories); ways

> to move *into and out of* rhetorics of authenticity … a systematic approach to the all-important concept of *cultural mediation.* (2012: 5)

Both hooks and Pratt stress holistic critical awareness of others and one own attitudes and actions. While hooks emphasizes self-actualization and personal responsibility, Pratt recognizes that these are linked to an individual's relationships with others. Pratt suggests exploring such connections through the 'exercise' of 'storytelling'; I do so through the analysis of food narratives. Because food communicates in ways other than inscribed forms, it redeems the oral and sensory way of sharing knowledge. The 'rhetorics of authenticity' and 'self-actualization', I argue manifest once we develop an 'authentic presence to food' which translates to 'a sense of candor', transparency, and openness to the food we eat; a simple willingness to face the reality of what we are willing to count as food; an 'accurate consciousness of the lives and the world from which food comes' (Curtin 129). I use this authentic presence to food to stress interdependence between diverse people*s* (producers, distributors, cooks, consumers), diverse geographical spaces of food productions (food industry, local farming, GMO, organic, etc.) diverse relationships with nature, and diverse knowledges. In class we examine these connections through Ruth L. Ozeki's *All over Creation* (2004), the work of Michael Pollan (2007, 2009), Vandana Shiva (2000), Gray Nabham (2009), and documentaries like *Food Inc.* (2008) and *Super Size Me* (2004).

M. Jacqui Alexander in *Pedagogies of Crossing* echoes hook's and Pratt's pedagogical convictions. She speaks of pedagogy as crossing 'over into a metaphysics of interdependence' by summoning 'subordinated knowledges that are produced in the context of the practices of marginalization in order that we might destabilize existing practices of knowing and thus cross the fictive boundaries of exclusion and marginalization' (2005: 7). Crossing such fictive boundaries, Alexander argues, takes us closer to Paulo Freire's 'ontological vocation to become more fully human' (2005: 6). From a theoretical standpoint, food can be used to make a similar claim as Alexander's assertion. With food we have an opportunity to ask (different) questions about the very nature of metaphysics and epistemology. Edited collections such as *Cooking, Eating and Thinking: Transformative Philosophies of Food* (1992) and *The Philosophy of Food* (2013) are good places to begin this exploration.

To explore the metaphysical and epistemological implications that food can afford us, food's embedded knowledge needs to be unearthed from its philosophical subordination. Michael Symons argues: 'Western scholars have largely complied [to Plato's warning] against an interest in cooks. [Yet] cooks have been in charge – [of] finding, sharing, and giving food meaning. We could not have survived without them. They have been everywhere, yet writers have hardly noticed' (2004: ix). If we are what eat, then 'cooks have not only made our meals, but … also made us. They have shaped our social networks, our technologies, arts, and religions' (xi). To not be critically conscious of how cooks (and by extension food) shape societies, technologies, the arts, religions, politics is to ignore a significant part of 'becoming more fully human'. It limits our awareness of how we have, do, and will engage in the world: through bodily knowledge*s* that are practical, embodied, spiritual, concrete, and forever temporal. Monique Truong in her novel *The Book of Salt*, which I have taught, illustrates these forms of knowledges through the main character, the Vietnamese cook employed by Gertrude Stein and Alice B. Toklas (2003). For him cooking *is* a 'thoughtful practice' that allows him to engage in the world through his senses, the temporal act of cooking and eating, his memory that guides his cooking, and his cooking that feeds his soul.

An engaged pedagogy that aims at achieving self-actualization, a classroom that acts as a 'contact zone of engagement' that illustrates our connection to others by stressing the 'metaphysics of interdependence' leads to the development of a critical social awareness. The kind of awareness that derives from engaging in an interdisciplinary theoretical analysis of food narratives is one I call food consciousness, which represents a form of an oppositional consciousness.

Oppositional Consciousness through Food Narratives

The fact that food narratives remind us that food finds expression beyond the limits of words represents an oppositional consciousness to inscribed knowledge. I recognize the paradox of this statement since I speak of written presentations of food. But the analysis of food passages is not purely a cognitive process but most often it is one that begins through the sensory recollections they evoke on the reader. Yet because historically we have undermined food's epistemological message, we have grown nearly deaf to food's communicative channels. This deafness has moved us away from a 'fuller and richer life'. But a food consciousness can move us toward such a life. In my conceptualization of how food narratives can lead to a form of oppositional consciousness, US Third-World feminist Gloria Anzaldúa's 'mestizo' consciousness is useful.

Anzaldúa's adjective '*mestiza*' to consciousness stresses not the purity of race, culture, gender, sexuality, or nationality, but how daily lives exist in the tensions, contradictions, and ambiguities created at the crossroads of multiple social and asymmetrical power encounters (2012). It is a process of labour that works 'to break down the subject-object duality that keeps' many prisoners; it also suggests possibilities for freedom.

> The answer to the problem between the white race and the colored, between males and females, lies in healing the split that originates in the very foundation of our lives, our culture[s], our languages [and] our thoughts. A massive uprooting of dualistic thinking in the individual and collective consciousness is the beginning of a long struggle … (80)

In teaching through food narratives, I explore this long struggle in the division between mind and body as well as the epistemological division between the cognitive senses – sight and hearing – and the bodily – smell, taste and touch (Korsmeyer 1999).

To engage in a critical discussion of these epistemological divisions, food narratives that address the history of anorexia nervosa and bulimia certainly remind us of the struggle between mind and body (Bordo 2003). A text I have taught to explore this issue is Frank Burni's *Born Round* (2009). It deals with his struggle between his ideals of what his middle-class, ethnic Italian, and gay body should socially represent and his ferocious appetite. Burni 'was a baby bulimic' who grew up to become *The New York Times*' restaurant critic (9). He frees himself from believing that he could control his body image by occasional periods of exercise, bulimic practices, and rigorous diets once he develops an honest relationship with 'the history of [his] own body' (347–8). Burni's honesty is made possible only after recognizing that his 'life-defining relationship' has been with his 'stomach' (5). Bruni's story offers an example of one kind of crossing over into 'the metaphysics of interdependence' where the mind and body's interlocking relationship becomes one of continuous balance not struggle.

Another example I have used in class of 'the metaphysics of interdependence' comes from Anzaldúa's text where she connects her body to the earth. Anzaldúa confronts the dichotomy of mind and body by embracing the ambiguities and contractions her mixed-ethnicity (Indigenous, Spanish, African, and Anglo), lesbian, and working-class body faces in a primary White, middle-class, and heterosexual world. Her shield of protection (and liberation) is conceptualized by metaphorically connecting her body with an ear of corn.

> Indigenous like corn … the *mestiza* is a product of crossroads, designed for preservation under a variety of contradictions. Like an ear of corn – a female seed-bearing organ – the *mestiza* is tenacious, tightly wrapped in the husks of her culture. Like kernels she clings to the cob; with thick stalks and strong brace roots, she holds tight to the earth – she will survive the crossroads. (81)

Corn is not a random metaphor in this survival. Its historical narrative as a sacred plan for Indigenous people of the Americas cannot be ignored (Abarca 2012). What this metaphor adds to Anzaldúa's *mestiza* consciousness that breaks the dualistic of mind and body is the element of spirituality.

Within the realm of Western philosophy, Anazldúa's and Bruni's food narratives (as only two examples) challenge what Theodor Adorno called the logic of identity: a constant struggle of mind over body (1973: 3–57). This logic of identity is based on a dichotomous conflict between mind (the intellect) and body (the material). The power of this seemingly unresolved conflict is evident in the (Western) dualistic worldview: mind versus body; self over other; culture before nature; logic above emotion; objective knowledge counter to subjective experience. Food's epistemological possibilities explore through food narratives rupture these perspectives. They suggest the logic of identity as one based on a symbiotic relation between mind and body, as Bruni shows in his culinary memoir, and between culture and nature, as Anzaldúa does by framing her subjectivity through the metaphor of corn. Food in these two food narratives, either as a literal consumption or a metaphor, is a catalyses of transformation that marks changes in Burni and Anzalúa's perception of their own personal, cultural and social identity that marks their food consciousness.

Food Consciousness as Theory of Transformation

Food is transformative. Cooking, after all, 'is the act that transforms a product "from nature" into something profoundly different' (Montanari 2006: 29). Warren Belasco aptly captures the transformative aspect of food when he states: 'Food Matters. It has weight, and it weighs us down' (2008: 2). To understand why food matters, why it has weight, and how it weighs us down, food must be de-familiarized. Yes, we all eat. But are we critically aware of how food's multiple narratives marks our lives? Defamiliarization means to critically read, analyse, reflect, rewrite, and perform the food narratives of our lives.

Food has the power to define us. If we are what we eat, as gourmand Jean-Anthelme Brillat-Savarin so declared, then cultural anthropologist David E. Sutton's pithy phrase holds true: we are what we ate (2001). Additionally, the next syntactical formulation becomes: we will become that which we eat. Belasco offers three paradigms that capture this idea of *food time* and its power to define us: classical, modernist, and recombinant.

> The classical future is a continuation and elaboration of the progress of the past – a future of ever bigger and better things made available largely through materialistic, qualitative, often imperialist expansions. In the classical vision, the new evolves seamlessly out of the old ... The modernist future, representing a distinct break with the past, is a radically new vision based on the very latest technologies and scientific breakthroughs, often producing a seemingly more efficient result ... The recombinant future ... envisions a world of neo-traditional foods mass-produced by modernist means ... Less confident in the new then the modernism, more eclectic and multicultural than classicism, the recombinant ... menu may reflect how many of us actually approach and experience the future: one foot forward, the other planted in an imagined, decontextualized past. (2006: xii)

These possibilities delineate how we might articulate our present food narratives. Classical narratives frame their plots around the polemics of authenticity, a rather contested term in food studies. The governing motif in modernist narratives is fragmentation as they rupture continuity to the past. The characters in recombinant narratives are at crossroads: feeling the pull of science and technology and the push of a past no longer conceptually known but still experienced through incorporated bodily knowledge and sensory collective memories (Abarca 2012).

As we develop a critical food consciousness, we become active agents and (re)formulate our relationship to these paradigms – perhaps even propose yet other options. Food consciousness is not just about a deeper understanding of food's weight and how it could weigh us down, but it also provides paths to other food narratives not controlled by the dominant food system. It help us develop a sensitivity to explore the history of hospitality, the social network of reciprocity, the connection and continuity to a diverse historical past, to an Epicurean theory of hedonism. For example, texts that I have taught such as Annia Ciezadlo's *Day of Honey: A Memoir of Food, Love, and War* (2011) and Diana Abu-Jaber's *The Language of Baklava* (2005) address all of these issues.

A food consciousness also presents challenges within the realms of politics, economics, and ecology. I bring this to students' awareness by exposing them to the range of arguments about sustainability, resources of animals, land and water, scientific and technological monopolies aided by political and financial capital. We read food scholars who expose contradictions and tensions of the food industry's practices that reveal unacknowledged and/or unrecognizable oppressions. Three documentaries to engage in these discussions are *Thirst* (2004), *Fast Food Nation* (2006) and *Food, Inc.* (2008).

To make these arguments relevant to students' personal lives, we read Claude Fischler's (1988) essay, 'Food, Self, and Identity', where he argues that the recipient of the food industry's unrecognized oppressions is the modern consumer (i.e. all of us). Fischler explains that this oppression manifests itself as a crisis of identity created by the modern food system. He offers four causes for the crisis: (a) the modern eater is 'merely a consumer' without knowledge of the history of food; (b) 'traditional culinary systems, which connect nature, food and community, have been considerably eroded by economic and technical changes'; (c) 'modern food is less and less identifiable by its consistency, flavor, smell, and texture', and (e) science and technology mask, imitate, and transform 'nature' or 'traditional products' with 'reconstituted proteins [and] artificial flavors' (289). This crisis of identity comes from a rupture from the past, a separation from nature, and a replacement of the concrete with the abstract. However, food consciousness derived from critical reflection of multiple food narratives, as I have been suggesting throughout this chapter, provides a path to discover ways of reconnecting with our past, to understand our interdependence with nature (and each other), and to find the concrete in the abstract.

Curtin (1992) in 'Food/Body/Person' shows how this sense of reconnection comes from a 'participatory' rather than an objective relationship with food. An objectified relation to food makes food 'other', and epistemologically reinforces the split of mind and body: 'food is understood merely as fuel that recharges the body while leaving the mind untouched' (11). A participatory relationship with food helps us understand food's 'weight': its power to define us through our relationships with it and others. A participatory self (or relational person) leads to a 'healthy personhood [that] comes from having the power to choose the relations through which one will be defined. Careful attention to the variety of food practices in which we engage highlights the ordinariness of this process' (1992: 17). A participatory self is holistic and fluid. Rather than compartmentalizing mind, body, and (I will add) spirit, it brings them together. Rather than breaking with the past, it connects with it to carve multiple paths towards the future.

Sutton adds the role the senses play in a participatory (relational) self. Rather than dividing and pitting the senses into two compartments of higher (sight and hearing) and lower (taste, smell, and touch), Sutton explains synesthesia, the crossing of different sensory registers, in the context of food memories as a process of '"returning to the whole"' (2001: 71). This process 'helps us understand the significance of food in the maintenance of identity' (2001: 17). The idea of 'whole' evokes a state of relatedness, conviviality, and an attempt to experience the self as a whole free of compartmentalization, disjointed possibilities, and/or fragmentation. The return to wholeness requires awareness of our historical continuity for 'memory can alter consciousness and consciousness can alter [the] institutionalized' intellectual neglect bestowed to food's power to define us (Moraga 2011: 7–8). The transformative possibilities that come from a critical food consciousness can take a 'student's individualized awareness,' the familiarity to his/her food narratives, and with such awareness a student can return to him/her collective, historical 'whole' through a de-familiarizing process of critically reflecting, analysing, and actively recreating their food narratives (Sutton: 76).

Food Consciousness in the Classroom

Since my desire has not been to suggest a paradigm to develop an engaged pedagogy that leads to food consciousness, I do not offer detailed lesson plans. To offer blueprints for lessons contradicts, as hooks states, the principle that 'engaged pedagogy recognize each classroom as different, that strategies must constantly be changed, invented, reconceptualized to address each new teaching experience' (10–11). While many changes do take place from one class to the next in my teaching, what remains constant in my literature undergraduate and graduate courses framed through the analysis of food narratives is my commitment to help students develop a food consciousness.

My engaged pedagogy works as a praxis of critical reflection of narratives and action in the form of students' assessments. The critical reflection results from the exposure of food's historical, social, cultural and theoretical implications embedded in the multiple forms of food narratives I teach; this critical reflection reveals how food and food narratives have the capacity to create significant transformative moments, and it illustrates how such transformations extend beyond intellectual understanding within the context of the class to the content of students' everyday life. The action takes place within a set of assignments that range from ethnographic research, culinary daily logs, electronic open class journals, bi-weekly ethical reflections, share meals, and a final research project. Often this final project is a research paper, but over the years students have created short documentary films about a family or community culinary practice. Once, six final projects became the central focus of a six-month museum exhibit, '*Mamá's Molcajete*: The *Mestizaje* of Mexican Cuisine', at the El Paso Museum of Archaeology.

The assignments themselves do not represent the transformative moments a food consciousness has the capacity to create, but the exploration and reflection they provide into students' own food narratives. The methodology for the ethnographic research is based on *charlas culinarias* (culinary chats) that resulted from my own process of consciousness while conducting food field research (Abarca 2006). Simply defined it is a methodology of decolonization. It is about speaking *with* others; it is about *collaborators* of knowledge*s*; it is about mutual comfort and trust. It is about intellectual humility. Linda Tuhiwai Smith defines humility in the content of academic research as awareness not to assume 'that we are the experts' and to recognize that 'we have a great deal to learn from others' (1999: 5).

In the classroom this ethnographic assignment appears as private and public grassroots research. As a class we select a number of food practices to investigate: a dish, an ingredient, a process, a commercial image, a ritual food, etc. Half of the students work on the private grassroots while the other half works on the public. The goal is to gather food narratives from students' own family and members of the community who create and provide a similar food. The requirements are that at least two students explore a similar food issue within the circle of their family and from their community at large. For the private fieldwork, they engage in culinary chats with at least three members of their family, ideally all from different generations; for the public, they converse with at least three food providers such as cooks in restaurants, grocers, growers, or food producers. About every three weeks, students brief each other on the status of their research to find similar themes or different approaches of the same practice. For example, *chile con queso* (chile with cheese) is a popular dish in the area where I teach, and one explored. Students find out whom in their family claims the best recipe, why recipes have been modified, who makes the hottest version, the creamiest, and on what occasions is best served. Others find out that the fame of *chile con queso* comes from the proximity of Hutch, New Mexico, the world capital producer of green chillies, and the influence of the Mennonites who live in the area (south of the US-Mexican border in the state of Chihuahua) and are known for their cheese making skills. Yet others discovered that Bhutanese enjoy a very similar dish. Discoveries such as this show students in concrete ways what Sutton theorizes about 'returning to a whole' as a means to reconnect with a historical (culinary) past.

The idea of juxtaposing these two approaches of grassroots ethnographic fieldwork is for students to see how culinary practices blur the divide between private and public spheres. But most importantly, they recognize that their 'ordinary' family cooking habits and geographical based food practices are part of a larger historical, social, and political content. The course final research project allows space to make such links by requiring students to theoretically contextualize aspects of their grassroots projects. Over the years titles of students' final projects exemplify these critical reflections: 'Discovering Myself through Critical Thinking'; 'A Culinary Journey of Self Discovery;' 'Traditions and Misinterpretations of Our Kitchen', and 'The Kitchen, a Woman's Prison. Says Who?'

The culinary daily logs, electronic open class journals and the bi-weekly ethical reflections are spaces for students to record their food practices, issues raised by the course reading material, and to examine the implication of their food practices in relation to their increased interdisciplinary textual awareness about foodways. The culinary log is kept daily only for the first three weeks and the last three weeks of the semester. It simply asks them to record what, when, where, and with whom they had breakfast, lunch, dinner, and (or) snacks. Of these three assignments, this is the only one that is kept private. The electronic journal and ethical reflections are open to the entire class, extending Pratt's notion of the classroom as a 'contact zone of engagement' into cyber space.

What students and I have witnessed through these assignments are seedlings of transformative moments that range from overcoming anxieties about eating, developing new rituals, supporting locally owned stores, giving up certain foods, and embracing others. These kinds of actions echoes Freire's notion of consciousness as a process of developing a critical awareness on one's social reality through reflection and action, where action becomes the method of changing that reality. It is possible for such transformations to take place during a semester because students, without often being fully aware, walk into class with the roots for such growth firmly planted. The learning community created in class through the open assignments, which affect as hooks rightly argues, 'our interest in one another, in hearing one another's voices, in recognizing one another's presence', function to nourish students' changes (8). This spirit is captured in a student's final journal during my first food narrative/ theoretical course in 2003:

> A lot has changed for me this year that in some way this class has given me the opportunity to put all the pieces together and find my true self. (Something that I was aware lived inside of me, yet I had been too busy to appreciate) … Each week we'd touch on a subject that would in some way tied into a personal realm I either hadn't deal with or had suppressed for other reasons … I learned much about my inner self and became capable of appreciating the individual I am … Thank you all for your companionship, for your encouragement, and for sharing yourselves!

This brings me to the last pedagogical aspect of my food consciousness courses: sharing meals. Since most of my classes are small, usually graduate courses and Women Studies courses, the shared meals take place at my home. The fact that I live five blocks from campus and teach one night a week for three hours facilities this arrangement. There are a number of objectives for this activity: to experience in concrete ways Heldke's theory of cooking as 'thoughtful practice', to move the analysis of food narratives into the realm of 'progressive [and] holistic education' by shifting the teaching setting from the classroom to the dining room of my home creating a greater sense of community throughout the semester (as the above student journal indicates). It introduces new forms of learning. Students literally have to cook for these meals. Assignments range from creating a dish with locally grown and produced products, to using a recipe presented in the food narratives (when they offered), to using an ingredient unfamiliar to them, to preparing a dish connected to a particular kind of memory about childhood, about traveling, about a holiday, or to create a dish that represents a theoretical concept studied in class such as cosmopolitanism. Some of the central arguments throughout this chapter have been that food communicates beyond the limits of written text, that food connects us to others outside our immediate cultural community and our own historical moment, that food involves political, aesthetic, and ethical choices. This assignment of shared meals provides a space to experience much of this in a concrete tangible and eatable moment.

In the most recent graduate food-based course I taught in 2012, 'Gastrographies: Food and Memory', the theme for the last shared meal was 'prospective memory' (Sutton 2001). Students prepared a dish that will enable remembering the course and each other in years come. I can think of no better way to conclude this chapter on developing a food consciousness through analysis of food narratives and self-reflection of food practices than to quote from a student's final journal as it exemplifies the core argument presented here: a food consciousness has the capacity to ignite transformation. The student expresses herself through what Jessica Hayes-Conroy and Allison Hayes-Conroy call the '*articulated bodily capacity to feel*' (2012: 6a), an expression of knowledge that is cognitive (inscribe), bodily (incorporated), and emotional:

> I decided to prepare lime celery Jell-O … for several reasons. First, my intention was to select a dish that somehow represents the course as a whole. Lime celery Jell-O (at least in my opinion) is not a very common way to prepare Jell-O; [it] looks different (visually), but once it is tasted it has a rich flavor that is quite exquisite. I apply the same principle to this course. When I first looked at the syllabus … I felt scared and uneasy because food studies was unfamiliar to me. Yet once I began reading the memoirs and philosophical articles I became enthralled and acquired a 'taste' for this type of literature.
>
> …
>
> Reflecting upon the course … I can undoubtedly assert that this class has definitely created many memories. I will forever remember our sharing meals, endless nights attempting to grasp the concept of subjectivity/objectivity, Kant's aesthetics … This class exposed me to new ideas and forms of thinking. Previous to this semester, I had never paid much attention to food, other than in a superficial manner. Now, I am more aware of food critical implications, the reflective capacity of taste, the way in which certain foods make me feel; how food can be seen in terms of time and space, and that we literally are what we

eat. Food has slowly become an essential part of my outlook on life. Of course food is essential as a nutrient, but food (at least for me) is now a way of looking at the world around me and in understanding my relationships in it.

References

Abarca, M.E. 2006. *Voices in the Kitchen: Views of Food and the World from Working-Class Mexican and Mexican American Women*. College Station, TX: Texas A&M University Press.

———. 2012. 'The Afro-Mestizo Tamal: Remembering a Sensory and Sacred Encounter'. In *Dialogues across Diasporas*, edited by M. Rohrleitner and S. Ryan. New York: Lexington Books, 157–73.

Abu-Jaber, D. 2005. *The Language of Baklava: A Memoir*. New York: Anchor Books.

Adorno. T. 1973. *Negative Dialectics*. New York: Continuum.

Alexander, M.J. 2005. *Pedagogies of Crossing: Meditations on Feminism, Sexual Politics, Memory, and the Sacred*. Durham, NC: Duke University Press.

Anzaldúa, G. 2012. *Borderlands/La Frontera: The New Mestiza*. Fourth Edition. San Francisco, CA: Aunt Lute Books.

Belasco, W. 2006. *Meals to Come: A History of the Future of Food*. Berkeley, CA: University of California Press.

———. 2008. *Food: The Key Concepts*. New York: Berg Publishers.

Bordo, S. 2003. *Unbearable Weight: Feminism, Western Culture, and the Body*. Berkeley, CA: University of California Press.

Brillant-Savarin, J.A. 1960. *The Physiology of Taste, or Meditations on Transcendental Gastronomy*. New York: Dover.

Bruni, F. 2009. *Born Round: A Story of Family, Food and a Ferocious Appetite*. New York: Penguin Books.

Ciezaldo, A.2011. *Day of Honey: A Memoir of Food, Love, and War*. New York: Free Press.

Counihan, C. and Van Esterik, P. (eds). 2013. *Food and Culture: A Reader*. Third Edition. New York: Routledge.

Curtin, D.W. 1992. 'Food/Body/Person'. In *Cooking, Eating, Thinking: Transformative Philosophies of Food*, edited by D.W. Curtin and L.M. Heldke. Bloomington, IN: Indiana University Press, 3–22.

Fischler, C. 1988. 'Food, Self, and Identity'. *Social Science Information*. 27 (2), 275–92.

Freire, P. 2000. *Pedagogy of the Oppressed*. Thirtieth Anniversary Edition. Boston, MA: Continuum.

Hayes-Conroy, J. and Hayes-Conroy, A. 2012. 'Veggies and visceralities: A political ecology of food and feeling'. *Emotion, Space and Society*, 30, 1–10.

Heldke, L. 1992. 'Foodmaking as a Thoughtful Practice'. In *Cooking, Eating, Thinking: Transformative Philosophies of Food*, edited by D.W. Curtin and L.M. Heldke. Bloomington IN: Indiana University Press, 203–29.

———. 2003. *Exotic Appetites: Ruminations of a Food Adventurer*. New York: Routledge.
hooks, b. 1994. *Teaching to Transgress: Education as the Practice of Freedom*. New York: Routledge.
Julier, A. and Lindenfeld, L. 2005. 'Mapping men onto the menu: Masculinities and food'. *Food & Foodways*, 13 (1–2), 1–16.
Kaplan, D.M. (ed.). 2013. *The Philosophy of Food*. Berkeley, CA: University of California, Press.
Korsmeyer, C. 1999. *Making Sense of Taste: Food and Philosophy*. Ithaca, NY: Cornell University Press.
Montanari, M. 2006. *Food Is Culture*. New York: Columbian University Press.
Moraga, C.L. 2011. *A Xicana Codex of Changing Consciousness: Writings, 2000–2010*. Durham, NC: Duke University Press.
Nabham, G.P. 2009. *Where Our Food Comes From: Retracting Nikolay Vavilov's Quest to End Famine*. Washington, DC: Shearwater Books.
Nestle, M. 2002. *Food Politics: How the Food Industry Influences Nutrition and Health*. Berkeley, CA: University of California Press.
Ozeki, R.L. 2004. *All over Creation*. New York: Penguin.
Pollan, M. 2007. *The Omnivore's Dilemma: A Natural History of Four Meals*. New York: Penguin.
———. 2009. *In Defence of Food: An Eater's Manifesto*. New York: Penguin.
Pratt, M.L. 1991. 'Arts of the contact zone'. *Professions*, 91, 33–40.
Shiva, V. 2000. *Stolen Harvest: The Hijacking of the Global Food Supply*. Cambridge, MA: South End Press.
Smith, L.T. 1999. *Decolonizing Methodologies: Research and Indigenous People*. New York: Zed Books.
Sutton, D.E. 2001. *Remembrance of Repasts: An Anthropology of Food and Memory*. New York: Berg Publishers.
Symons, M. 2004. *A History of Cooks and Cooking*. Chicago, IL: University of Illinois Press.
Truong, M. 2003. *The Book of Salt*. New York: Mariner Books.

Chapter 13

Of Dialectical Food Pedagogies and Political Economies: Taking Debates Forward in an Afterword[1]

Michael K. Goodman

As framed by this volume and its multiple contributions, we are in the midst of a series of pedagogical 'moments' with respect to food in the UK. Foodbanks,[2] literally unheard of before I moved here a decade ago, are now spreading like wildfire. The Trussell Trust which runs the majority of foodbanks in the UK, handed out close to a million food parcels in 2013 which is almost a third more than the previous year and a tenfold increase since 2010 (Trussell Trust 2014). At the same time, there has been rapidly massive growth in all forms of food media, from television to print to the Internet and social media. In effect, food has colonised literally all of the niches in the media ecologies that make up post-industrial societies, and not merely in the guise of cheeky or swear-prone celebrity chefs. As I put it in a forthcoming piece, 'through numerous popular media ecologies and forms, we are concerned about food and its place in our lifeworlds now more than ever: we celebrate it and are entertained by it, we deplore, explore, historicise, voyeurise, fictionalise and document food in every possible guise' (Goodman forthcoming). Indeed, one of the more key roles of this rise of food media has been to investigate and 'teach' us in numerous ways what is actually in the food that we eat (Freidberg 2004); importantly, these food 'detective stories' form the core evidence for a number of recent political movements to shame or at least pressure food and consumer-goods corporations to drop the use of rainforest-destroying, orang-utan-killing palm oil in their products, for example (Short 2013).

1 I'd like to thank David Goodman, Emma-Jayne Abbots, Ben Coles and Colin Sage who read and commented on earlier drafts of this afterword. Thanks also to Elaine and Rick for their patience and guidance in getting this piece into the wonderful book they have worked to assemble.

2 While operating slightly differently in the UK than in the US, foodbanks provide the needy access to food they would not otherwise have access to through either a referral system (UK) or more informal means (US). Foodbanks are typically run by civil society/third sector organisations, charities, community and/or church-affiliated groups and have taken hold in both the US and UK as 'normal' features of the foodscape for many of the poor and marginal.

The detective story of the 'Horsemeat-Gate' forms yet a third important, recent pedagogical moment for food in the UK. Here, illegal sources of horsemeat where found, in trace to massive amounts (e.g. 95 to 100 percent), to be masquerading as beef in processed products from lasagne to beefburgers to meatballs and sold in supermarkets, fast-food joints and even Ikea. Throughout the after-the-fact investigative reporting on the topic, much of it done by the ever-relentless and sharp-penned Felicity Lawrence at the *Guardian* newspaper (Lawrence 2014), it was shown that not only was out and out fraud responsible for putting ol' Seabiscuit on our plates, but that it was also due to the roll-back regulatory effects of the neo-liberalism that casts its long, dark shadow over the industrialised food system (Abbots and Coles 2014). The apogee of neo-liberalism known as a 'self-regulating market', in this case, meant the incorporation of the cheapest beef-like protein available, i.e. horsemeat that not only looked and tasted like beef, but could, of course, not be satisfactorily un-incorporated from oneself. In addition – and rather scandalously – there was literally only one, single commentator – the aforementioned Lawrence – who sketched out the direct line between the power of supermarkets sourcing goods at increasingly cheaper costs and this 'sneaky' use of horsemeat which, in response to supermarket power, was designed to ultimately keep prices low on the various goods it came to be incorporated in.

So what might these pedagogical moments tell us about the contemporary status of food in the UK? At one level, they tell us about the place of food within contemporary UK society: that access to it is unequal and this inequality is deepening under the auspices, politics and political economies of Tory-led austerity that has similarly failed to address the overall real wage declines that started in the 1970s and 1980s (Allen 2014). For a large segment of the population, or at least the food-obsessed media, food is something we watch, communicate and know – and often know in (material) excess. Moreover, it makes a great deal of money for its stars and their associated cookbook- and media-producing corporations. At the same time, weak regulation combined with the continuing 'super' power of supermarkets virtually guarantees that some might have to continue to cross their fingers when eating in the near future. In essence, if indeed one has enough to eat, many watch Jamie Oliver and his ilk prepare local, seasonal free-range/organic meals – that they then can afford to purchase and make – while the less fortunate are lucky if they get to actually eat what it says they are buying on the tin. Thus, at a broader level, as these separate food moments combine into one over-determined moment in the style of Althusser, a number of food-based contradictions have begun to sit relatively comfortably side by side: inequality and questions of having enough food to eat are positioned right next to those of eater-tainment, eating to excess and being 'worried well' about questions of food quality. In short, what I am trying to argue here is that these pedagogical moments articulate and frame the contemporary relationalities of food and society under the current auspices of UK-flavoured austerity capitalism.

In light of the fascinating chapters in this book, it is clear that critically analysing food pedagogies and the pedagogies of food – what crudely I like to think of as those implicit and explicit attempts to define what and how we should eat, prepare and provision our food – must sit front and centre to understanding not merely the relationalities of food/society, but how we got to these relationalities in the first place, how they been made durable and, as necessary, how we might 're-flavour' them to create more just foodscapes. As this book has opened up through its innovative empirical analysis and new theory building, understanding foods' pedagogies means we are all but required to ask *who* has the power to create and circulate food pedagogies, the cultural-economic *resources* to incorporate and/or resist these food pedagogies and even *who* has the power and/or resources *to be in on* these relational pedagogies in the first place. Similarly, those fundamental concerns – or better yet struggles over – having the 'right' and 'correct' food pedagogies taught to us must also come in for extensive critical analysis. Here then, building off of Flowers and Swan (2012) and the contributions developed in this volume, it is crucial to ask a series of linked, far-reaching, yet also ongoing questions: *who* is articulating *what* food pedagogies, *how* are they being taught and *whom* are they for?

If we turn back to my pedagogical moments, then, as understood in the broad, anti-essentialist manner suggested in Flowers and Swan's introduction in Chapter 1, these moments undoubtedly contain and are surrounded by a set of multiple and complex answers to these questions. Without the space to get into too much detail, several different and indeed divergent possible pedagogically inflected interpretations emerge from the rise of foodbanks in the UK. For critics on the left – much like my analysis above – this is an expression of how more and more people in the UK must access food to survive under the current regime of austerity, continuingly decrepit economic opportunities for the middle and lower classes and historically depressed wages (Butler 2014). Not so for the right, though, who characterise foodbanks as merely the expression of an economy of never-to-be-satisfied demand seeking greater supply in the form of 'takers' and 'skivers' pouncing on a free lunch, many of whom have failed to learn the skills to cook, let alone hold down a job (Bennett 2014). And while this version from the right couldn't really be further from the truth as actual, real, on the ground research is beginning to show in both the UK (Lambie-Mumford 2014), US (Pine, forthcoming) and across the EU (Oxfam 2013), what these divergent pedagogies say about the same event is that, when specifically performed and interrogated in the media-ted, public sphere, foods' pedagogies are and always will be politicised and embedded within much wider political agendas.

With the continuing rise of food media, and particularly the increasing prevalence of show, after show, after new show for celebrity chefs, it seems as if this might be a real and substantial space that audiences, people and society look to for food pedagogies. Intuitively this does indeed make sense: more shows, more media, more celebrity chefs and so more opportunities and sources for quantitatively and qualitatively *more* food pedagogy to 'take place'. And yet, when we actually speak to and ask audiences about their multiple engagements with celebrity chefs and food programmes, we begin to see the layered complexity that makes up these food pedagogies and the indeterminate relationships of information provision, knowledge and pedagogy. This complexity is revealed by an online survey (n = 600) designed to explore audience engagements with chefs and food programmes. Christine Barnes and I (Barnes, forthcoming) have found that when asked why our respondents regularly watch food programmes, three-quarters of the total said they watched for entertainment, a little over half stated that the programme just happened to be on and just under a half said they have an interest in food or cooking. Interestingly only 40 per cent said they watched food programmes and celebrity chefs because they wanted to learn or cook new food. And, when asked where they most regularly look for information about food – what and how to eat – respondents' top three choices in descending order were friends and family, food labels and the Internet. Food programmes and TV came fourth, yet no single response scored highly, suggesting that respondents tended to get information about food from a large spectrum of different sources, including NGOs, food brands, advertisers and the government. When asked in a different question about who they trusted to inform them about what and how to eat, friends and family again came top of the list of responses with food labels next and food programmes third. In the qualitative responses to this question, many indicated that 'chef programmes are enjoyable … so [they] enjoyed the food porn aspect of them' and that watching was mostly about getting new ideas and inspiration. This last point was one that echoed across the whole of the survey: most people had an already existing interest in food and so many watched food programmes to either get *new* knowledge or inspiration for food they already prepared and ate. What this says is that – while fruitfully engaged here through several of the book's chapters (i.e. Robert Chapter 6; Sandlin, Quiroga, and Redmon-Wright Chapter 4) – we have much more work to do to understand the relationships of entertainment and inspiration to those of pedagogy, affect and behavioural change as everyday food cultures are increasingly media-ted through the lenses of popular culture and the 'cultural vanguard' of the celebrity chef.

In food media in the UK, the 'for whom?' question has really risen to the top. Indeed, it might very well be argued that a great deal of what Jamie Oliver does now in the public sphere is a form of pedagogy pointed directly at government officials (see Bell et al., forthcoming) as well as indirectly to the government through audience pressure.[3] This was surely the point of *Jamie's School Dinners* which was about getting healthy food into schools and showed Jamie meeting and talking to those in power in the context of school food provisioning across the UK (see Harrison, Kelly and Campbell, Chapter 5, for Jamie's pedagogies of 'neo-liberal passion' in his restaurant Fifteen). Hugh Fearnley-Whittingstall's *Fish Fight* – a series of multi-year TV shows and social networking campaign created to bring attention to the amount of wasted by-catch from EU fishing boats (*Fish Fight* 2014) – was designed with a number of different audiences in mind, much

3 Although this latter point has yet to be empirically shown, it might yet be through further extensive audience studies.

beyond the 'viewers at home'. Specifically, it targeted the European Parliament, which makes EU fishing policy, as well as supermarkets and food corporations, who could begin to supply more sustainably sourced fish. The *Fish Fight*'s pedagogical aim and effect was one that began with audience-consumers who applied pressure through petitions, social media and guerrilla shopping, and ended by influencing European fishing policy through its campaign to educate and enrol Parliamentary members. In this, celebrity chefs – who are more often than not these days acting as investigative journalists – and their associated food pedagogies are no longer merely for those 'at home' audiences wishing to get inspired. These very broad and more far-reaching pedagogical foodscapes of celebrity chefs and food programmes now strategically cross numerous technological and communication platforms from their very inception, and like the suggestion made above for further and greater audience studies, deserve much more sustained critical investigation given the vastly elevated voice of so many of these important, mediating figures.

The pedagogies of the horsemeat scandal were certainly designed to teach the consuming public about how the beef chain had been contaminated by substances that should not have been in these foods in the first place. Pursued by some of the best 'follow the thing' (Cook et al. 2004) narrating around, multiple spider-like diagrams were used to effectively uncover and illustrate beef/horsemeat supply chain nodes involved in bringing industrial meat to market across the EU. Beyond the newspaper-reading, television-watching and other media-engaged public, this case again raises the question about whom these pedagogies were for. If these food pedagogies were intended for supermarkets, then what it really reveals is that they have little idea about their supply chains they themselves source from. As the head of Tesco put it in response to the investigations, 'I have asked my team to review our approach to the supply chain, to ensure we have visibility and transparency, and to come back with a plan to build a world-class traceability and DNA testing system' (*The Guardian* 2013). What this statement suggests is that, in the first instance, they don't have full visibility nor transparency of the food they are selling to us and we are eating, which is a particularly striking pedagogical moment if ever there was one.

If these pedagogies were directed to the government, then they have really missed their mark as little to nothing has been done as yet, except for the shadow Environment Secretary echoing the statements of Tesco about the need for further transparency, which of course, will be voluntary and left in the hands of supermarkets themselves to provide, police and articulate for consumers (Mesure 2013). But even asking supermarkets to further regulate themselves seems to be going a step too far as another supermarket CEO argued that all this transparency and checking of meat supply chains would, of course, raise the price of meat for *all* consumers (Hough 2013). And, even if these food pedagogies were designed to inform the public of what they were eating – and here it should be said mostly those in the working and lower classes who tend to eat the cheaper food items that contained the horsemeat – it was all too little, too late: the horsemeat ingested could not be un-ingested. Indeed, for some of the most callous commentators, as described in Abbots and Coles (2013), the poor really should have expected this and should consider themselves lucky to be eating any sort of protein, horse or no, fraud or no and regardless of their right to choose what it is they eat. Here then, we must add another core concern to the pedagogies of food and food pedagogies: their temporal context matters and matters in vastly important ways, especially in the context of knowing beforehand about what it is we are actually choosing or not choosing to incorporate into our bodies.

I wish to take this current discussion further, however. In my reading of the chapters of this book – one of the first, it must be said, that moves from the rhetorical use of pedagogy and learning in food studies to a closer examination of processes, practices and their political effects – an overarching question has come to the fore: what exactly are food pedagogies *about*? For me, they are about contradiction, they are about paradox, they are and can be opposed and/or parallel and/or be complementary and mutually supportive. In this, these contradictory, oppositional, parallel and/or complementary pedagogies are relational and are intimately related. They are, in a word, *dialectical*: the notions and pedagogies of what constitutes 'good food' are a case in points here (Goodman et al. 2010). Indeed, if we investigate contemporary foodscapes, I think we can begin to see that there are particular contexts where food pedagogies are in 'actually existing' (cf. Castree 2005) opposition and complementarity. Simultaneously, however, there are oppositional and complementary pedagogies that are full of 'potential' but have yet to be uncovered, fulfilled, or come together. What all this says, first and foremost – as documented empirically through the different, international sites presented by the chapters in this volume – is that food pedagogies must be contextualised, and contextualised in both time and space for them to literally *be* pedagogical. At the very same time, analysis, too, must be equally temporally and spatially contextualised to allow us to understand food pedagogies in any useful empirical and theoretical sense.

In order to briefly work through this question of what food pedagogies are about, I focus on three potentially oppositional but also intimately related and indeed dialectical characteristics of contemporary food pedagogies. I work through them here, not as an attempt to seek resolution or to say that we must overcome what many might see as a set of dualisms, but rather to suggest, as many in this book have done, that these dialectics are already on offer in food pedagogies, we *should*, specifically, work through them and should continue to do so as we carry on speaking truth to food (pedagogical) power. Indeed, some of these characteristics can *work* for those in power, others can work as *resistances* to those in power and other can just *simply work*. Thus, I am not looking to provide answers here or *the* definitive statement about what food pedagogies are about but rather very briefly point to their multiple and complex characteristics to open up further space for discussion and debate.

In any case, my first response to thinking about what food pedagogies are about goes something like this: they can be about *control* as much as they can be about *opportunity* and/or instances of *resistance*. Starting with control first, everything – from public healthy eating programmes to reduce obesity and other (relative) diseases of affluence, to celebrity chef recipes for healthy meals, to the shaming discourses surrounding those who use foodbanks, to the knowledge embedded in family food traditions that says what is 'proper' to prepare and eat – contain an element of attempted/successful control of what sorts of food we ingest. Indeed, recent public health campaigns, from those in Ireland (Sage 2014) to the recent utterances of Jamie Oliver (Campbell 2014; see also Green 2014), have begun to show how the control of food is intimately related to the control of space through proposed changes in zoning laws to keep unhealthy food away from schools.

At the very same time, however, food pedagogies can be about opening up opportunity and possibilities in food engagements all the way from the individual to the global scale. Jamie 'watchers' might shift to more home cooked, quick, cheap meals for the family or investigative food documentaries could bring shifts to environmental and social policy or change supermarket supply chain governance for the better. Food pedagogies can also provide resistance-focused grist for potentially more healthy and sustainable eating in local food movements as a form of push-back against the environmentally and socially problematic food from the 'global nowhere' (Campbell 2009; Carolan 2011) or even resistances to these movements as their racial and class-based nature begin to be more thoroughly investigated (Guthman 2008a,b; Hayes-Conroy and Hayes-Conroy 2010; Slocum 2006, 2007; Slocum and Saldanha 2013). These resistances might even be seen in those one-off or ongoing conscious decisions to eat even more junk food or even eat nothing at all (Lavis, forthcoming) as a desire to remain outside the so-called 'normal' eating regimes of society (Abbots and Lavis 2013). Actually what, how and for whom these pedagogies control, open or resist contemporary food cultures and materialities are very important stories that need to be told and, so, must be pursued through more and greater ethnographies of the food pedagogies that are intended for or serendipitous engaged with by differing publics.

Secondly, food pedagogies bring into focus and, so, are about the *pedagogues* themselves but also their *audiences* and/or *learners*. Pedagogues can range from family, to friends, to various forms of media, to food corporations, supermarkets, NGOs, nutritionists and other scientists and, of course, the state. In particular, the role of supermarkets as food pedagogues is woefully under-explored at the moment (but see Dixon et al. 2014; Isaacs and Dixon Chapter 8); Johnston 2008) especially given their powerful role in our everyday engagements with them both in the real and virtual senses. Moreover, as our survey suggests, the highly charged, moralistic tales about the decline of family involvement in food cultures that are circulating at the moment might need to be seriously re-thought and re-moralised. Audiences and learners also, obviously vary, indeed often doing so in terms not only of the context of time and space, but also as related to the various identities and roles we taken on, slough off or shift over time and space; clearly questions of race, class and gender are overtly pertinent as well as critical here as addressed by Pike and Leahy (Chapter 9) and Flowers and Swan (Chapter 3).

Crucially, pedagogues and audiences only really emerge out of their fluctuating and contingent relationalities formed through those equally fluctuating and contingent relationalities of attention (Rousseau 2012), socio-economic status, media programming and consumer access.

The third set of intimately related characteristics involve the ways that food pedagogies are about both the *visceral* and *affective* – how one feels about food and its taste – as well as the *political economic* – those processes and structures that bring good/bad foods to our plates, mouths and stomachs. Learning what tastes 'good' and/or 'bad' and how we feel about it after eating is an intimate process that is equally shaped by social and cultural relationships (see Rich and Evans Chapter 2; Flowers and Swan Chapter 3). There is always that element of trial and error that can be as exciting as it can be fraught, all of which involves the kinds of boundaries about what is acceptable or 'supposed' to taste good/bad from within one's own food culture. And, yet, taste and the visceralities of food are almost invariably shaped by political economy, whether it is one's personal circumstances that shape access and ability to choose/not choose particular foods or the wider political economies of how various foods make their ways to us. Here, learning about these political economies – i.e. where industrially produced meat comes from – can turn to 'distaste' and so shift diets along the spectrum to either vegetarianism or the sourcing of more friendly meat products. Thus, as Hayes-Conroy and Hayes-Conroy (2008) have it, taste and its visceralities is political and has – and should have – the potential to be at the forefront of more sustainable food movements looking to 'do' food in more alternative and socially just ways. In both the organoleptic and cultural senses, taste has the potential to shift political economies and, at the same time, political economies have the potential to shift those relationalities, experiences and visceralities of taste. Food pedagogies, as explored by Robert (Chapter 6) and Rich and Evans (Chapter 2), no matter if explicit or implicit, hidden or stated, or targeted or opportune will invariably contain the dialectic of food's visceralities and its political economies.

To conclude my afterword to this insightful volume, there are several crucial questions – mixed in with the others articulated above – I wish to end with. The first, while also broached in a number of the chapters in the volume (i.e. Jubas Chapter 7; Flowers and Swan Chapter 3; Isaacs and Dixon Chapter 8; Robert Chapter 6; Rich and Evans Chapter 2), brings forth the concerns I have about the problematics of either engaging with or pursuing food pedagogies *only* along the planes of knowledge. In short, where are the everyday, lived experiences with food and food pedagogies as – through food pedagogies – we learn and perhaps learn anew about how and what to eat? How do foods' pedagogical visceralities, affects and tastes modulate, mediate and mix with its learning, knowledge, media and marketing? Second, as introduced by Abarca (Chapter 12) and Sumner (Chapter 11), what might a more emancipatory and/or democratic food pedagogy *actually* look and *perform* like? And the follow up question, of course, is this: how might we go about bringing these more social justice-focused pedagogies about in the realms of food? These are merely a few of the very important questions that, in this era of growing inequalities in both food access and access to food pedagogies, this book has begun to raise and do so in rather auspicious and prescient ways.

References

Abbots, E. and Coles, B. (2014) Horsemeat-gate: The discursive production of a neoliberal food scandal. *Food, Culture and Society*, 16(4): 535–50.

Abbots, E. and Lavis, A. (eds) (2013) *Why We Eat, How We Eat: Contemporary Encounters between Foods and Bodies*. Farnham: Ashgate.

Allen, K. (2014) Official data shows longest fall in living standards for 50 years. *The Guardian*. http://www.theguardian.com/business/2014/jan/31/official-longest-fall-wages-living-standards-50-years.

Barnes, C. (forthcoming) Navigating good food, politics and power with Jamie Oliver. *Geoforum*.

Bell, D., Hollows, J. and Jones, S. (forthcoming) Campaigning culinary documentaries and the responsibilization of food crises. *Geoforum*.

Bennett, A. (2014) Edwina Currie says 'pernicious food banks make people poorer'. *Huffington Post UK*. http://www.huffingtonpost.co.uk/2014/01/28/edwina-currie-food-banks-_n_4680965.html.

Butler, P. (2014) Families turn to food banks as last resort 'not because they are free'. *The Guardian*. http://www.theguardian.com/society/2014/feb/20/food-bank-review-undermines-ministers-claim.

Campbell, D. (2014) Jamie Oliver calls for crackdown on junk food being sold near schools. *The Guardian*. http://www.theguardian.com/lifeandstyle/2014/apr/25/jamie-oliver-crackdown-junk-food-schools.

Campbell, H. (2009) Breaking new ground in food regime theory: Corporate environmentalism, ecological feedbacks and the 'food from somewhere' regime? *Agriculture and Human Values*, 26(4): 309–19.

Carolan, M. (2011) *Embodied Food Politics*. Farnham: Ashgate.

Castree, N. (2005) The epistemology of particulars: Human geography, case studies and 'context'. *Geoforum*, 36: 541–44.

Cook et al. (2004) Follow the thing: Papaya. *Antipode*, 36: 642–64.

Dixon, J., Hattersley, L. and Isaacs, B. (2014) Transgressing retail: Supermarkets, liminoid power and the metabolic rift. In M. Goodman and C. Sage (eds), *Food Transgressions: Making Sense of Contemporary Food Politics*. Farnham: Ashgate.

Fight, F. (2014) Hugh's fish fight. http://www.fishfight.net/.

Flowers, R. and Swan, E. (2012) Introduction: Why food? Why pedagogy? Why adult education. *Australian Journal of Adult Learning*, 52(3): 419–33.

Freidberg, S. (2004) The ethical complex of corporate food power. *Environment and Planning D: Society and Space*, 22: 513–31.

Goodman, M. (forthcoming) Food geographies I: Of relational foodscapes and the busyness of being more-than-(a)-food(ie). *Progress in Human Geography*.

———, Maye, D. and Holloway, L. (2010) Ethical foodscapes?: Premises, promises and possibilities. *Environment and Planning A*, 42: 1782–96.
Green, C. (2014) With one fast food restaurant for every 1,100 people, Birmingham takes a stand against the takeaway. *The Independent*. http://www.independent.co.uk/news/uk/home-news/with-one-fast-food-restaurant-for-every-1100-people-birmingham-takes-a-stand-against-the-takeaway-9231132.html.
Guthman, J. (2008a) Bringing good food to others: Investigating the subjects of alternative food practice. *Cultural Geographies*, 15: 431–47.
——— (2008b) 'If they only knew': Color blindness and universalism in California alternative food institutions. *Professional Geographer*, 60(3): 387–97.
Hayes-Conroy, A. and Hayes-Conroy, J. (2008) Taking back taste: Feminism, food and visceral politics. *Gender, Place and Culture*, 15(5): 461–73.
——— (2010) Visceral difference: Variations in feeling (slow) food. *Environment and Planning A*, 42: 2956–71.
Hough, A. (2013) Horsemeat scandal: Food prices 'may rise', Tesco boss admits. *The Telegraph*. http://www.telegraph.co.uk/foodanddrink/foodanddrinknews/9896756/Horsemeat-scandal-food-prices-may-rise-Tesco-boss-admits.html.
Johnston, J. (2008) The citizen-consumer hybrid: Ideological tensions and the case of whole foods market. *Theory and Society*, 37: 229–70.
Lambie-Mumford, H., Crossley, D., Jensen, E., Verbeke, M. and Dowler, E. (2014) Household food security in the UK: A review of food aid final report. *Defra*. https://www.gov.uk/government/uploads/system/uploads/attachment_data/file/283071/household-food-security-uk-140219.pdf.
Lavis, A. (forthcoming) Eating, feeding and starving in cyberspace: Affect and the visceralities of virtual food. *Geoforum*.
Lawrence, F. (2014) Felicity Lawrence at *The Guardian*. http://www.theguardian.com/profile/felicitylawrence.
Mesure, S. (2013) Horsemeat – special report: Public confidence drops as food goes untested. *The Independent*. http://www.independent.co.uk/life-style/food-and-drink/news/horsemeat – special-report-public-confidence-drops-as-food-goes-untested-8498246.html.
Oxfam (2013) A cautionary tale: The true cost of austerity and inequality in Europe. *Oxfam Briefing Paper*. http://policy-practice.oxfam.org.uk/publications/a-cautionary-tale-the-true-cost-of-austerity-and-inequality-in-europe-301384.
Pine, A. (forthcoming) *Community and Scarcity: Empowerment, Community and the State in the Alternative Economies of Community-based Food Programs*. Farnham: Ashgate.
Rousseau, S. (2012) *Food Media: Celebrity Chefs and the Politics of Everyday Interference*. London: Berg.
Sage, C. (2014) No fry zones around schools. *News Talk Ireland*. http://www.newstalk.ie/player/shows/Lunchtime/48490/no_fry_zones_around_schools.
Short, A. (2013) 5 ways to stop junk food co's from profiting from death and destruction caused by an excess ingredient. *Alternet*. http://www.alternet.org/

environment/orangutans-may-go-extinct-just-so-consumers-can-save-few-pennies-junk-food-5-ways-you.

Slocum, R. (2006) Anti-racist practice and the work of community food organizations. *Antipode*, 38: 327–49.

——— (2007) Whiteness, space and alternative food practice. *Geoforum*, 38: 520–33.

——— and Saldanha, A. (eds.) (2013) *Geographies of Race and Food Fields, Bodies, Markets*. Farnham: Ashgate.

The Guardian (2013) Horsemeat scandal: 'We will never know how many have eaten horse'. *The Guardian*. http://www.theguardian.com/uk/2013/feb/16/horsemeat-scandal-how-many-ate-meat.

Trussell Trust (2014) Latest foodbank figures top 900,000: Life has got worse not better for poorest in 2013/14, and this is just the tip of the iceberg. http://www.trusselltrust.org/foodbank-figures-top-900000.

Index

Note: Page numbers in **bold** indicate tables.

Abarca, Meredith E. 18–19
abuse 123, 125, 126
accretive learning 7
Adorno, Theodor 220
adult education 1, 8, 131, 143, 206
adult learning 132, 133, 135, 143
advertisements 16, 114, 117, 118, 119, 120, 121–2, 127, 143, 191
advertising myths 113
affective learning 7, 16, 120, 123
alcohol abuse 123, 125
alcohol advertising 113, 114, 123–5, 127
  health warnings 123, 124–5, 126
  Loi Evin 16, 113–14, 115, **116**, 116–17, 118–19, 120–122, 126, 127
Alexander, M. Jacqui 19, 218
Ali, Suki 55–6, 67
alimentary pedagogy 8
alternative chefs 15, 78–80, 81–3, 84–5, 86–7, 88–9, 90
alternative cooking shows 15, 20, 77, 78–9, 83, 89–90
  PPK 77, 78–9, 81, 83, 84, 85, 86, 87, 88, 89
  TCS 77, 79–80, 82, 83, 85, 86, 87, 88, 89
alternative food 21, 90
alternative food activism 8
alternative food pedagogies 11, 21, 22, 87, 89–90
Anderson, Zoe 57
Angela (Filipino migrant) 56, 58–9, 61–2, 63, 64–5
animal welfare 142, 189 90, 191
Ankeny, Rachel A. and Bray, Heather J. 18
ANPAA (Association Nationale de Prévention en Alcoologie et Addictologie) 119
anti-obesity media 9, 10, 17, 124
Anzaldúa, Gloria 19, 219, 220, 221
ascetic pleasure 43–4, 45
Australia 57–9, 149, 169, 185–6, 189–90, 191; *see also* Shepparton
  food labels 185, 186, 189, 191, 192
  GM foods 192–3
  school food 169, 170
  supermarkets 17, 149, 151, 157, 158, 160, 165
  'White Australia Policy' 56–7, 58
authenticity 218, 221
authorities 75, 76, 83–5

Belasco, Warren J. 221
Berliner, David 49–50, 51, 53, 69
Beucler, Pascal and Favreau, Fanny 117, 122
Biggest Loser 76–7
'bio-pedagogy' 9
black box of pedagogy 6, 68
bodies learning 35, 41, 63, 67, 69
body pedagogies 9, 14, 32, 34
boundary objects 18, 188, 196
Burdick, Jake and Sandlin, Jennifer 4–5, 6
Burni, Frank 220, 221

capacitisation 76
celebrity chef cooking shows 15, 75, 77, 80–81, 83, 85–6, 87, 89, 90
celebrity chefs 12, 77–8, 81, 83–4, 86, 87–8, 231–2, 233
celebrity culture 84, 101
children 8, 9, 20, 56, 98–9, 179
  health risks 1, 31, 32, 40
  meal times 50, 53, 54
  obesity 31, 34, 169
Chinese food 60, 61–2, 64, 67–8

citizen-consumers 150, 151, 164
collective learning 206
Collins, Kathleen 77–8
comfort food 63, 68
commensality, learning through 8, 63
communal food 82, 87
community 17, 82, 152–3
congeries of education 1, 69
congeries of methods of learning 69
congeries of modes of learning 69
constraints 76, 117, 127
constructivists 132
consumerism 85, 89, 90, 133, 140, 143, 195, 196
consumerist lifestyles 15, 75, 89
consumption 32, 35, 78, 81, 83, 89, 133, 144, 164, 178
  ethical food 15, 16, 18, 20–21, 189–90, 195
consumption-focused learning 89
'contact zone of engagement' 19, 216, 217–18, 219, 225
control 234–5
convenience foods 11, 81
conversationally pedagogic 69
conviviality 75, 89, 90, 223
cookbooks 67
Cooking Show con Karimi & Comrades, *see* TCS
cooking shows 7, 11, 12, 15, 75, 86–7, 231–2; *see also* alternative cooking shows; celebrity chef cooking shows
corporate food 81, 204
corporeal learning 8, 35
Coveney, J. and Bunton, R. 36, 37, 39, 40, 44, 45
Coveney, John 8–9, 36
critical food consciousness 222, 223
critical food pedagogies 201, 203, 204–5, 206, 209, 210, 211
critical learning 144
critical pedagogy 6, 203–4, 206
critical theory 18, 19, 215, 216
Cronin, Anne 113, 118, 119, 120
cultural pedagogy 3, 6–7, 8
cultural transmission 49–50, 51, 53, 54, 55, 56, 60, 68–9
cumulative learning 7
Currie, Dawn 131
Curtin, D.W. 222–3

De Solier, Isabelle 12, 13
Dean, Mitchell 172, 178
DeVault, Marjorie 52, 54, 59
diabetes 82
discipline 107–8, 109
disciplined pleasure 39, 40, 43, 44, 45
disgust 17, 41, 65–6, 176
disgusting pedagogies 10
Dixon, Jane 149
Dovid (*Jamie's Kitchen Australia*) 97, 101, 102–4, 105, 106, 107, 108, 109
drinking, *see* alcohol abuse; moderation; responsible drinking
dynamic learning 5

Eden, Sally 188
education
  adult education 1, 8, 131, 143, 206
  congeries of education 1, 69
  education studies 3, 8
  educational discourses 3, 14, 54
  educational effects 3, 6–7, 14, 113, 114, 118
  educational force 172, 176
  educational sites 6, 10, 31, 169
  everyday education 132, 143
  feminist education 3, 6, 10, 211
  feminist popular education 211
  food education 1, 10, 11, 19
  formal education 1, 8, 32, 132, 134
  gastronomic education 12
  health education 8, 170–171, 172, 175, 179
  holistic education 217, 225
  incidental education 1, 132, 143
  informal education 1, 9, 11, 132, 143
  lifestyle education 14, 16, 31, 34
  material education 12
  middle-class education 11, **33**, 33–4
  nutritional education 8–9, 172–5, 176–7
  post-secondary education 134
  progressive education 217, 225
  self-education 143

sensory education 8, 21
sustainable education 8
taste education 8, 21, 54
education studies 3, 8
educational discourses 3, 14, 54
educational effects 3, 6–7, 14, 113, 114, 118
educational force 172, 176
educational sites 6, 10, 31, 169
eggs, free range 189, 190
El Mero Cocinero, *see* Karimi
Elder, Catriona 56–7, 58
embodied learning 7, 14, 68
embodied racial practices 51, 61
embodiment 7, 14, 33, 34, 35, 42
engaged pedagogy 19, 216, 217, 219, 223
ethical food 18, 185, 186–7, 188, 189, 194–5, 196
GM foods 192, 193
ethical food consumption 15, 16, 18, 20–21, 189–90, 195
ethnic food 10–11
ethnographies of learning 50
Evans, Bethan; Colls, Rachel and Horschelmann, Kathrin 9–10
Evans, John and Rich, Emma 10, 14, 236
everyday education 132, 143
everyday life pedagogies 3, 5–6
experiential learning 206

fair trade 133, 136, 138, 142, 144, 208, 210
Fairley's supermarket 158
family 50, 52, 54, 56, 69
family food 49, 50, 52–3, 55–6, 68–9
racial practices 60, 61, 63, 67, 68
farmers' markets 135–6, 158, 165
Shepparton 159, 161, 162, 165
fast food 176
feeding work 52–3, 54, 59, 60, 64, 68
feminist education 3, 6, 10, 211
feminist popular education 211
feminists 3, 5–6, 36, 50, 52, 203–4
Fifteen programme, *see Jamie's Kitchen*; *Jamie's Kitchen Australia*
Filipino food 61–4, 65–6
Finger, Matthias 203, 204
Fischler, Claude 222
Fish Fight 232–3
fishing policy, EU 232–3
fixed modes of learning 50
Flowers, Rick and Swan, Elaine 14–15, 20, 35, 76, 141, 187–8, 202, 203, 205, 231
FNB (Food Not Bombs) 204
food 1, 19, 31, 32, 49, 99–101, 107, 215, 217, 218–19, 221, 229
alternative food 21, 90
communal food 82, 87
convenience foods 11, 81
corporate food 81, 204
ethnic food 10–11
fast food 176
food consumerism 85, 89, 139, 195
food porn 232
food practices 14, 32, 45, 49, 50, 53, 68, 224–5
food preparation 80–81, 83
food production 18, 133, 154–5, 157, 165
food security 1, 134, 186, 204
food shopping 16, 131–2, 133, 134, 135–6, 138–42, 144
globalised foods 54, 204
home-grown food 96, 157
junk food 176, 195, 235
local food 150, 151, 152–3, 155, 159–60, 165
material food 19, 66, 68, 69
material properties 66, 68, 69
organic foods 133, 134, 137, 138, 139, 142, 188, 189
pleasurable food 32, 41, 43, 87
political food 8, 19, 21, 81, 87
pre-industrialised food 99
pre-packaged foods 81, 82, 100
regional food 101, 165, 185, 207
sensory food 14, 66, 68, 69
slow food 20, 96, 98
sustainable food 8, 16, 142, 154, 186, 236
symbolic food 19, 62, 63
twenty-first century food 101
urban food justice 80
vegan foods 79, 81–2, 84, 85, 87, 90
food activism 8, 10
food beliefs 35–6

Food/Body/Person (Curtin, 1992) 222–3
food-centred nostalgia 67, 68
food consciousness 19, 215, 216, 219, 222–3, 224, 225, 226
food consumerism 85, 89, 139, 195
food diaries 17, 176–7, 178
food education 1, 10, 11, 19
food ethics, *see* ethical food
food labels 18, 138, 185, 186–7, 188, 189, 190–`91, 194–5, 196–7
  GM foods 192–3, 194
food learning 7, 13, 150
food media 9, 10, 17, 119, 124, 229, 230, 231, 232, 233–4
food narratives 18–19, 215–16, 217, 218, 219–21, 222, 223–6
Food Network (US show) 77, 78, 81, 83, 86, 87–8
Food Not Bombs, *see* FNB
food pedagogies 1–2, 13, 19–20, 21–2, 35, 169, 202–3, 211, 230–231, 234–5, 236–7
  critical 201, 203, 204–5, 206, 209, 210, 211
food pedagogues, *see* pedagogues
food porn 232
food practices 14, 32, 45, 49, 50, 53, 68, 224–5
food preparation 80–81, 83
food production 18, 133, 154–5, 157, 165
food rejection 65–6
food security 1, 134, 186, 204
Food, Self, and Identity (Fischler, 1988) 222
food shoppers 16, 133, 134–7, 142–3, 144
food shopping 16, 131–2, 133, 134, 135–6, 138–42, 144
foodbanks 229, 231
foodiesm 11–12
formal education 1, 8, 32, 132, 134
formal learning 1, 16, 132
Foucault, Michel 9, 96, 105, 106, 171, 177, 178
France 113, 125, 126–7
  health warnings 123, 124–5, 126
  Loi Evin 16, 113–14, 115, **116**, 116–17, 118–19, 120–122, 126, 127
free range products 189, 190, 191
Freire, Paulo 18, 204, 210, 225

gastronomic education 12
gender 2, 20, 138–40
genetically modified foods, *see* GM foods
Gilbert, David 55, 67
Girgarre market 161, 165
Giroux, Henry A. 4, 6, 115, 118, 202
Glenn, Cathy B. 191
globalised foods 54, 204
GM (genetically modified) foods 18, 185, 191–4
Gordon's London Dry Gin (adverts) 121–2
government 171–2, 175, 176–7
Gramsci, Antonio 132, 133
Greek kitchens 11
green consumerism 195
Guthman, Julie 11, 21, 22, 195, 210, 211

Haiven, Max 143–4
Harrison, Lyn; Kelly, Peter and Campbell, Perri 15–16
Harvey, David 209, 210
Hayes-Conroy, Allison 8, 37, 45, 67
Hayes-Conroy, Jessica 8, 21
Hayes-Conroy, Jessica and Hayes-Conroy, Allison 35–6, 226, 236
health 8, 31, 32, 82
health education, schools 8, 170–171, 172, 175, 179
  life skills 174–5, 176, 178
  nutritional education 173–4, 175, 176–7
  'Supersize Me' 172–3, 175, 176
health pedagogies 10, 16, 20, 125
health risks 32, 38, 44, 122, 175
  alcohol abuse 114, 123
  children 1, 31, 32, 40
  obesity 31, 36, 41, 42
health warnings 113, 114, 115, 116, 127
  responsible drinking 123–5, 126
healthy lifestyle 14, 31, 34
Heinz factory 157
Heldke, Lisa M. 215, 217
Hickey-Moody, Anna; Savage, Glen and Windle, Joel 3, 6, 114–15, 117–18
Highmore, Ben 8, 60, 69
Hodgson, Godfrey 118

holistic education 217, 225
holistic learning 132
home-cooking, learning through 11
home-grown food 96, 157
hooks, b. 19, 140, 141, 216, 217, 218, 223, 225
'Horsemeat-Gate' 230, 233–4

identity 9, 14, 55, 56–7, 187, 220–221, 222
  food shopping 131, 133, 138–42
  mixed-race families 61, 64, 66, 67–8, 69
imagined pedagogies 113–14, 127
  Loi Evin 114, 118, 119, 120, 121, 122, 123, 126
immigration 55, 57–9
incidental education 1, 132, 143
incidental learning 1, 16, 132
informal education 1, 9, 11, 132, 143
informal learning 1, 11, 132, 206
informal pedagogies 8, 187, 196
'information transfer' pedagogies 122–3
Isaacs, Bronwyn and Dixon, Jane 16–17, 18
iterative learning 7, 211

Jackson, Peter 54
Jamie's Italy 98, 100, 101
Jamie's Kitchen 95, 96, 98, 99
Jamie's Kitchen Australia 95–6, 97, 98, 101, 102–5, 106, 107–8, 109–10
Jamie's School Dinners 31, 98–9, 232
Japanese food 11
Johnson, Richard 77
Johnston, Josee and Baumann, Shyon 11, 12
Johnston, Josee and Goodman, Mike 13
Johnston, Josee and Szabo, Michelle 150, 163
Jubas, Kaela 16
junk food 176, 195, 235

Kahn, Richard 195
Karimi, Robert 79–80, 81, 82, 83, 84, 85, 86, 87, 88, 89, 90
Kimura, Aya H. 11

Lawrence, Felicity 230
Lawson, Nigella 12, 87
Leahy, Deana and Pike, Jo 10, 17, 36
learning
  accretive learning 7
  adult learning 132, 133, 135, 143
  affective learning 7, 16, 120, 123
  bodies learning 35, 41, 63, 67, 69
  collective learning 206
  congeries of methods of learning 69
  congeries of modes of learning 69
  consumption-focused learning 89
  corporeal learning 8, 35
  cumulative learning 7
  dynamic learning 5
  embodied learning 7, 14, 68
  ethnographies of learning 50
  experiential learning 206
  fixed modes of learning 50
  food learning 7, 13, 150
  in foodeism 12
  formal learning 1, 16, 132
  holistic learning 132
  incidental learning 1, 16, 132
  informal learning 1, 11, 132, 206
  iterative learning 7, 211
  learning ideologies 1
  learning processes 1, 2, 5, 6–7
  lifelong learning 202, 206
  macro discourses 3
  middle-class learning 12
  multidimensional learning 132, 143
  from newspapers 11
  non-cognitive learning 5
  programmatic learning 1, 171
  psychologistic models of learning 50
  relational learning 5
  rule learning 107
  sensory learning 14, 68
  shopping-as-learning 16, 144
  sites of 1, 6, 31, 54, 202
  social learning 54, 206
  social movement learning 21, 202
  technologies of 187, 202
  through commensality 8, 63
  through home-cooking 11
  through social occasions 1, 43
  transformative learning 206
  unpredictable learning 5

learning ideologies 1
learning processes 1, 2, 5, 6–7
learning sites 1, 6, 31, 54, 202
learning technologies 187, 202
Lewis, Tania 12–13
life skills 174–5, 176, 178
lifelong learning 202, 206
lifestyle education 14, 16, 31, 34
Lingard, Bob 3
Lipson, Leslie 204
Littler, Jo 144
livestock production 189–90, 191
local community markets 159–60, 161–3, 164, 165
local food 150, 151, 152–3, 155, 159–60, 165
Loi Evin, France (1991) 16, 113–14, 115, **116**, 116–17, 118–19, 120–122, 126, 127
  health warnings 123, 124–5, 126
Luke, Carmen 5–6, 10, 53–4, 55
Luke, Carmen and Carrington, Vicki 55
Lupton, Deborah 31, 39

macro discourses 3
Margaret (Chinese migrant) 56, 57, 58–9, 60, 61
marketing 117, 118, 120
material education 12
material food 19, 66, 68, 69
material properties 66, 68, 69
material racial practices 51
meal times 49, 50, 52, 53, 54, 60, 68–9
  racial practices 60, 61, 63, 67, 68
meat, free range 190, 191
memories, *see* nostalgia
'*mestiza*' consciousness 219, 220
middle-class education 11, **33**, 33–4
middle-class learning 12
Miller, Peter and Rose, Nikolas 172
mixed-race families 20, 50–51, 53, 54–6, 69
  identity 61, 64, 66, 67–8, 69
mixed-race family, Australia 14, 56–7, 59
  Angela 56, 58–9, 61–2, 63, 64–5
  Margaret 56, 57, 58–9, 60, 61
  Oscar 56, 60, 61, 62, 64, 66–8, 69
  Steven 56, 60, 61, 62, 63, 64, 65, 66, 69
moderation 114, 116, 124, 126
Moore, D. and Valverde, M. 176
Morgan, David 52, 56
Moskowitz, Isa Chandra 78–9, 81–2, 83, 84–5, 86, 87, 88, 89, 90
mothers 1, 10, 20, 54, 85, 138–9
multidimensional learning 132, 143
multiple pathways 75, 76

National Association for the Prevention of Alcoholism and Addiction, *see* ANPAA
neoliberalism 10, 143, 201, 209, 210
New Zealand 157, 170, 179, 192
newspapers, learning from 11
Next Food Network Star 78
NHMRC (National Health Medical Research Council) 169
Noble, Greg 6–7, 64
non-cognitive learning 5
non-verbal racial food practices 51–2
nostalgia, food-centred 67, 68
nutritional education 8–9, 172–5, 176–7

obesity 31, 32, 34, 36, 41, 42–3, 169, 171, 175
  schools 14, 17, 31, 169–70
Oliver, Jamie 12, 15–16, 31, 95–6, 97–9, 100–101, 107, 109, 232
opportunity 234, 235
organic foods 133, 134, 137, 138, 139, 142, 188, 189
Oscar (mixed-race family) 56, 60, 61, 62, 64, 66–8, 69
overweight 31, 41, 169, 175, 178
owner-operated shops 136, 158–9, 160

parents 9, 10, 53, 54, 160, 170
Parker, Christine 191
participatory self 222–3
passion 15–16, 96, 97, 105, 106, 107, 108, 109
pedagogical authorities 16–17, 150, 151, 153, 157, 164, 165–6
pedagogical turn 3, 202
pedagogies

alimentary pedagogy 8
'bio-pedagogy' 9
black box of pedagogy 6, 68
body pedagogies 9, 14, 32, 34
conversationally pedagogic 69
critical food pedagogies 201, 203, 204–5, 206, 209, 210, 211
cultural pedagogy 3, 6–7, 8
disgusting pedagogies 10
engaged pedagogy 19, 216, 217, 219, 223
everyday life pedagogies 3, 5–6
food pedagogies 1–2, 13, 19–20, 21–2, 35, 169, 202–3, 211, 230–231, 234–5, 236–7
health pedagogies 10, 16, 20, 125
imagined pedagogies 113–14, 127
'information transfer' pedagogies 122–3
pedagogical turn 3, 202
'pedagogies of everyday life' 3, 5–6
pedagogues 2, 6, 12–13, 19, 21, 40–41, 101, 152, 235–6
Pedagogy of Food 8, 18, 201, 205–8, 209–10, 211
pedagogy studies 54
post-human pedagogies 5
public pedagogy 3, 4–5, 6, 9, 10, 114–15, 117–18
relational pedagogies 5
school food pedagogies 14, 178–9
sensory food pedagogy 14
transfer pedagogies 5
'pedagogies of everyday life' 3, 5–6
pedagogues 2, 6, 12–13, 19, 21, 40–41, 101, 152, 235–6
pedagogy 3, 7–11, 13, 40–41, 54, 187, 201–2
Pedagogy of Food (course) 8, 18, 201, 205–8, 209–10, 211
pedagogy studies 54
pig's blood stew 65–6, 69
Pike, Jo and Leahy, Deana 36
pleasurable food 32, 41, 43, 87
pleasure 14, 32, 33–4, 35, 36–7, 38, 39–43, 44, 45, 82–3, 87
ascetic 43–4, 45
disciplined 39, 40, 43, 44, 45
political food 8, 19, 21, 81, 87
post-human pedagogies 5
post-secondary education 134
PPK (*Post Punk Kitchen*) 77, 78–9, 81, 83, 84, 85, 86, 87, 88, 89
Pratt, Louise 19, 217–18, 225
pre-industrialised food 99
pre-packaged foods 81, 82, 100
problematisation 76, 80–82
productive constraints 117, 127
programmatic learning 1, 171
progressive education 217, 225
'proper meal' 53, 59, 61, 63, 64, 65, 69
psychologistic models of learning 50
public health 9, 10, 32, 44, 115–16, 118, 122, 125
public health policies 14, 31, 35, 36, 44, 45, 186, 235; *see also Loi Evin*
public pedagogy 3, 4–5, 6, 9, 10, 114–15, 117–18
advertisements 118, 119, 120, 127

race 14, 51, 54, 55, 140–141
racial practices 51–2, 55, 60, 61, 63, 67, 68
embodied racial practices 51, 61
family food 60, 61, 63, 67, 68
material racial practices 51
meal times 60, 61, 63, 67, 68
non-verbal racial food practices 51–2
sensory racial food practices 51–2, 60, 61, 67
visceral racial food practices 51–2, 63, 67
white food racial practices 61
racialisation 10–11, 14, 20, 21, 51, 55, 58, 61, 66
Ray, Rachael 84, 86
reflexivity 144, 150
regional food 101, 165, 185, 207
relational learning 5
relational pedagogies 5
relationality 9–10, 231, 236
resistance 4, 186, 234, 235
responsible drinking 113, 114, 116, 123–5, 126–7
rice 62–3, 64
Rich, Emma 123–4
risk 175, 176, 178, 179

risk culture 31, 32, 35, 36, 38, 40, 41, 42–3, 44
Robert, Julie 15, 16, 236
Rose, Nikolas 75, 76, 151, 172
Rose, Nikolas and Miller, Peter 151
Rousseau, Signe 83–4
rule learning 107

Sandlin, Jennifer A. 133, 143, 144
school food 10, 14, 31–2, 98–9, 169–70, 178, 232
school food pedagogies 14, 178–9
schools 10, 17, 34
  health education 8, 170–171, 172, 175, 179
  life skills 174–5, 176, 178
  nutritional education 173–4, 175, 176–7
  obesity 14, 17, 31, 169–70
  'Supersize Me' 172–3, 175, 176
  UK 14, 31–2, **33**, 33–4, 37–9, 40–43, 44
self 37, 45, 76, 106, 108, 109, 151, 177–8, 222–3
  technologies of 15, 96, 105, 106, 107, 108–9
self-actualization 218, 219
self-education 143
self-formation 175, 176–7, 178
self-government 76, 178
sensory education 8, 21
sensory food 14, 66, 68, 69
sensory food pedagogy 14
sensory learning 14, 68
sensory racial food practices 51–2, 60, 61, 67
shared meals 225–6
Shepparton, Australia 153–4, 155–6, 157–60, 164–6
  farmers' markets 159, 161, 162, 165
  local community markets 159–60, 161–3, 164, 165
  local food 150, 151, 152–3, 155, 159–60, 165
  supermarkets 149–50, 151, 153, 156, 157–8, 159, 160, 161–3, 165
Shepparton Processing Cooperative, *see* SPC
shopping, *see* food shoppers; food shopping
shopping-as-learning 16, 144
Short, Frances 11
Slocum, Rachel 21, 51
slow food 20, 96, 98
Slow Food Movement 8, 133, 142
social entrepreneurship 99, 101
social learning 54, 206
social movement learning 21, 202
social occasions, learning through 1, 43
sovereignty 107
SPC (Shepparton Processing Cooperative) 153, 154–5
Spurlock, Morgan 172–3, 175, 176
Steven (mixed-race family) 56, 60, 61, 62, 63, 64, 65, 66, 69
Stewart, Liz and Casswell, Sally 118
subjectification 151
subjectivities 34, 37, 75, 76, 83, 106
'sugar junkies' 38
Sumner, Jennifer 8, 18
supermarkets 2, 16–17, 18, 149, 150, 152–3, 154, 155–7, 164, 235
  Australia 17, 149, 151, 157, 158, 160, 165
  'Horsemeat-Gate' 230, 233
  Shepparton 149–50, 151, 153, 156, 157–8, 159, 160, 161–3, 165
'Supersize Me' 172–3, 175, 176
sustainable education 8
sustainable food 8, 16, 142, 154, 186, 236
Sutton, David E. 11, 221, 223, 224
symbolic food 19, 62, 63
Symons, Michael 149, 218–19
synesthesia 223
Szkupinski-Quiroga, Seline; Sandlin, Jennifer A. and Redmond Wright, Robin 15, 20

taste education 8, 21, 54
TCS (*The Cooking Show con Karimi & Comrades*) 77, 79–80, 82, 83, 85, 86, 87, 88, 89
teachers 17, 38–9, 45
  pleasure 14, 32, 33–4, 39–43
technologies 75, 76, 85–6

technologies of the self 15, 96, 105, 106, 107, 108–9
Todd, Anne Marie 191
transfer pedagogies 5
transformative learning 206
transmission, *see* cultural transmission
True Food Guide 193
Truong, Monique 219
twenty-first century food 101

UK (United Kingdom) 35, 54, 170, 179, 229, 230, 231
  'Horsemeat-Gate' 230, 233–4
  public health policies 14, 31, 35, 44, 45
  school food 14, 31–2, 98–9, 232
  schools 14, 31–2, **33**, 33–4, 37–9, 40–43, 44
unpredictable learning 5
urban food justice 80

Valentine, Gill 52, 54
Vancouver, Canada
  food shoppers 134–7, 142–3, 145
  food shopping 131–2, 134, 135–6, 138–9, 140–141, 142–3
vegan foods 79, 81–2, 84, 85, 87, 90
vegetarian cooking 79, 82
visceral racial food practices 51–2, 63, 67

Watkins, Megan; Noble, Greg and Driscoll, Catherine 6, 7, 8
'White Australia Policy' 56–7, 58
white food culture 8, 20, 21, 59, 60–61
white food racial practices 61
whiteness 14, 20, 60–61
women 2, 20, 138–40
Woolworths supermarket 17, 160
Wright, Jan and Harwood, Valerie 9

young people 31, 32, 34, 35, 37–9, 43–4, 54, 99, 178
  Jamie's Kitchen Australia 95–6, 97, 99, 106, 109
  pleasure 14, 32, 33–4, 39–43, 44, 45

www.ingramcontent.com/pod-product-compliance
Ingram Content Group UK Ltd.
Pitfield, Milton Keynes, MK11 3LW, UK
UKHW020012200926
475702UK00014B/1846
* 9 7 8 1 1 3 8 5 4 7 3 9 1 *